T0228254

The Risks of Medical Inr

Questions of risk and safety have increasingly gained significance in the development of biomedicine in the past two hundred years, but the way dangers involved in medical innovations are portrayed and discussed has varied, often being highly dependent on context.

The Risks of Medical Innovation studies specific cases of medical innovation in their respective contexts, including X-rays, the Pill and Thalidomide. Cases are looked at through the lens of a particular set of shared questions concerning risk, highlighting differences, similarities, continuities, and changes, and offering a historical sociology of risk. Particularly important is the re-conceptualization of dangers in terms of risk, a numerical and probabilistic approach which allowed for seemingly objective and value-neutral decisions. However the historical examples show that the political dimension inherent in any decision about medical innovation does not simply disappear by reframing it in terms of risk.

Read together, these papers add to the current debate about risk and safety by providing a comparative background and a set of generally applicable criteria for analysing and evaluating contemporary issues around medical innovation.

Thomas Schlich is Canada Research Chair in the History of Medicine at the Department of Social Studies of Medicine at McGill University, Canada.

Ulrich Tröhler heads the Institute for the History of Medicine of the University of Freiburg, Germany.

Routledge Studies in the Social History of Medicine

Edited by Joseph Melling
University of Exeter and
Anne Borsay
University of Wales, Swansea

The Society for the Social History of Medicine was founded in 1969, and exists to promote research into all aspects of the field, without regard to limitations of either time or place. In addition to this book series, the Society also organises a regular programme of conferences, and publishes an internationally recognised journal, *Social History of Medicine*. The Society offers a range of benefits, including reduced-price admission to conferences and discounts on SSHM books, to its members. Individuals wishing to learn more about the Society are invited to contact the series editors through the publisher.

The Society took the decision to launch 'Studies in the Social History of Medicine', in association with Routledge, in 1989, in order to provide an outlet for some of the latest research in the field. Since that time, the series has expanded significantly under a number of series editors, and now includes both edited collections and monographs. Individuals wishing to submit proposals are invited to contact the series editors in the first instance.

1 **Nutrition in Britain**
   Science, scientists and politics in the twentieth century
   Edited by David F. Smith

2 **Migrants, Minorities and Health**
   Historical and contemporary studies
   Edited by Lara Marks and Michael Worboys

3 **From Idiocy to Mental Deficiency**
   Historical perspectives on people with learning disabilities
   Edited by David Wright and Anne Digby

4 **Midwives, Society and Childbirth**
   Debates and controversies in the modern period
   Edited by Hilary Marland and Anne Marie Rafferty

5 **Illness and Healing Alternatives in Western Europe**
   Edited by Marijke Gijswit-Hofstra, Hilary Maarland and Has de Waardt

Also available in Routledge Studies in the Social History of Medicine series:

The Risks of Medical Innovation

Risk perception and assessment in historical context

Edited by
Thomas Schlich and Ulrich Tröhler

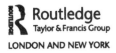
Routledge
Taylor & Francis Group

LONDON AND NEW YORK

First published 2006
by Routledge
2 Park Square, Milton Park, Abingdon, Oxfordshire OX14 4RN

Simultaneously published in the USA and Canada
by Routledge
711 Third Avenue, New York, NY 10017

Published 2014 by Routledge

First issued in paperback 2014

Routledge is an imprint of the Taylor & Francis Group, an informa business

Transferred to Digital Printing 2006

© 2006 Editorial matter and selection, Thomas Schlich and
Ulrich Tröhler; individual chapters, the contributors

Typeset in Garamond by Taylor & Francis Books

British Library Cataloguing in Publication Data
A catalogue record for this book is available from the British Library

Library of Congress Cataloging-in-Publication Data
A catalog record for this book has been requested

ISBN 978-0-415-33481-5 (hbk)
ISBN 978-1-138-86794-9 (pbk)

T&F informa

Taylor & Francis Group is the Academic Division of T&F Informa plc.

Contents

Illustrations

Figures

Tables

Contributors

Silke Bellanger studied contemporary history, sociology and public law in Freiburg and Milan. Together with Aline Steinbrecher, she worked and published on the history of brain death in Switzerland from 1960 until 2000. She is currently finishing her PhD project, a sociological analysis of contemporary strategies of exhibiting science and technology.

Christian Bonah, MD and PhD (History and History of Science) presently heads the Département d'Histoire des Sciences de la Vie et de la Santé at the Medical Faculty of the Louis Pasteur University in Strasbourg, France. Following his book *Instruire, Guérir, Servir: Formation, Recherche et Pratique Médicales en France et en Allemagne Pendant la Deuxième Moitié du XIXe siècle* (Strasbourg, Presses Universitaires de Strasbourg, 2000) and a collective volume edited with Etienne Lepicard and Volker Roelcke *La Médecine Expérimentale au Tribunal : Implications Éthiques de Quelques Procès Médicaux du XXe Siècle Européen* (Paris, Editions des Archives Contemporaines, 2003), he is now working on the history of therapeutics and therapeutic agents in a comparative perspective and on the history of human experimentation in France during the twentieth century.

Ian Burney is a Wellcome Research Lecturer at the University of Manchester's Centre for the History of Science, Technology and Medicine. His latest project, *Poison, Detection and the Victorian Imagination*, will be published in the University of Manchester Press's "Encounters" series in 2005.

Alberto Cambrosio is Professor of Social Studies of Medicine at McGill University in Montreal. He specializes in the sociology of biomedical practices and innovations at the interface between laboratory and clinical activities. His publications include: *Exquisite Specificity: The Monoclonal Antibody Revolution* (New York: Oxford University Press, 1995) and *Biomedical Platforms: Realigning the Normal and the Pathological in Late-Twentieth-Century Medicine* (Cambridge, MA: MIT Press, 2003), both co-authored with Peter Keating.

Arthur Daemmrich is a policy analyst at the *Chemical Heritage Foundation* in Philadelphia. He holds a PhD in Science and Technology Studies from Cornell University and has published on biotechnology policy and politics, the sociology of medicine, and pharmaceutical drug regulation. In his research, he brings long-range perspectives to bear on the analysis of globalization, risk, health, and environmental policy. Daemmrich has held fellowships from the Social Science Research Council/Berlin Program for Advanced German and European Studies, and the Kennedy School of Government at Harvard University and the Chemical Heritage Foundation. He is the author of *Pharmacopolitics: Drug Regulation in the United States and Germany*.

Monika Dommann received her PhD in History from the University of Zürich in 2002. She is the author of *Durchsicht, Einsicht, Vorsicht: Eine Geschichte der Röntgenstrahlen.* (Zürich: Chronos Verlag, 2003). Currently, she is working on her habilitation project under the working title "Legal Instruments: Technological Change and the Rise of Copyright (19th and 20th Century)", funded by the Swiss National Foundation. During Winter 2004/2005 she was Research Fellow at IFK (Wien) and in the summer of 2005 Visiting Scholar GHI (Washington DC).

Sarah Dry is a Gates Cambridge scholar and a doctoral student in the Department of History and Philosophy of Science, Cambridge University. Her research is on science, safety, and control in mid-to-late nineteenth-century Britain. She is the author of *Curie: A Life* (London: Haus Press, 2003), a biography of Marie Curie.

Jean-Paul Gaudillière is researcher at the Institut National de la Santé et de la Recherche Médicale (France). He has been working on the history of biomedical research after World War Two in France and in the United States. He is currently writing a history of biological drugs with a special look at the changing relationship between biomedical researchers and the industry. He is the author of *Inventer la Biomédecine: la France, l'Amérique et la Production des Savoirs du Vivant, 1945–1965* (Paris: La Découverte, 2002), (English translation forthcoming, Yale University Press).

Christoph Gradmann studied history and German at the universities of Birmingham (UK) and Hannover, where he earned his DPhil in 1991. He is employed at the Institute for the History of Medicine of Heidelberg University. He has published extensively on the history of German medical bacteriology, the cultural history of medicine and medical biography. The biographical dictionary *Ärzte-Lexikon* (with Wolfgang U. Eckart, Heidelberg: Springer, 2001 (1996)) is heading for its third edition. His book *Robert Koch. Bakterien, Krankheit und Medizin* (Göttingen: Wallstein-Verlag) will be published in 2005. His current work is on post-World War Two medical bacteriology.

Peter Keating is professor of history at the Université du Québec à Montréal where he teaches the history of science and medicine. He is also a member of the Interuniversity Research Center for the Study of Science and Technology (CIRST) located at the same institution. He has recently published, with Alberto Cambrosio, Biomedical Platforms: Realigning the Normaland the Pathological in Late Twentieth Century Biomedicine (MIT Press, 2003). He specializes in the history and sociology of post World-War Two biomedicine.

Valerie Leiter received a joint PhD in Sociology and Social Policy from Brandeis University in 2001. She is an Assistant Professor of Sociology and director of the Society and Health program at Simmons College. Her work focuses on the social construction of childhood disability and the relationship between familial and formal systems of care for children with disabilities.

Lara Marks received her DPhil (History of Medicine) from Oxford University in 1990. She is presently a visiting senior academic at Cambridge University and the London School of Hygiene, as well as a senior research partner at Silico Research. Following her book *Sexual Chemist: A History of the Contraceptive Pill* (New Haven: Yale University Press, 2001) she is now expanding her research into the biopharmaceutical industry.

Thomas Schlich is Canada Research Chair in the History of Medicine and associate professor at the Department of Social Studies of Medicine at McGill University in Montreal, Canada. His most recent book is *Surgery, Science and Industry: A Revolution in Fracture Care, 1950s–1990s* (Houndsmills, Basingstoke: Palgrave, 2002). He is now working on standardization and objectivity in twentieth-century medicine and on a book project, the *Rise of Modern Surgery, 1800–2000*.

Aline Steinbrecher studied history, educational science and social and economic history in Zürich. Her PhD thesis is a social history of madness in Zürich during the seventeenth century. Together with Silke Bellanger she worked and published on the history of brain death in Switzerland from 1960 until 2000.

Carsten Timmermann worked as a biochemist before he turned, in 1995, to the history of science and medicine. He holds an MA and a PhD from the University of Manchester, where he still works as a Wellcome Research Fellow. After writing on the history of hypertension treatments he is now researching the history of lung cancer, as part of a larger project on the history of cancer research and cancer services in Britain since World War Two.

Stefan Timmermans is professor of sociology at UCLA. He is the author of *Sudden Death and the Myth of CPR* (Philadelphia: Temple University Press, 1999) and *The Gold Standard: The Challenge of Evidence-Based Medicine and Standardization in Health Care* (with Marc Berg: Philadelphia: Temple University Press, 2003). His book *Suspicious Death* is forthcoming from the University of Chicago Press.

Ulrich Tröhler received his MD and PhD (History of Science) from the Universities of Zürich (1972) and London (1979) respectively. He presently heads the Institute for the History of Medicine of the University Freiburg, Germany. Following his book *"To improve the evidence of medicine": The Eighteenth Century British Origins of a Critical Approach* (Edinburgh, Royal College of Physicians, 2000), he is now expanding this field under the working title *"Methods, numbers, obligations": New Alliances and Procedures in Medical Statistics, Pharmacology and Drug Regulation in Germany 1930–1985.*

Preface

Ulrich Tröhler and Thomas Schlich

The idea for this book stems from a simple but intriguing personal experience that Ulrich Tröhler had some forty years ago: the discussions around the proposed treatment of a fracture resulting from a skiing accident in Switzerland. At this time, the use of metal implants (osteosynthesis) was hotly debated, not only within the Tröhler family but also among doctors themselves. While some saw osteosynthesis as an injury added to an injury and therefore a risky procedure, or even one that should not be performed under any circumstances, others focused on the gain in time and functionality associated with the procedure. Since then, the method has become standard practice and no longer arouses much discussion. How and why did this change in attitude come about? Was it due to better (post-) operative management in general? In other words, did the risks change and, if so, what evidence was there for arguing that they had changed? Or, do patients, the public and doctors today simply perceive these same "risks" differently? Did the criteria for safety change, or did the burden of proof shift from the theoretically and empirically well-founded method *per se* to the individual surgical practitioner, or even to the patient? When Thomas Schlich set out to answer some of these questions,[1] we wondered whether they had been dealt with in the professional world of medicine and law, by the public and in politics, when earlier medical inventions had first been introduced, then later widely implemented and accepted. Had these innovations elicited the same questions and responses, or had specific inventions elicited specific reactions related to the type of invention, the cultural setting and/or the timing of the innovation? Finally, were there any constant features that could be observed over a longer time period?

In order to learn about these issues, and to place our own work in context, we organized two workshops on risk and safety in medical innovations. The first one was held in Freiburg, Germany, in 2001, and the second in Philadelphia, USA, in 2003 (with the help of Arthur Daemmrich of the Chemical Heritage Foundation). They met an enthusiastic response from colleagues and in the press. Therefore, the contributions to these workshops constitute the basis for this book.

There have been mixed feelings about medical innovations since the 1960s,[2] and one can identify an increased interest in risk issues in recent times.[3] This is understandable given the high risk of medical treatments: adverse drug reactions range between the fourth and sixth most frequent cause of death in the United States. In a systematic review of the international literature, adverse drug reactions that were so dramatic as to warrant discontinuation of treatment or therapeutic countermeasures were found to affect some 7 percent (95 percent confidence interval, 5.2–8.2 percent) of hospitalized patients. Although the majority of such drug reactions are due to dosage errors or treatments no longer necessary due to the patient's current health status, and are thus potentially preventable, they still have to be included among the risks confronting both patients and medical practitioners today.[4] Besides providing new historical information, the interest in reading this book lies in the fact that its objective parallels the current relevance of the perception, assessment, and management of risk for healthcare professionals, policy-makers and economists, as well as for all citizen-patients.

Our project has received funding from a variety of sources. We would like to thank the AO/ASIF Foundation in Davos, Switzerland, especially its former president Peter Matter, and the German Research Foundation, DFG, in Bonn, Germany, for supporting the Freiburg conference. We owe thanks to the Chemical Heritage Foundation in Philadelphia for funding the meeting there, and in particular Arthur Daemmrich for splendidly organizing it. We are also grateful to participants in both conferences, in addition to the contributors of this book, who have inspired us: Darrell Salk gave the keynote speech in Philadelphia; David Cantor, Tom van Helvoort, Norbert Paul, John Pickstone, Christoph Rehmann-Sutter, Claudia Wiesemann and Eberhard Wolff were engaged in various ways in the Freiburg meeting and provided input when we conceived its structure.

We are also much indebted to Jonathan Simon for the excellent job he did in copy-editing and translating the chapters of those authors whose first language is not English. Margaret Andergassen's language assistance and Natascha Beyer's indispensable coordination work during the editing process are also gratefully acknowledged.

Ulrich Tröhler and Thomas Schlich
Freiburg and Montreal
September 2004

Notes

1 Thomas Schlich, *Surgery, Science and Industry: A Revolution in Fracture Care, 1950s–1990s*, Houndsmill, Basingstoke: Palgrave, 2002 (Series: Science, Technology and Medicine in Modern History).

2 John V. Pickstone, "Introduction", in John V. Pickstone (ed.), *Medical Innovations in Historical Perspective*, Houndmills, Basingstoke: Macmillan, 1992, 1–16; Ilana Löwy, "Introduction: Medicine and Change", in Ilana Löwy (ed.), *Medicine and Change: Historical and Sociological Studies of Medical Innovation*, Les Editions INSERM, Paris, 1993, 1–19.

3 Gerd Gigerenzer, *Reckoning with Risk: Learning to Live with Uncertainty*, London: The Penguin Press, 2002.

4 Jason Lazarou, Bruce H. Pomeranz and Paul N. Corey, "Incidence of Adverse Drug Reactions in Hospitalized Patients: A Meta-analysis of Prospective Studies", *Journal of the American Medical Association*, 279 (1998), 2000–5.

1 Risk and medical innovation

A historical perspective

Thomas Schlich[1]

Medical innovations do not always turn out the way they are supposed to. Any therapeutic, diagnostic, or preventive measure can have unexpected and undesired effects, making uncertainty inherent in medicine. As the sociologist Renée C. Fox states, "clinical advances change the content of medical uncertainty and alter its contours, but they do not drive it away."[2] Advances even create new uncertainties. To the extent that modes of diagnosing and treating disease and illness have become more powerful, they have also grown more dangerous, exposing patients to more potential harm through anticipated and unanticipated negative consequences. Doctors, patients, state authorities, and others have developed strategies for dealing with this problem. Most importantly, they have increasingly framed the problem in terms of risk. Using the notion of "risk" implies a specific strategy for dealing with uncertainty, based on the calculation of probabilities.[3] Probability-based logic has been employed "to approach the uncertainties of diagnosis, therapy, and prognosis, and the clinical judgment that lies at their heart" since the eighteenth century.[4]

The term "risk" is derived from the French word "risque" and first appeared in its anglicized form in England in the early nineteenth century. It was originally used in a neutral way in order to refer to a wager made by individuals after taking the probabilities of losses and gains into account. In more recent times it has come to refer exclusively to negative outcomes; to the likelihood of some adverse effect of a hazard.[5] Social scientists acknowledge the fuzziness of the term with its range of synonyms like "gamble, hazard, danger, probability, uncertainty, and odds ratio".[6] Technically, one can speak of risk when the probability estimates of an event are known, or at least knowable, while "uncertainty", by contrast, implies that these probabilities are inestimable or unknown. In the real world, however, the distinction is not so sharp, and risk and uncertainty are better conceived of as poles on a continuum, with "risk" being used as shorthand for forms of technology and social organization that have the potential to harm people.[7] Despite its fuzziness, the notion of risk is typically linked to the particular purpose of reducing, modifying, or anticipating the extent or nature of uncertainty in decision-making processes.[8] Thus, using the term "risk" implies human agency. According to Niklas Luhmann one speaks of "dangers" if the potential damage is attributed to causes outside one's own control, as is the case, for example, with natural disasters. "Risk" implies that damage is perceived as being the consequence of one's own decision, and could be prevented by using, for example, technologies of risk control.[9]

In contemporary medicine the issue of risk has become so common that social scientists speak of a veritable "risk epidemic" in the medical literature since the 1960s.[10] The concept of risk has also been employed in different ways in this later period, but is most often used to refer to the likelihood of falling ill. Again, the notion of risk carries with it the connotation of human agency in the origin of illness, as opposed to fate or nature, and this has made it easier to apply the risk concept to medical intervention. Since the mid-twentieth century new technologies, procedures, and drugs have increasingly been evaluated in terms of risk.[11] Because of the fear of the risks involved, medical innovation has often been perceived as a mixed blessing.[12] This general disillusionment with the advances of science and technology has led sociologists like Ulrich Beck to proclaim a new phase of "reflexive" modernity in which "progress" is increasingly problematized by the production of risks that pervade and transform modern societies.[13]

The contributions to this volume explore the historical dimension of the issue of risk in medical innovation. They look at how, in the nineteenth and twentieth centuries, historical actors have dealt with the uncertainty associated with medical innovations in different contexts. Medical innovation is understood as the process of introducing a new medical technique or drug, a process during which both the context and the technology itself may change. Therefore, sharp distinctions between invention and discovery, innovation and diffusion threaten to oversimplify the complex process of the technology's acceptance.[14] Risk plays a key role in this process, since whether a medical novelty gets accepted or not is, in part, the result of a process of negotiating its potential benefits and dangers.[15] Considerations of risk belong to the "real, messy, contested and complex debates by which, over time, some procedures were accepted in preference to others"[16] and thus changed the face of modern medicine.

As will be evident from the case studies presented in this volume, different kinds of innovations resulted in diverse strategies for increasing certainty. Highly visible surgical procedures required a different logic from other therapeutic modalities such as new drugs whose effects cannot be immediately identified. Preventive measures like vaccination, lifestyle drugs such as the contraceptive pill, life-saving measures for cancer, medicines for pain management, or diagnostic techniques for ascertaining brain death have all been associated with distinctive rationales of risk management. What all the examples have in common is the attempt by developers, users or regulators to make the consequences of innovation more predictable and controllable using documentation, calculation, and regulation. It is also obvious that the mathematical control of uncertainty by using techniques such as probability functioned primarily as an ideal, serving as a model or as a rhetorical device, but only rarely put into practice in a comprehensive manner. The approach was apparently taken from the context of theories about disease causation and then applied to the problem of medical innovation. This seems to have happened around the middle of the twentieth century, when the notion of risk became more widespread in various areas of society, but this is still an open research question. However, elements of the fully developed risk concept such as quantification, calculation, and probability-logic were adopted much earlier from fields such as life insurance and population studies and used for the purpose of regulating medical innovations. In the following passages I aim to provide a short historical survey of the origins of these elements.

Creating certainty

From a historical perspective, strategies for dealing with uncertainties in medical knowledge and practice that involve applying mathematical methods can be traced back to the period of the Enlightenment.[17] The idea of risk first emerged in an economic context of new, extended and more internationalized markets. Risk referred to the danger of losing money in business, especially on loans, in gambling and in insurance, and was related to attempts to hedge one's bets.[18] The earliest application of risk to health issues took place in another business context, namely when life insurance companies needed a basis to decide on the acceptance of applicants for a policy. This was again a quantified and calculable precaution for predicting and, if possible, avoiding financial loss. As early as 1762, the first life insurance company, The Equitable in England, charged extra premiums for applicants with gout, a hernia, and no history of smallpox.[19] The companies were able to use mortality tables as a basis for determining their policy. The technique of drawing up mortality tables goes back to vital statistics, a field of enquiry that produced knowledge about the statistical regularity of health conditions within populations. As raw material for these statistics, investigators used records of births, deaths, and often marriages in a locality or country. The first examples are the bills of mortality published in 1562 by the City of London to keep track of plague deaths.[20]

Vital statistics became more sophisticated when the mathematics of business practices were applied to them. In the seventeenth century, the London merchant John Gaunt started applying commercial accounting practices to those mortality lists, and the resulting tables were published in 1662 under the title "Natural and Political Observations Made Upon the Bills of Mortality". They enabled a systematic comparison between parishes and city neighborhoods, causes of death and gender specificities, as well as the past and present states of affairs. British physicians subsequently started to use this type of procedure for dealing with other medical and public health questions as well.[21]

Taking up the vital statistics approach and broadening their perspective beyond the traditional individualistic approach of medicine, doctors and administrators could now focus on the well-being of specific groups within the population – such as the laboring poor, soldiers, women, and children, rather than considering only the individual patient. Thus, doctors assumed a role in Enlightenment population politics, an increasingly important area for strengthening and stabilizing the nation state. Starting in the 1830s, statistics also contributed to public health measures. In his 1829 textbook on vital statistics, *Elements of Medical Statistics*, Francis Bisset Hawkins predicted that the application of statistics to medicine would permit not only the determination of the effectiveness of treatments, and provisions of a basis for reliable diagnoses, but also the evaluation of the impact of living conditions on life, health, and labor.[22]

In this way medicine became one of many areas in which counting and accounting constituted an important way of thinking. The population-based mathematical approach was broadened to cover more medical fields of application, including accounting for the efficiency of new medical institutions. The British hospital and dispensary movement, for example, induced doctors and lay sponsors alike to establish recovery and death rates within these institutions and so to calculate the success rates of specific cures. The evaluation of clinical experience was another new field of application for numerical calculations. An analysis of British medical journals from 1733 to 1829 shows the gradual reduction in dependence on single case reports and a growth in the publication of larger series, some of which were even analysed by what can be called proto-statistical methods. Especially in eighteenth-century Britain, doctors perceived the need for the empirical evaluation of remedies by comparative trials with results expressed in numbers. These physicians wanted to base clinical medicine on elementary numerical analysis of compilations of cases and observations made on distinct groups of patients, not on individuals. For them, arithmetic calculation was a way out of the maze of contradictory observations. As a result, by the first decades of the nineteenth century a more or less tacit acknowledgment of the utility – and even necessity – of numerical observations in clinical medicine emerged in the British medical literature.[23]

The strategy of making the potential dangers of medical innovation calculable and controllable by the quantification and calculation of probabilities can be observed early on in the disputes over smallpox inoculation in the eighteenth century. Smallpox inoculation had its own hazards: patients could die from it, and they could also spread the disease by infecting others with inoculated smallpox. This made contemporaries wonder whether the benefit outweighed the risk. The discussions on that topic, for example those between Daniel Bernoulli and Jean le Rond d'Alembert in the 1760s, are considered classics in the history of probabilistic thinking.[24] In England, the physician Thomas Nettleton (1683–1742) introduced a particular approach to this problem, using what he called "Merchants Logick". Merchant's logic argued that physicians should calculate the utility of particular practices by summing up the costs and benefits among a population of patients. Nettleton's was only one of various forms of merchant's logic that cropped up in eighteenth-century medical literature, especially around the question of smallpox inoculation. Most often, the numerical arguments were aimed at establishing the balance of profit and loss in terms of public good, which was measured by gross smallpox mortality or the proportion of smallpox mortality compared to total mortality, and in terms of private benefit, measured by the risk of dying from inoculation.[25]

The British case is just one example of a more general trend, of which the most famous advocate was the noted French physician Pierre Charles Louis (1787–1872). Louis proposed the general application of a numerical method that quantified the available facts in order to achieve statistical measurement and the comparison of benefits of particular treatment methods.[26] Generally speaking, the use of statistics in therapeutics was part of the process of objectification through which science entered medicine.[27] In the late nineteenth and early twentieth centuries statistical methods were being used to help with a number of medical problems, ranging from evaluating tests for the efficacy of medical treatment to determining the heredity of tuberculosis. Statistics now appeared to be the handmaid of medicine, as Karl Pearson characterized it.[28] In the later decades of the nineteenth century the proliferation of medical expertise and the accelerated pace of medical discoveries gave further impetus to the integration of mathematical statistics into medical research and innovation. After World War Two, with the rise of the randomized clinical trial, rigorous monitoring and control of therapeutic advances became the order of the day and "mathematical statistics came into its own as an accepted regulator of medical research".[29]

Risk factors

The general perception of risk in medical contexts was very much shaped by the notion of the risk factor, which emerged in its modern sense in the 1950s and 1960s, when probability calculation came into use in the epidemiology of chronic disease.[30] Its origins go back to the use of the technological approach embodied in vital statistics and mortality tables for the prediction of illness. Speculations on who would fall ill with particular illnesses, and for what reasons, had been an element of medical literature for a long time, although, as Patricia Jasen shows in her historical study on breast cancer, the word "risk" was only occasionally used in eighteenth- and nineteenth-century case histories.

The risk factor concept is an example of how scientific statements about risk embody, and at the same time, often obscure underlying moral values and implicit political decisions. The concept emerged as life insurance companies devised a new statistical approach to predicting chronic diseases for the purpose of selecting policy holders. The companies identified personal characteristics that increased the probability of premature mortality, and they required the physicians whom they employed as medical examiners to measure these characteristics in their examinations of applicants. By 1911, life insurance companies had not only determined a number of medical and non-medical factors, but had also quantified the statistical risk of excess mortality associated with each. At this stage, the factors included physical build, family history of disease, insanity, stroke, premature death of parents and siblings, physical condition, personal and medical history and habits, and occupation. In the area of medical diagnostics, urinalysis and blood pressure measurement also proved to be of predictive value.[31]

Medical measurements like blood pressure provided a focus for a new type of risk-factor approach. This new concept of *medical* risk factor (as opposed to the older life-insurance risk factor) was embodied by the influential Framingham study. This investigation was initiated in 1947 to survey the population of a typical American city over 20 years for coronary heart disease (CHD) and its possible causes. Framingham, a Massachusetts town with a population of 28,000, was considered to be representative of the American urban way of life. The first Framingham reports were published in 1957 and they claimed that high blood pressure, along with obesity and hypercholesterolemia, were associated with a high incidence of CHD.[32] The Framingham study introduced the risk factor into medical research, but at the same time changed its character in a number of ways: whereas the old life-insurance risk factor was conceived in terms of a gradient of risk, depending on its level, the new medical risk factors tended to be dichotomized into healthy and unhealthy levels. Each life-insurance risk factor was related to all other risk factors; by contrast, each of the medical risk factors was usually considered separately. Finally, whereas the life-insurance risk factor emphasized both the social and the medical characteristics of the applicant, medical risk factors were restricted to medical characteristics.[33] The medicalization of the risk-factor approach went even further. Subsequently, some risk factors were treated like straightforward diseases, as was the case with hypercholesterolemia and hypertension. In these conditions, precise quantitative levels defined disease entities and the need for specific drug therapy.[34] At the same time, and also in keeping with the predominant medical approach to understanding disease, risk-factor discourses illustrated a tendency to personalize the responsibility for any illness, constructing risk as the consequence of "lifestyle" choices made by individuals and emphasizing the need for self control.[35]

Risk factors have become a central part of modern clinical, public health and financial strategies for predicting and managing individual variation in disease predisposition and experience. The overwhelming success of the medical version of the risk factor approach can probably be explained by its technological character. Its relative simplicity made it attractive in the context of a kind of medicine that was increasingly modeled after reductionist laboratory science: medical risk factors reduce complex social relationships to discrete and measurable physiological phenomena that take place within the individual (even though, ironically, this brand of individualism is rationalized and legitimated by aggregate data and a focus on populations). Thinking in terms of risk factors instead of causes might well appear to be a major attempt to shift the focus from monocausal, reductionist approaches to a more holistic outlook, but, as Robert Aronowitz explains, "the discrete, quantitative contributions of these factors to CHD, the emphasis on specificity and mechanism, and the growing tendency to view risk factors as diseases in their own right, are reductionist features" that link it to the mainstream technocratic approach in medicine.[36] Again, the concept of risk can be understood as a tool for dealing with uncertainty, but, like any other tool, it is a tool that already embodies a whole range of political and moral values.

Risk politics

Whatever the context, framing the uncertainties of technical innovation in terms of calculable risk is intended to provide an objectified and neutral assessment. In general, numbers and the techniques that are used to manipulate them are appreciated for their ostensible neutrality in situations where values clash and consensus is elusive.[37] However, despite their appearance of objectivity and neutrality, processes of risk assessment and management always involve value judgements.[38] Science and technology are not politically neutral and thus cannot replace political decision-making. In the case of low-level radiation, as described by Sarah Dry in this volume, for example, scientific data was not merely insufficient but *irrelevant* for decisions on safety. At the end of the day, any decision about the acceptability of risk is political in nature, and even the decision to base one's assessment on science is inherently value-laden. As Deborah Gordon explains, reliance on science privileges a particular approach to reality that is as committed to a particular set of values as any other approach and selects for certain specific measurements while other types of information are rendered unimportant or irrelevant.[39]

The technological rationale inherent in the statistical approach to the dangers of medical innovation was criticised from the start. Critics rejected the merchant's logic in the eighteenth-century debates on smallpox inoculation and disapproved of the population-based, utilitarian approach they embodied. "Numbers were persuasive because they were impersonal," Andrea Rusnock writes,[40] "but, by the same measure, they were also insensitive because they valued the welfare of the population over the welfare of the individual." Opposition to population-based reasoning on the basis of a preference for individualizing clinical practice became a recurring theme in modern medicine. In the early nineteenth century, opponents of Pierre Louis's "numerical method" feared that his approach threatened the authority of the clinician and his freedom to treat patients on an individual basis.[41] One-and-a-half centuries later, as Thomas Schlich's chapter in this volume shows, opponents of operative fracture care in the 1960s and 1970s rejected statistical data because they could neither predict the outcome of the individual case nor appropriately represent the individual tragedy of a complication for a patient.[42] Obviously, statistical reasoning fails to convince those who do not appreciate the generalized type of information it yields. Such fundamental differences in worldviews testify to the "ethical clash" that historians of modern medicine have identified between those doctors who endorsed "professional values centered on the individual" and others who advocated "the statistical necessity of taking averages".[43]

In discourses on risk, the non-neutral character of scientific knowledge also manifests itself in the fact that talking about risk involves talking about responsibility.[44] This is a fundamentally political issue, since it involves ascribing the mandate and attributing the power to act on behalf of others. Changes in the way risks are conceptualized lead to a redistribution of "responsibilities for risks, change the locus of decision making and determine who has the right – and who has the obligation – to 'do something' about hazards."[45] It makes a big difference whether the responsibility for unwanted side effects is seen to lie with the drug users, for example, or the manufacturers, or the doctors who prescribe them. Thus, risk discourses can be analysed in terms of their specific ways of distributing responsibility and ascribing trust. In the cases of osteosynthesis and Interleukin-2 that are discussed in this volume, the responsibility for bad outcomes was shifted from the inventors of the technique towards the medical practitioners. This redistribution of responsibility made these new and risky treatment methods acceptable on a larger scale. The regulations for the reintroduction of Thalidomide, as described by Timmermans and Leiter in Chapter 15, emphasized the responsibility of women users, who were conceived as being basically unreliable and unpredictable, instead of focusing on possible actors within the system, such as the doctors. Thus, while controlling the use of the drug rendered the risk of birth defects manageable and acceptable, it also established inequalities in the power relationships between the actors.

While the ostensibly neutral concept of risk helps to turn politically charged problems into technically manageable ones, the way political issues are translated into technical ones is not always accepted by all those who are involved. The very act of quantifying "actual risk", for example, necessarily ignores all kinds of *qualitative* features that may be relevant for the social actors affected, such as the involuntary or unfamiliar character of "exposure".[46] This is particularly significant because the recognition of who can legitimately accept or reject risks is unevenly distributed: if laypeople reject the expert view, scientists patronizingly tend to describe public reactions as subjective and irrational. Public opposition to nuclear power seems to be caused by a misunderstanding of "the 'real' risks as known to science".[47] Scientists tacitly assume that scientific knowledge is always useful and relevant in the layperson's own social context.[48] They often ignore the fact that laypeople may have good reasons for their rejection of scientific rationales because the complexity and multidimensional variability of everyday-world problems in fact require a more comprehensive kind of rationality than that of purely statistical reasoning.[49] In the extreme case this can mean that laypeople ignore expert opinion on safety altogether. As Lara Marks notes in Chapter 11, some women were prepared to use the contraceptive pill "whatever the costs were to [their] health". In their individual risk–benefit calculations the pill was by far the preferable choice. Marks describes taking the pill or not as "a very individual decision, based on the kind of relationship a woman had, her family circumstances, her medical history and the alternative contraceptives available to her". Pill users thus appropriated choices about taking risks on an individual level. In his book *Impure Science*, on the case of HIV/AIDS, Steven Epstein has examined how differences in priorities between experts and laypeople were played out on the collective level of an organized social movement when severely ill patients insisted on using new drugs even at the risk of grave side effects. The appropriation of knowledge and power by organized self-help groups resulted in a new pattern of claims to regulatory control.[50]

As Arthur Daemmrich argues in Chapter 14, state authorities like the U.S. Food and Drug Administration (FDA) now have to acknowledge that the "comparatively simple calculus of gauging whether a new medication would benefit more patients than it might harm from side effects" had to be supplemented by regulations "to accommodate patients with fatal diseases clamoring for medicines as well as greater publicity of even interim testing results". Ironically, the measures that were enacted by experts in order to protect the patients in the first place were now attacked by a particular group of patients. It is obvious that differences in risk evaluation are not merely "subjective" or perceptual. Those differences rather point to the fact that cognitive frameworks for risk evaluation are rooted in differences of interest and social relations of power.[51] Disputes over risk decisions are about the distribution of the burden of uncertainty and about who are to be the victims of risks imposed by others.[52]

However, medical technologies are not purely socially or culturally constructed, they are also material. They transfer politics into the material objects that are involved and the bodies that are affected. As science and technology studies have shown, technologies are "intricate systems that weave together the technical and the social".[53] Thus, technologies help shape risk concepts and vice versa: "Perceptions of risk are not things that get tacked onto technology at the end of the day. Definitions of risk get *built into* technology and shape its evolution,"[54] so that "risks are constructed constantly as technological networks evolve."[55]

Risk of medical innovation

The individual case studies in this book examine a range of strategies used to deal with uncertainty involving different modes of knowledge production and regulation. Ulrich Tröhler starts off with a number of examples from the eighteenth through to the twentieth century. In Chapter 2 he analyses his cases as to the use of two ideal types of strategy in dealing with medical innovations. The first approach consists in the evaluation of potential dangers and benefits of an innovation for the patient. The second strategy is to try to avoid the dangers altogether by improving the innovation itself.

In the third chapter of this volume, Ian Burney looks at how the ideal of ridding decision-making of its arbitrary, idiosyncratic, and subjective dimension by using numbers, statistics, and probabilities[56] was pursued in the context of the introduction of anaesthesia. In the 1840s the introduction and the selective use of anaesthetics was accompanied by quantified risk–benefit calculations, giving rise to what the medical historian Martin Pernick (1985) has described as a "calculus of suffering".[57] In an article from 1847, James Simpson, the British surgeon and advocate of anaesthesia, embraced the emergent "numerical method" as the best means of setting anaesthesia on secure, rational grounds. Numerical cost–benefit analysis gave medical utilitarians like Simpson a means of objectively managing the "passions and anxieties" provoked by the new technology of anaesthesia and construct an "ideology grounded in technical, rationalistic calculation", as Burney concludes in his chapter.

As opposed to the cautious attitude displayed towards anaesthesia, the announcement in the 1890s that Robert Koch had found a cure for tuberculosis was greeted with widespread enthusiasm. However, as Christoph Gradmann shows in Chapter 4, the supposed wonder-drug tuberculin not only proved to be ineffective but also dangerous for many patients. In the ensuing discussions the issue of danger was closely connected to the question of effectiveness. Despite the use of quantification for the documentation of the clinical experience, the notions of probability and risk did not enter into the discussion. At that time, the term "risk" was still restricted to the financial and commercial domain. The word "danger" that was used instead did not have the associations with calculability and controllability that risk had. The tuberculin scandal seems to have left traces in the profession's collective memory, becoming a standard ingredient of later critical considerations of the side effects of drugs. New drugs were now viewed with more suspicion and often triggered controversial discussions about their effectiveness and inherent dangers.

In Chapter 5, Christian Bonah deals with another milestone in the history of medical innovation, the Lübeck vaccination scandal of 1931–2. In this northern German town, inoculation against tuberculosis with an unsafe batch of *Bacille Calmette-Guérin* (BCG) caused the death of 76 new-born babies. Since BCG is a live vaccine, the procedure itself could cause tuberculosis. In order to evaluate the danger, the statistical risk of dying from BCG vaccination had to be balanced against the statistical risk of dying from naturally occurring tuberculosis. Because of this, evaluation of both efficacy and safety required long periods of observation and remained to some extent uncertain. BCG is an example of how different types of knowledge enter into those discussions. Deterministic knowledge produced in the laboratory was combined or countered with probabilistic knowledge derived from clinical research, providing much opportunity for disagreement about methodology and interpretation. The court trial of those who conducted the Lübeck inoculations not only sheds light on the legal and forensic dimension of the issue of risk, it also demonstrates how considerations of risk involve the distribution of responsibility and how decisions about risks are always made within the framework of particular value choices. The trial triggered public discussion of medical ethics in Europe, and it catalysed the establishment of the German state regulations for medical research on human beings, the first in the Western hemisphere.

Regulations and the authority to enforce them also feature prominently in the case of X-rays. The question of who is in charge of controlling risk thus determined power relationships on a range of levels and created new social realities. In Chapter 6 Monika Dommann describes how regulation transformed the perceived danger of X-rays in twentieth-century Switzerland into calculable and controllable risks. The creation, enactment and control of regulation raised the question of competence and legitimation. Up until the 1960s, Swiss radiologists had successfully avoided state regulation by establishing their own system of self-control. For them, the expertise necessary for controlling the new technology provided a nucleus for their particular specialization.[58] The radiologists were one of several groups of experts that could professionalize themselves around new dangers, and so for them managing risk was a professional resource. On a more general level, the risks linked to X-rays were also used to draw a boundary between physicians and laypeople. When the Swiss rules governing X-ray procedures defined the use of X-rays as a medical activity, non-physicians were excluded from the practice, outlawing, for example, the use of X-rays for fitting shoes. The subsequent struggle between chiropractors and doctors over the use of X-rays also illustrates how drawing these boundaries was a contested issue.

Another expression of scientific authority is the setting of standards, such as radiation standards. Establishing quantified limits is part of converting incalculable dangers into calculable risks. In Chapter 7, on the controversies over low-level radiation in the 1950s, Sarah Dry analyses the way in which those limits resulted from negotiations to find a compromise between avoiding danger and benefiting from the usefulness of the new technique. Standards are thus a matter of politics and values. Already the choice of the type of standards to be used – "tolerance dose" versus "maximum permissible dose", for example – involves implicit decisions concerning values. The discussions over the risk of radiation demonstrate the essentially political character of any decisions on environmental risk-taking, even if they are expressed in technical scientific terms. One can see how reifying potential harm as risk and delegating decisions to experts makes risks appear to emerge from the technical properties of things rather than from the power relationships between people.[59] This naturalization of risk in turn shapes social relationships and attributions of responsibility.

Bonah's and Dry's chapters furthermore demonstrate how modern medicine tries to deal with uncertainty by using science. Different kinds of scientific knowledge help to construct networks of causality and probability that identify and assess risks and link innovations to a putative harmful consequence in a specific way.[60] Ever since the nineteenth-century "laboratory revolution",[61] the experimental laboratory has been a privileged space for creating medical knowledge. In the field of risk evaluation, animal experiments, for example, were used early on for determining the hazards of new surgical interventions. Later they became an important tool to study the carcinogenic nature of new drugs.[62] Sarah Dry describes how, for laboratory scientists, the ultimate ideal of objectifying risk is a quantified and calculable causal relationship between the medical intervention and unwanted side effects. Its embodiment is the "dose-response-curve", which in the case of radiation is the "graphical representation of the relationship between a given dose of radiation and subsequent disease". Other practitioners, for example in epidemiology and public health, are often wary of this type of reductionism. They criticise laboratory scientists for using idealized concepts that are appropriate to highly controlled laboratory conditions but are not well suited to the assessment and analysis of "real-world" risks.[63]

In general, doctors have to consider how much and what kind of evidence they need before they start using new vaccines, drugs or procedures on humans. However, results from clinical and epidemiological research are equally underdetermined and always require further interpretation in order to apply them to a risk problem.

The evaluation and combination of laboratory and epidemiological evidence was also significant for the introduction of antihypertensive drugs, as analysed by Carsten Timmermann (Chapter 8). Here, considerations about the risk of medical innovation were linked to a risk-factor discourse since the new drugs were not used for a manifest disease but against a risk factor: doctors were balancing the risk of not treating chronic mild hypertension against the risk of drug treatment. In practice this meant that the cost for avoiding the risk factor of hypertension was to subject individuals who were not yet sick to the risks of new treatments.

When in the 1970s treatment of women with diethylstilboestrol (DES) was linked to an increased occurrence of breast cancer, the dangers of this new therapy were clearly framed in what we would now call "terms of risk". Jean-Paul Gaudillière traces the discussions on the hazards of sex steroid treatment back to Germany in the 1930s, in which risk as a probability-based category was not yet present. However, the occurrence of cancer was seen as preventable through the creation of knowledge and regulation. Scientists and doctors first aimed at creating and applying scientific knowledge about toxicity and dosage in the laboratory, and, second, aimed at controlling the use of hormones through medical experts. This case also shows how the context of drug use shapes the perception of its risk; whether hormone treatment was seen as dangerous or not depended on the context of its use. As long as steroids were used against the symptoms of menopause, the cancer problem was discussed as a serious issue; when the same hormones were used later on to treat cancer, the fact that they themselves might induce cancer disappeared from sight.

In Chapter 10, Thomas Schlich analyses the introduction in the 1960s and 1970s of a new surgical technique for fixing broken bones called osteosynthesis or internal fixation. The benefits of this method were not only balanced against its risks, but also against the risks and benefits of the established conservative method of treating fractures. The Swiss-based surgical association, the Association for Internal Fixation (AO/ASIF), which succeeded in introducing the new method into the standard surgical repertoire, tried to limit the risks by exerting an unprecedented degree of control over the levels of production and clinical use of the technology. At the same time, the AO managed to shift the locus of risk from the procedure itself to the individual surgeon by attributing the blame for complications to the surgeon's (lack of) competence. The AO's remedy was the strict standardization of surgical competence and practice, a strategy that was resisted by those surgeons who wanted to preserve their professional autonomy. These surgeons also opposed the strategy of dealing with risk through probabilistic calculations of a risk–benefit ratio at the level of populations. This example shows that such a strategy only makes sense for those willing to accept the de-individualizing approach involved in risk considerations and the associated changes in relations of authority and power.

Lara Marks's chapter on the contraceptive pill, Chapter 11, deals with a drug that considerably reshaped the regulation and social perception of medication and risk in the second half of the twentieth century. Taken by healthy women of reproductive age for long periods of time, the drug raised questions about its potential for harm in terms of fertility and long-term health. Part of the context of assessing this medical innovation was the postulation of the "natural" risks of pregnancy and childbirth as a background against which to assess the new, "artificial" risk. As Lara Marks makes clear, this distinction is hypothetical, since the risk of childbirth depends to a large degree on man-made factors such as social status. Despite its artificiality, the contextualization of the risk of medical innovation against the background of supposedly "natural" risks went even further when proponents of the pill compared the risk of taking it with "lifestyle risks" and argued that the hazards associated with oral contraceptives were minimal compared to other activities such as traveling by air, car, or motorbike, rock climbing, smoking, domestic accidents, or playing soccer. The fact that many of these activities were typically male recreational activities further underscores the culture dependency of these supposedly natural risks.

Nature and culture are also integral to another source of medical uncertainty, the pronouncement of death.[64] The introduction of the brain death concept in the 1960s resulted in serious uncertainties and the perceived risk of diagnosing death prematurely. Silke Bellanger and Aline Steinbrecher examine in Chapter 12 how in Switzerland the objectifying strategies of quantification and visualization transformed brain death into a standardized object of knowledge and practice. Standardization of practices was used to decrease uncertainty and cancel out individuality and subjectivity in the diagnosis of brain death. Eventually, however, individuality and subjectivity were explicitly addressed and subjected to new forms of *self*-regulation in order to decrease the heterogeneity of individual attitudes towards the issue of brain death.

In Chapter 13, Peter Keating and Alberto Cambrosio analyse risk in clinical cancer trials from the 1950s to the 1990s. As a new approach for generating biomedical knowledge, these trials produced certain forms of risk at the same time. One risk consists in the toxicity of new treatments. Since patients in cancer trials are seriously ill, this is regarded as a relative risk which has to be balanced against potential benefits. A second kind of risk is that, by participating in a clinical trial, an important feature of which is comparison of an older therapy to a new therapy, cancer patients might be forgoing another more effective treatment. A third risk concerns the risk of invalidating the trial itself: the trials had in some way to be protected against their premature cessation at the moment when first results emerged that seemed to indicate the superiority of one of the treatments tested. For this purpose, specific mechanisms were built into the trial design in order to protect the knowledge-generation process and thus future patients who would benefit from that knowledge. In clinical trials, research and testing are thus interwoven in ways that tie, in the authors' words, risk issues "to the same seamless web of material, organizational and socio-cognitive elements", a fact that "makes the management of cancer trial risks different from risk management in other fields of biomedical research".

As Arthur Daemmrich shows in Chapter 14, control of application was the most important strategy for dealing with risk when Interleukin-2 was introduced into cancer therapy in the 1990s. The producer of this new therapeutic agent claimed to be able to mitigate at least some of its negative side effects through standardization and an extremely precise treatment regimen. By contrasting the use of the new treatment in the USA and Germany, Daemmrich demonstrates the significance of technical issues of application for the production, perception and evaluation of risk. Such cross-national comparisons[65] of drug regulation strikingly illustrate the fact that, as Sheila Jasanoff states, "evaluations of risk by technical experts frequently take color from their social context"[66] and that the certification process of drugs and chemicals in different countries is conditioned by larger cultural assumptions about risk. In addition to the differences in healthcare systems and risk regulation, Daemmrich's chapter also looks at the differences in business cultures and in political climate in the two countries and concludes that a new form of "BioRisk" emerged in each country, driven by different patterns of medical risk assessment, approaches to clinical testing, financial invest-ment, and public response to visions of the future of therapeutic approaches.

Historically, the most important reforms of drug regulation occurred in the wake of the Thalidomide disaster. The sedative was withdrawn from the market in 1961 when it became known that several thousand children worldwide had been born with incomplete arms and legs after their mothers had taken Thalidomide during pregnancy. Highly publicized lawsuits and the subsequent re-examination of the legal mechanisms of drug regulation turned Thalidomide into a cultural symbol for the risks associ-ated with legal drugs.[67] This is why it is of particular interest to look at what happened when Thalidomide was re-introduced in the 1990s. In Chapter 15 Stefan Timmermans and Valerie Leiter have analysed the highly regulated re-launch of the drug in terms of the interests and meanings for physicians, patients, the Thalidomide victims' organization, and the FDA. One main strategy to deal with this problem was standardization and control on many different levels. In this way, a previously unacceptable risk could be reframed as a permissible, "residual" risk. Their symbolic-interactionist perspective allows the authors to understand how this system could be established by negotiating control and autonomy, attributing blame and responsibility among the actors involved, and how this shapes them in particular ways.

Historiography of risk in medicine

The different chapters of this book examine their respective cases from a variety of perspectives. Despite these differences they all show that history contributes in a specific way to a better understanding of how people deal with potential health dangers. Thus, historical case studies point beyond rational choice theory and show that risk-taking behaviour cannot be explained by notions of preference and rationality in any simple way. They also transcend psychological explanations of risk perception. Historical evidence supports the idea that decision-making on risks must be under-stood as a social and relational phenomenon.[68] Even when decisions on medical innovations had been made by individuals, "they were usually part of some formal or informal political process, matters of alliances or enmities, of professional co-operation or rivalry", as John Pickstone emphasizes, pointing out that "historical case studies can then help to illustrate how the political frameworks have varied and how they have tended to change over the last century or so in medicine".[69] History also helps us to understand risk perceptions "in terms of plural social constructions of meaning which are culturally framed".[70] This has been formulated by Mary Douglas and Aaron Wildavsky[71] in their influential anthropological essay on risk in which they state that "what needs to be explained is how people agree to ignore most of the potential dangers that surround them and interact so as to concentrate only on selected aspects". The choices people make reflect their beliefs about values, social institutions, nature, and moral behaviour. Risks are exaggerated or minimized according to the social, cultural, and moral acceptability of the underlying activities.

Based on the assumption that medical knowledge and practice are products of human activity and that, according to Ilana Löwy, "medicine should be studied simultaneously as a body of knowledge, a practice, a profession, a cultural and social phenomenon and a political issue",[72] it makes sense for historians to use concrete case studies for analysing risks as being culturally produced in specific periods and places. They examine "how perceptions and judgment arise from a host of complex factors, including historical trends, underlying values, ideological currents, and the nature of social, cultural, economic, scientific, and political institutions at specific points in time and in specific spaces".[73]

Historical investigation is therefore an excellent way of doing justice to the socially and culturally contingent character of risk realities. This is not a purely academic exercise: an analysis along these lines can help to develop an alternative to the various technical and regulatory approaches to risk assessment and management, and it can reveal "the socially constructed or framed nature of health risks and the various plural rationalities involved".[74] History demonstrates that the tools for dealing with uncertainty already contain political decisions on values that, in a democratic society, should be up for public discussion rather than being relegated to experts. A historically informed understanding of decision-making on risks thus provides the background information for finding appropriate strategies for coping with the uncertainties surrounding potential threats to health, whether they are seen as originating in the environment, individual behaviour or in medicine itself.

Notes

1 Acknowledgments: I want to thank Silke Bellanger, Alberto Cambrosio, Katherine Frohlich, Jonathan Kimmelman, Ulrich Tröhler, and George Weisz for their valuable comments on earlier versions of this chapter.
2 R. C. Fox, "Medical Uncertainty Revisited", in G. L. Albrecht, R. F. and S. D. Scrimshaw (eds), *Handbook of Social Studies in Health and Medicine*, London, Thousand Oaks and New Delhi: Sage, 2000, pp. 407–25; see p. 409.
3 J. F. Short and L. Clarke, "Social Organization and Risk", in J. F. Short and L. Clarke (eds), *Organizations, Uncertainties, and Risk*, Boulder: Westview Press, 1992, pp. 309–21; see pp. 317–18.
4 Fox, *Uncertainty*, pp. 410–11.
5 J. Gabe, "Health, Medicine and Risk: The Need for a Sociological Approach", in J. Gabe (ed.), *Medicine, Health and Risk: Sociological Approaches*, Oxford: Blackwell, 1995, pp. 1–17; see p. 2; M. V. Hayes, "On the Epistemology of Risk: Language, Logic and Social Science", *Social Science and Medicine*, 1992, vol. 35, pp. 401–7; see p. 403.
6 John-Arne Skolbekken, "The Risk Epidemic in Medical Journals", *Social Science and Medicine*, 40, 1995, pp. 291–305; see p. 292.
7 J. F. Short and Lee Clarke, "Social Organization and Risk"; see pp. 317–18.
8 Hayes, *Epistemology*; see p. 401.

9 N. Luhmann, *Risk: A Sociological Theory*, New York: Aldine de Gruyler, 1993, pp. 1–31.

10 Skolbekken, *Epidemic*.

11 Skolbekken, *Epidemic*, pp. 295–6.

12 J. V. Pickstone, "Introduction", in J. V. Pickstone (ed.), *Medical Innovations in Historical Perspective*, Houndmills, Basingstoke: Macmillan, 1992, pp. 1–16; I. Löwy, "Introduction: Medicine and Change", in I. Löwy (ed.), *Medicine and Change: Historical and Sociological Studies of Medical Innovation*, Paris: Les editions INSERM, 1993, pp. 1–19.

13 U. Beck, *Risikogesellschaft: Auf dem Weg in eine andere Moderne*, Frankfurt: Suhrkamp, 1985.

14 T. Schlich, *Surgery, Science and Industry: A Revolution in Fracture Care, 1950s–1990s*, Houndmills, Basingstoke: Palgrave-Macmillan, 2003, p. 241.

15 A number of studies on the history of medical innovation focus on the benefit side. There is less on the negative side of dangers and risks that made new techniques harder to accept for contemporaries. On the resistance to innovation, see J. Stanton (ed.), *Innovations in Health and Medicine: Diffusion and Resistance in the Twentieth Century*, London, and New York: Routledge, 2002.

16 Pickstone, *Introduction*; see p. 16.

17 E. Magnello and A. Hardy, "Preface", in E. Magnello and A. Hardy (eds), *The Road to Medical Statistics*, Amsterdam, New York: Rodopi, 2002, pp. iii–xi; see p. iv.

18 G. Gigerenzer *et al.*, *The Empire of Chance: How Probability Changed Science and Everyday Life*, Cambridge: Cambridge University Press, 1989; see pp. 20–6.

19 W. G. Rothstein, *Public Health and the Risk Factor: A History of an Uneven Medical Revolution*, Rochester: University of Rochester Press, 2003; see pp. 61–2.

20 Gigerenzer *et al.*, *Empire*, pp. 20–1.

21 A. Rusnock, " 'The Merchant's Logick': Numerical Debates over Smallpox Inoculation in Eighteenth-Century England", in E. Magnello and A. Hardy (eds), *The Road to Medical Statistics*, Amsterdam, New York: Rodopi, 2002, pp. 37–54; see pp. 40–50.

22 Magnello and Hardy, *Preface*, vi–viii.

23 U. Tröhler, *"To Improve the Evidence of Medicine": The 18th Century British Origins of a Critical Approach*, Edinburgh: The Royal College of Physicians of Edinburgh, 2000; see pp.16–21, 69–72, 115–24.

24 Gigerenzer *et al.*, *Empire*, pp. 17–18.

25 Rusnock, *Logick*, pp. 38–51.

26 G. Weisz, *The Medical Mandarins: The French Academy of Medicine in the Nineteenth and Early Twentieth Centuries*, New York, Oxford: Oxford University Press, 1995, pp. 159–188; J. R. Matthews, *Quantification and the Quest for Medical Certainty*, Princeton NJ: Princeton University Press, 1995.

27 Gigerenzer *et al.*, *Empire*, p. 47.

28 E. Magnello, "The Introduction of Mathematical Statistics into Medical Research", in E. Magnello and A. Hardy (eds), *The Road to Medical Statistics*, Amsterdam, New York: Rodopi, 2002, pp. 95–123; see pp. 107–8.

29 Magnello and Hardy, *Introduction*, pp. ix–x.

30 R. A. Aronowitz, *Making Sense of Illness: Science, Society and Disease*, Cambridge: Cambridge University Press, 1998, p. 111; P. Jasen, "Breast Cancer and the Language of Risk, 1750–1950", *Social History of Medicine* , 2002, vol. 15, pp. 17–43; see p. 17.

31 Rothstein, *Public Health*, pp. 50–70, 261.

32 See Carsten Timmermann, Chapter 8 in this book.

33 Rothstein, *Public Health*, pp. 279–85.

34 Aronowitz, *Making Sense*, pp. 127–41.

35 Gabe, *Health*, p. 3; S. Hilgartner, "The Social Construction of Risk Objects: Or, How to Pry Open Networks of Risk", in J. F. Short and L. Clarke (eds), *Organizations, Uncertainties, and Risk*, Boulder: Westview Press, 1992, pp. 39–53; see p. 47.

36 Aronowitz, *Making Sense*, pp. 112–18, 131–5; quote from p. 112.

37 Gigerenzer *et al.*, *Empire*, pp. 236–7.

38 S. Jasanoff, "Cultural Aspects of Risk Assessment in Britain and the United States", in B. B. Johnson and V. T. Covello (eds), *The Social and Cultural Construction of Risk: Essays on Risk Selection and Perception*, Dordrecht: D. Reidel, 1987, pp. 359–97; see p. 359.

39 Gordon 1988, p. 283.

40 Rusnock, *Logick*, p. 49.

41 J. R. Matthews, "Almroth Wright, Vaccine Therapy and British Biometrics: Disciplinary Expertise Versus Statistical Objectivity", in E. Magnello and A. Hardy (eds), *The Road to Medical Statistics*, Amsterdam, New York: Rodopi, 2002, pp. 125–47; see pp. 135–41, Weisz, *Mandarins*, pp. 159–88.

42 See Chapter 10 by Thomas Schlich in this book.

43 Gigerenzer *et al.*, 1989, p. 261.

44 Aronowitz, *Making Sense*, p. 132.

45 Hilgartner, *Social Construction*, p. 47.

46 L. Levidov, "De-Reifying Risk", *Science and Culture*, 1994, vol. 20, pp. 440–56; see pp. 442–3.

47 Wynne 1995, p. 363.

48 Wynne 1995, p. 363.

49 Wynne, 1995.

50 Epstein, Steven: *Impure Science: AIDS, Activism, and the Politics of Knowledge*, University of California Press, Berkeley, 1996.

51 Levidov, *De-Reifying Risk*, p. 449.

52 James F. Short, Jr., "Defining, Explaining and Managing Risks", in James F. Short and Lee Clarke (eds), *Organizations, Uncertainties, and Risk*, Boulder: Westview Press, 1992, pp. 3–2; see p. 10.

53 Stephan Hilgartner, "The Social Construction of Risk Objects: Or, How to Pry Open Networks of Risk", in James F. Short and Lee Clarke (eds), *Organizations. Uncertainties, and Risk*, Boulder: Westview Press 1992, pp. 39–53; see p. 43.

54 Hilgartner, *Social Construction*, p. 39.

55 Hilgartner, *Social Construction*, p. 52.

56 Gigerenzer *et al.*, *Empire*, p. 288.

57 M. S. Pernick, *A Calculus of Suffering: Pain, Professionalism and Anesthesia in Nineteenth-Century America*, New York: Columbia University Press, 1985.

58 More generally on this see G. Weisz, "The Emergence of Specialization in the Nineteenth Century", *Bulletin for the History of Medicine*, 2002, vol. 77 (2003), pp. 536–75.

59 Levidov, *De-Reifying Risk*, pp. 440–1.

60 Cf. Hilgartner, *Social Construction*.

61 A. Cunningham and P. William (eds), *The Laboratory Revolution in Medicine*, Cambridge and New York: Cambridge University Press, 1992.

62 J. Abraham, "Scientific Standards and Institutional Interests: Carcinogenic Risk Assessment of Benoxaprofen in the UK and US", *Social Studies of Science*, 1993, vol. 23, pp. 387–444; see pp. 392–404.

63 Abraham, *Standards*, p. 417.

64 On nature and culture in the pronouncement of death, see T. Schlich, "Tod, Geschichte und Kultur", in T. Schlich and C. Wiesemann (eds), *Hirntod: Zur Kulturgeschichte der Todesfeststellung*, Frankfurt a.M.: Suhrkamp, 2001, pp. 209–35.

65 See also A. Daemmrich, "A Tale of Two Experts: Thalidomide and Political Engagement in the United States and West Germany", *Social History of Medicine*, 2002, vol. 15, pp. 137–58.

66 Jasanoff, *Cultural*, p. 359.

67 Daemmrich, *Tale*; B. Kirk, *Der Contergan-Fall: eine unvermeidbare Arzneimittelkatastrophe? Zur Geschichte des Arzneiwirkstoffs Thalidomid*, Stuttgart: Wissenschaftliche Verlagsgesellschaft, 1999.

68 L. Clarke, "Context Dependency and Risk Decision Making", in J. F. Short and L. Clarke (eds), *Organizations, Uncertainties, and Risk*, Boulder: Westview Press, 1992, pp. 27–38.

69 Pickstone, *Introduction*, p. 11.
70 Gabe, *Health*, p. 7.
71 M. Douglas and A. Wildavsky, *Risk and Culture. An Essay on the Selection of Technological and Environmental Dangers*. Berkeley, Los Angeles, London: University of California Press, 1982, p. 9.
72 Löwy, *Introduction*, pp. 1–2.
73 V. T. Covello and B. B. Johnson, "Introduction: The Social and Cultural Construction of Risk: Issues, Methods, and Case Studies", in V. T. Covello and B. B. Johnson (eds), *The Social and Cultural Construction of Risk*, Dordrecht: D. Reidel, 1987, pp. vii–xiii; see p. xii.
74 Gabe, *Health*, p. 11.

2 To assess and to improve

Practitioners' approaches to doubts linked with medical innovations 1720–1920

Ulrich Tröhler

Introduction

While most chapters of this book focus on innovations in modern medicine from the 1850s to the 1990s, the present contribution takes account of the fact that there were innovations in healthcare well before 1850: eighteenth-century examples that come to mind are inoculation of human smallpox,[1] the obstetric forceps,[2] the use of digitalis,[3] the introduction of the "lateral" method for the surgical treatment of urinary bladder stones, lithotomy, the flap method for amputation,[4] and the extraction of the ocular lens for the treatment of cataracts.[5] For us an innovation would imply comparison to an earlier situation. However, very little is known, historically, about how practitioners presented and perceived these new interventions, either in terms of gains ("advantage" and "benefit" were the concurrent terms) or losses ("harm" or "danger") *for the patient and/or society*, or in terms of *medical* safety. Attempting a systematic view from a long-term perspective, this chapter looks at the histories of inoculation and of a few eighteenth and nineteenth-century obstetrical and surgical innovations, and seeks to highlight the conceptual origins of what was later called "risk".

Doubts about inoculation in the eighteenth century

The case of inoculation against smallpox constitutes a noteworthy exception and an appropriate starting point, in that it has been historically well researched.[6] It was applied in the West on the basis of reports of empirical experience that it prevented this often fatal disease, but in the absence of any rational, "scientific" understanding of its functioning. Yet inoculation, besides not "functioning" as expected, could also lead to propagation of the disease and directly to death. These facts gave rise to several debates about its medical value and moral admissibility. These discussions included one of the earliest examples of a medical problem being tackled academically with the aid of mathematical estimates of probabilities, in a famous contest that took place in the 1760s between two academic experts, Daniel Bernoulli in Basle and Jean Le Rond d'Alembert in Paris.[7] However, forty years earlier, two practitioners, Doctors Zabdiel Boylston (1680–1766) in Boston and James Jurin (1684–1750) in London, had already calculated the "dangers in [naturally acquired smallpox] and the reasonable expectation they [people] have of doing well [following inoculation]". Using his own records, Boylston estimated this probability to be one in seven (14 per cent) in the former population, versus one in forty-six (2 per cent) in the latter.[8] Note that neither Boylston nor Jurin, nor the many others who treated this question throughout the eighteenth century, used the term "risk". Jurin noted in 1724: "People do not easily come into a Practice, in which they apprehend any Hazard, unless they are frightened into it by a greater Danger."[9] It is true "risk" is a nineteenth-century concept term. But Boylston and Jurin used the notion of danger differently than we do today, when it means, according to sociologist Niklas Luhmann, "potential damages … being attributed to causes outside one's control":[10] By their retrospective determination of the "dangers" of the procedure in quantitative terms that were meant to be of use prospectively, they in fact attempted to transform an incalculable "danger" into a calculated "risk" *avant la lettre*.

Such calculation of outcomes was interesting for policy-makers, indeed for any kind of authority – maybe even for enlightened parents with respect to the treatment of their children.[11] The different mortalities together with actual experience were the medical argument in favour of inoculation.[12] But there were also medical doubts. Did it really produce permanent immunity? Did this artificial disease not weaken the body? Might other diseases not be co-inoculated? Other objections were socially, philosophically, religiously and emotionally motivated.

Social objections centred on the argument of propagation by contagion, potentially leading to unsought infection of a whole community.[13] Expert philosophers argued whether there was a moral duty to inoculate smallpox or whether putting oneself deliberately into danger was a breach of the moral duty to oneself as a physical body.[14] More emotionally unsettling for many were probably the religious objections, deeply rooted in a traditional belief that "fear of disease was a happy restraint to men" and that one should neither inflict oneself nor one's children, nor interfere with God's will. It was with him that the power to inflict disease rested, "as a Trial of our Faith, or for the Punishment of our Sins".[15] Identical arguments were used against another eighteenth-century innovation, the lightning rod. Others considered inoculation diabolic or, given its oriental origins, "heathenish". Taken together,

> [t]hese were all spontaneous and logical doubts arising inevitably from the current state of medical knowledge and from accustomed religious thought.[16]

This atmosphere of controversy caused advocates of inoculation to interpret this oriental folk practice according to current occidental medical theories and consequently to introduce accompanying measures to render it "safer". These included new techniques for treating and new devices for applying the variolous matter. Furthermore, people were prepared by bleeding, purging and reduction of food intake, and they were isolated once they had been inoculated in order to prevent propagation of the disease. Thus, proponents aimed to reduce the "dangers" for both individuals and society. However, these measures could not be applied in times of an epidemic and were in all events restricted to the wealthier segments of the population.[17] Finally, enthusiastic promotion and blind opposition gave way to regulation by legislative action in England, the American colonies and later in Paris.[18] While the new emotional "dangers" of propagation and death associated with the invention persisted and were evidently perceived as a concrete threat to the individual, the calculated "advantage" and the medical safety were obviously tangible enough at this time to persuade enlightened individuals and authorities responsible for groups. In 1749 even the conservative editor of the classical works of Thomas Sydenham (1624–89) noted that:

> ... the practice is now so well establish'd, and become so general, many physicians and surgeons inoculating their children, that the safety, expediency, and advantages of it, cannot with any colour of reason be called in question.[19]

This example shows that (i) the outcome of an empirical folk treatment was assessed in terms of gains and losses, and (ii) that theoretically deduced medical measures were taken in order to increase the technical safety of the intervention. At the same time, leading propagators brought the individually perceived danger on an abstract level by quantification and by relating the individual outcome to the whole population. The intervention was finally adopted by regulations aimed at reducing these dangers, or, in other terms, at making the intervention *safe in medical terms*, while keeping the advantage of its *benefits for the people*.

Patients' versus doctors' perspective

The eighteenth-century example of smallpox inoculation suggests two ideal types of approach that can be distinguished in the way practitioners dealt with innovative interventions. One approach consisted in assessing (we can put the questions of criteria and evidence aside for the moment) whether the innovation did more good than harm *to the patient and/or to society*, while the other consisted in making the new intervention safer *from a technical, i.e. doctors' point of view*. Albeit closely intertwined and aiming ultimately at the same end, namely rendering the results of the innovation reliable, these two approaches involved different strategies. The "assessment" approach was concerned with the outcome of a given method in terms of patient "advantage" or "danger", implying its clinical testing in its present technical incarnation at any given time. The other approach focused on the medical safety of the new method, on eventually technically modifying it, implying that the "improved" method would give better results in the future until, ideally, it would exhibit only the originally intended beneficial effects of the innovation. It may therefore be called the "improvement-and-safety" approach. In the end, some kind of outcome assessment, implicit or explicit, cannot be evaded in this approach either, but the criteria for defining and assessing benefit, harm and danger on one hand and safety on the other may depend on the perspective of those concerned, and the criteria may vary with time. In the case of smallpox they were relatively simple – survival or death.

Whilst in eighteenth-century inoculation both these ideal approaches converged, the following three examples from the eighteenth and nineteenth centuries illustrate cases of predominance of the "improvement-and-safety" approach.

The obstetric forceps

Another eighteenth-century innovation, the obstetric forceps, was altogether different from the preventive intervention of smallpox inoculation, for two reasons: (i) the use of the instrument initially was only meant to be considered when the lives of both mother and child were immediately threatened; and (ii) the forceps was introduced by doctors as an *ultima ratio* not on empirical, but on logical, theoretical grounds, following insight into the mechanical physiology of the birth process.

The *ultima ratio* has since become a typical situation for the introduction of many inventions. In the eighteenth century, however, lay-people saw this differently, as they were not yet accustomed to the idea that medicine could successfully intervene in a terrifying situation that they attributed to fate or to God's inexorable will. The English obstetrician, William Smellie (1697–1763), one of the advocates of the forceps, summarized the situation in 1752:

> ... women ... observed that, when recourse was had to the assistance of a man-midwife, either the mother or child, or both, were lost. This censure ... could not fail of being a great discouragement to male practitioners. [But now] a more *safe* [my italics] and certain expedient for this purpose has been invented ... so that if we [i.e. man-midwives] are called in before the child is dead, or the parts of the woman in danger of a mortification, both the *Foetus* and mother may frequently be happily saved. This fortunate contrivance is no other than the forceps.[20]

Three generations later, the Göttingen professor of obstetrics, Johann Friedrich Osiander (1787–1855) could write, "that in order to recommend the forceps – if this is deemed at all necessary – one needs only to say that they have rendered *male* (italics in original) obstetrics humane", making its formerly cruel interventions of cutting the foetus into pieces (embryotomy) almost superfluous.[21] However, as was the case with inoculation, this development was not achieved without weighing individual and social benefits against dangers. But there were no calculations. There were medical arguments, as there were religious and emotional ones of fate and fear. And again, technical measures were taken to render the innovation medically "safer", with the result that Smellie's forceps were shorter and lighter than the models used by some of his contemporaries. Furthermore, he covered the blades with leather because he believed that this would reduce the danger of injuring mother and/or child. In fact, this was his chief reason for these coverings.

But the coverings led in turn to medical criticism on rational grounds: was not the leather responsible for bringing the contagion of childbed fever from one mother to the other? Early opponents also attributed the possible transmission of "*lues venereae*" and other "*morbi contagiosi*" to these leather-bound instruments.[22]

The new dangers were not calculated. Yet, aware of the objections, Smellie recommended as an improvement "that the blades of the forceps ought to be *new* [my italics] covered with stripes of washed leather, after they have been used, especially in delivering a woman suspected of having an infectious distemper".[23]

Yet there was still another aspect. Smellie also looked at his innovation from the perspective of the parturient and those surrounding her. In his *Treatise on Theory and Practise of Midwifery* (1752) he wrote: "The forceps are covered with leather, and appear so simple and innocent ... At any rate ... women are commonly freightened at the very name of an instrument."[24] Consequently we find the following instructions for the young practitioner:

> ... when he sits down to deliver, let him spread the sheet that hangs over the bed, upon his lap, and under that cover, take out and dispose the blades [of the forceps] on each side of the patient; by which means he will often be able to deliver with the forceps, without their being perceived by the woman herself, or any other assistants. Some people pin a sheet to each shoulder and throw the other end over the bed, that they may be the more effectually concealed.[25]

The forceps could sometimes prevent apparently certain death in childbirth – of the child and/or the mother. This was certainly an advantage for all concerned. But, as was the case with inoculation, this innovation created new problems: transmission of disease, injury and fright that might in turn lead to further consequences for mother and/or child. Since they were iatrogenic, as in inoculation, these problems concerned the practitioner, particularly if he had little experience.[26]

Appropriate technical and behavioural measures were recommended, albeit with entirely qualitative arguments at first, for Smellie gave no quantitative data on the success with his new forceps. Not until later, in the eighteenth century, were some results published in the simple statistical form of survivals.[27]

Furthermore, in the view of its propagators, the negative medical and emotional consequences of this innovation might be controlled by training with obstetric models and other teaching aids[28] as well as with *in vivo* cases of normal birth. Indeed, this became customary in some midwifery hospitals in the second half of the eighteenth century, particularly in Germany.[29] All these measures intended to render male obstetrics – an innovation in itself – technically and emotionally safer and thus more humane, at least from the doctors' point of view.

By fostering a judicious use of the forceps, Smellie actually represented a middle line among man-midwives, for there were adherents of the inventors of the forceps, the Chamberlen family, who thought it to be useful in nearly all cases. Since the *mechanical* physiology of normal delivery, the movements of the child in the birth canal, were well understood by then, was it not reasonable to assist nature regularly with a *mechanical* device, the forceps? Others pleaded for nature to have her way, that is for expectative, at most hand-assisted, obstetric care. This was not primarily a gender issue, for midwives were not forbidden to use this innovation, and historians still debate why midwives ultimately never did.[30] Rather, there were controversies among man-midwives about the indication for its use. These still went on around 1800, and they were European. While the French tended to favour a widespread use of the forceps, the British remained sceptical. William Hunter (1718–83), a prestigious London personality in the field, opposed it.[31] In German-speaking countries, the dispute between the interventionist Professor Friedrich Benjamin Osiander (1759–1822) in Göttingen and his colleague, Lukas Boër (1751–1835), in Vienna was notorious. While the former used the forceps in 40 per cent of all his hospital births (sometimes just for teaching), his Viennese counterpart, defending the concept of "natural birth" with equal consequence, did so in only 0.4 per cent of his cases.[32] Thus the forceps, introduced as a last hope in emergencies, later became the object of ideological considerations, giving an early example of a theory-driven, rather than outcome-driven innovation, featuring the "improvement-and-safety" approach to medical innovation more prominently than the "assessment" approach.

The "improvement" approach, in the case of the forceps, modified both the instrument and the modalities of its application, contributing to a slow process of cultural change, in which male, i.e. "scientific" and in part interventionist practice, gradually superseded traditionally female, i.e. "experience"-based midwifery.[33] In this process, the medical and lay concepts of the dangers of the use of the forceps would change too. A similar process would also occur when many new surgical interventions were introduced in the increasingly instrument-oriented nineteenth century, which was more eager for progress than its precedent had been.[34]

Nineteenth century radical surgery

Conceptual, technical as well as professional changes contributed to the development of this new surgery that features routine therapeutic interventions within the body – rather than on its surface only – based on the triumvirate of pathological anatomy, anaesthesia, anti- and asepsis.[35] Quite unlike the case of purely empirical inoculation, the new surgical operations were backed up by scientific theories that came to be widely accepted. They are epitomized by Rudolf Virchow's cellular pathology and Robert Koch's and Louis Pasteur's germ theory of infections. One of the world's leading surgeons of this highly innovative period was the Swiss, Theodor Kocher (1841–1917).[36] Among other achievements, he was internationally known to be the most innovative goitre surgeon of his time. For him in 1882, thyroidectomy, a once dreaded procedure, was so "safe", with an operative lethality of 14 per cent, that he even recommended it for aesthetic reasons. Twenty-seven years later, in his Nobel lecture of 1909, he could report on the one thousand operations – actually his fourth thousand – that he had performed between 1906 and 1909. He proudly announced that, due to his in many ways improved methods, lethality had decreased to 0.7 per cent.[37]

These "improvements" had once included his technique for *total* thyroidectomy. Now, he no longer spoke of it, although he had performed this operation at an increasing rate in the late 1870s. The reason was that in 1883 he had realized in retrospect the damage he had been doing for years with this innovation, and he had since abandoned it and restricted himself to partial excisions. Still it was a perfectly logical consequence of Virchow's localistic theory.[38]

This case shows, as that of the forceps suggested, that an innovation founded on a well-accepted theory may lend itself in terms of practitioners' handling of its dangers to the "improvement-and-safety" approach. The idea is to have rendered the innovation technically "safe" – at any rate – before it might eventually be dropped because of persistent unsatisfactory results. In the meantime, the criteria for that safety may change.

A further example of the priority given to the "improvement" approach was Kocher's therapy of bone and joint tuberculosis. Again in line with localistic concepts of pathology, he greatly fostered the excision of tuberculous foci – it was the only rational therapy promising a cure. When, in around 1900, high alpine heliotherapy was developed as an alternative, Kocher recalled the last decades of the nineteenth century as:

> ... the time of the prodigious rise of the operative therapies. Based on the fact that Koch's bacillus was the essential cause of tuberculosis of the joints, we set ourselves the task of eradicating the pathogenic agent from the body, and the operative elimination of the affected ... tissues under continuous perfecting of the techniques dominated the field.[39]

Thus the most recent operations promised, according to him, long-term outcomes better than those previously known that had inevitably resulted from the former, by then outdated techniques. This continued extrapolation from theory to practice was fuelled partly by real technical improvements, partly by the evolution of Kocher's own safety criteria.

Kocher eventually admitted the better functional results of tissue-saving heliotherapy as compared to his excisions. Indeed, the latter treatment often was followed by recidivation after the operation, thus leading surgeons to propose further mutilating interventions and even amputation.[40]

Accordingly, he wrote: "We surgeons have to confess that we did not always take the dangers of an operation sufficiently into consideration."[41] And one of his assistants stated:

> [We have to avow] that after an operative therapy, where every diseased part has been radically removed, there is more recidivation than with conservative treatment. Could not the operation itself through traumatic damage even increase the disposition to new infections?[42]

This question, formulated as a fact by the conservative heliotherapists,[43] recalls the eighteenth-century doubts about inoculation and the criticism of Smellie's "improved" forceps: all three innovations were denigrated for (potentially) propagating the disease they were meant to contain.

Documenting technical change

Albeit anecdotal, these cases of thyroidectomy and "tuberculosectomy" illustrate (i) that a "safe" treatment (by surgeons' standards!) does not actually tell us anything about its value for the health of a patient, and (ii) that "scientific" theories do not always lead to practice that is helpful for the patient. This is a lesson that medicine as well as patients are still reluctant to learn, given the traditional self-perception of many doctors as well as of the public.

With these unilateral results Kocher lost his scientific innocence, yet he did not realize that he might have prevented damage, at least partially, had he used a comparative "assessment" approach to take into account the dangers of his innovation. Indeed, he had acted without any explicit comparative test of the outcome of his procedures. Maybe such testing seemed superfluous at first, when the natural course of the disease was assumed to be worse – on a more or less anecdotal basis. A "fair" test was a frequently used expression in the debates about smallpox, and recent historical research has revealed the difficulties and tensions Jurin and others had experienced in producing their numerical data. Attempting to produce "fair" evidence about the outcome of Kocher's surgical innovations would have required an understanding of some statistical principles, the solution of difficult logistical problems as well as humility and courage. Yet, the leading academic figures among Kocher's contemporaries saw themselves as rational scientists. Their therapeutic innovations were logical consequences of widely shared scientific theory, and/or the argument of the "only last hope" used already when innovating the obstetric forceps 100 years earlier provided sufficient rationale.

Failures called for technical improvement in order to make the new logical invention medically "safer", rather than for an assessment of harm to patients. Comparisons were made between old and new *operations*, rather than between *types of treatment*, and the natural course of a disease was implicitly seen as worse than under any treatment. As outlined above, assessment of one kind or another is also implicit in this approach: Kocher's examples were rather typical of the then usual, merely one-sided way of assessing the outcome of an innovation within the "improvement-and-safety" approach. He (and his peers) documented, in fact, technical change.[44] But when the priority lay with improvement and safety of an innovation, technical standards, the determinants of its safety, were of necessity never comparable over time.

Explicit, implicit or no comparisons

With respect to the "assessment" approach to medical innovation as such, it has been recognized for centuries that making comparisons is an important way toward obtaining the kind of knowledge required, that is, to evaluate whether an intervention does more good than harm. In the history of therapeutics, the famous Renaissance surgeon, Ambroise Paré (1510–90), provides two early examples of decisions about an innovation based on comparative observations. He had accidentally performed an experiment when comparing the outcome of a group of amputated soldiers treated *lege artis* with boiling oil to that of a few others, for whom no oil was left: unexpectedly, the latter did much better. Open-minded and trusting his own observation more than theory and authoritarian teaching, Paré "resolved never again so cruelly to burn poor men wounded with arquebus shot".[45] When he heard an old woman had extolled the qualities of a folk-remedy for the treatment of burns, he tested it in what we now call a "prospective trial":

> ... a German of the Guard was very drunk and his [powder] flask caught fire and caused great damages to his hands and face, and I was called to dress him. I applied onions to one half of his face and the usual remedies to the other. At the second dressing I found the side where I had applied the onions to have no blisters nor scarring and the other side to be all blistered; and so I planned to write about the effect of these onions.[46]

These examples of *explicit comparison* were quite exceptional, for in medicine it has long seemed difficult to understand the need for comparisons.[47]

People may recover from illness without having received any specific treatment. Nature is a great healer. But, although the doctrine of the healing power of nature had a secular tradition that goes back to classical antiquity,[48] it was not until the eighteenth century that doctors clearly formulated the idea that the progress and outcome of illness without treatment should be taken into account when evaluating traditional treatments or testing new ones.[49] Thus, the result of a treatment may show that it improves – or that it worsens – the outcome that would have occurred without treatment.

The debates about smallpox inoculation were just one example of this sceptical attitude about claims that the outcome of a medical intervention could improve on nature's outcomes. Again the history of innovations in eighteenth-century surgery affords some instances of its application. The treatment of cataracts illustrates these comparative and unprejudiced points nicely, particularly since it was widely discussed in the medical field and even in the political sphere. At the very beginning of the eighteenth century, the famous French surgeon to King Louis XIV, Pierre Dionis (1718), wrote in the introduction to his *Course of Chirurgical Operations*:

> [T]he Certainty of Chirurgery is manifestly proved by the wonderful Effects which it produces ... in Couching of Cataracts, it instantly restores the Sight of the Blind ... In short, nothing is more certain than what it does ...[50]

Some 42 years later, when Dionis's book was out in its fifth French edition, Jacques Daviel (1696–1762) presented his new operation for cataracts to the *Académie Royale de Chirurgie* in Paris. Some six months later, in June 1753, a veritable surgical tournament was organized at the *Hôtel Royal des Invalides* in Paris, featuring nineteen patients and three surgeons. The first surgeon operated on six patients according to the old method, the tried and tested one known since antiquity, i.e. the couching of the lens. His two colleagues operated using the new method, i.e. the extraction of the lens. The result was ambiguous, since three out of the first six patients and seven out of the remaining thirteen regained their sight.[51] This was a reason to continue the discussion about the value of the new operation right through the eighteenth century. In 1825 the French surgeon Anselme-Barthélémy Richerand (1779–1840) concluded in his *Histoire des Progrès Récens de Chirurgie* (History of Recent Progress in Surgery):

> In order to escape from such a lot of contradictory opinions and finally to determine such an important point of doctrine in surgery, there is only one way: under the supervision of the Academy, a certain number of patients should be brought together in a suitable place and be operated on comparatively, placing the individual patients in the same circumstances as far as is possible. Only an academic body, whose sole interest is truth can undertake and successfully pursue such an experiment.

For a surgeon alone, be he the most capable and striving for truth, upright with the utmost candour, will never be free of a multitude of prejudices, the existence and impact of which he is often ignorant of himself.[52]

While the idea was there, we do not know yet whether such a trial ever took place. However, recent historical research has yielded quite a few placebo-controlled, single and even double-blind trials involving another medical innovation starting around 1800, Samuel Hahnemann's (1755–1843) homeopathy. Such trials were performed starting in the 1810s and throughout the nineteenth century, with and without some form of bias.[53]

Sometimes comparisons were simply made in the doctors' heads, as they sensed that patients were responding differently to a new treatment compared with the way that apparently similar patients in the past had responded to another or no treatment. The obstetric forceps in its beginnings was a case in point of such *implicit comparison*. Clinical impressions of this kind were sometimes followed up by an analysis of patients' case records to compare the experiences of patients given a new treatment with the experience of previous patients or other current patients who had received different treatments. Such treatment comparisons provided reliable information, but only in the rare circumstances where treatment effects were dramatic, as was the case of the forceps when used in emergencies. Examples of implicit comparisons included – to remain in the eighteenth century – opium for pain relief,[54] cinchona bark around 1700 for intermittent fevers ("malaria");[55] examples of record-based comparisons were the mid-eighteenth century trials of a new versus the traditional operation for cataract (see above), of immediate versus delayed amputation after a battle injury, the "historical" comparison of the new method of immediate versus delayed union of wound edges, or William Withering's adoption of the foxglove (digitalis) for certain kinds of "dropsy".[56]

It is tempting to speculate about the changing significance and relevance of comparison in medicine. There is a link to innovation: where there is nothing new, there is nothing to compare either, the only exception being precisely the comparison of a traditional treatment with "the unassisted effort of nature", as one eighteenth-century author put it.[57] Therapeutic innovations were indeed rare before that period. A new procedure might result from sheer necessity, as when Paré ran out of oil; it might be due to imports from foreign countries, such as the smallpox inoculation or Peruvian bark for intermittent fevers; it might be derived from (new) pathophysiological theory, as was the question of timing for amputations[58] or for some eighteenth-century drugs;[59] it might come from folk medicine and simply be submitted to empirical trial and error, such as inoculation or the foxglove.

The history of new eighteenth-century drugs shows, however, that explicit comparison was by no means always deemed indispensable. There were other methods of testing innovations, such as *in vitro* studies and uncontrolled animal as well as human experiments.[60] But, as the examples of smallpox, obstetric forceps and surgery showed, they were also judged by social and religious criteria. On the other hand, such cultural influences and factors other than innovations must have also played a role when comparison was used, as the example of smallpox showed. Certainly a sceptical empirical bent could be found among some doctors during the European Enlightenment, particularly in Britain.[61]

Most medical treatments did not, however, have such dramatic beneficial effects as inoculation or the forceps, especially in chronic situations such as in goitre or tuberculous bones. For reasons discussed elsewhere,[62] it was realized in the eighteenth century that in these common circumstances the "assessment" approach to the uncertainties associated with medical innovation was extremely important and that it should ideally involve explicit comparison. Authors also saw the need for reducing the misleading influences of prejudices – what we would now call "biases" – and of the "play of chance" when assessing the outcome of innovative procedures.

As the examples of the forceps and of new surgical techniques show, albeit anecdotally, innovators tended to be biased in favour of their invention and a small number of selected observations confirmed them. They were quite capable of selecting favourable ones and/or explain away ones that did not fit. This has been common practice for a long time.

"Fair" comparison

In order to prevent doctors from misjudging the outcome of an innovation, certain measures were propagated in eighteenth-century Britain, such as the "compare-like-with-like" rule. Comparisons of two treatments were considered unfair, for instance, if relatively healthy patients received one of the treatments and relatively sick patients the other, or if the patients allotted to different treatments differed in the localisation of their injury, or in their age. This was implemented, for example, when assessing various remedies for scurvy, treatment of bladder stones and a new method for amputating limbs by making musculo-cutaneous flaps to cover the wound instead of leaving it open.[63] This problem was also overcome by comparing different treatments given at different times to the same patient in an early example of what is today called a "cross-over" study.[64]

In order to understand mere psychological influences, an even more sophisticated application consisted in intentionally leaving the patient ignorant about the treatment he was receiving. This method was used during trials made by a French Royal Commission with the collaboration of the famous chemist Antoine Lavoisier, and the physicist Benjamin Franklin, later an American President, in Paris in 1784. They investigated whether Anton Mesmer's claims about the beneficial effects of "animal magnetism" (mesmerism) were due to any real [physical] force, or to "illusions of the mind".[65]

This trial design was further refined by a group of British doctors who, around 1800, used a placebo in addition, i.e. a treatment that is in fact physically inert. The idea was that, even though such a placebo treatment was not expensive, it was worth knowing whether it was safe and had no physically mediated harmful adverse effects.[66]

Other sources of misjudgement, namely those of prejudiced selection from the available evidence, and of the play of chance were also clearly recognized in the eighteenth century. In his 1792 summary of many previous authors, John Ferriar (1761–1815), a physician at the Manchester Infirmary, emphasized that the method "so fashionable at present of publishing single cases, appears not well calculated to enlarge our knowledge, either of the nature or cure of diseases".

He realized that the way to reduce the likelihood of being misled by the play of chance was to consider a sufficiently large number of outcomes experienced by the people participating in tests of medical treatments. But he maintained that even serial observations would become reliable only if they were written down in a journal, regularly updated, and included both the favourable and unfavourable outcomes of a treatment. This was "absolutely necessary" if the physician wanted to avoid the false conclusions he would arrive at "if he trusted memory alone". Furthermore, data obtained in this way could and must be compared with those of other physicians.[67]

Although his contemporaries did not always follow Ferriar's programme for objectifying outcome assessment with consistent action,[68] enlightened authors clearly criticised that, by ignoring some criteria for "fair" comparison and/or biases – or by sometimes unscrupulously exploiting them – people would persuade themselves or others that a new treatment was better than an existing one when it was not. But, whether biases were inadvertent or deliberate, the consequences were the same: unless tests of treatment were "fair", some useless or harmful treatments would appear to be useful, while some useful treatments would appear to be useless or harmful.

Methodical empirical scepticism has many facets that, albeit they were recognized individually much earlier, were only seldom brought together in complete combination before the end of the nineteenth century.[69] Furthermore, as pointed out above, this was only one type (with many sub-types) of the "assessment" approach in the perception and management of doubts linked with medical inventions. For many reasons it was not even a very frequently used type, either, until the end of the twentieth century.[70]

Conclusion: doubts in the short run

Clearly, while solving some problems, medical innovations have created new ones. This seems at first a trivial statement, but it is less banal to ask precise questions about the gains and losses in a specific process.

For nearly three centuries practitioners have tackled the associated doubts in terms of assessment of gains, losses and linked dangers as well as in terms of improvements and safety of a new method. This has never been straight-forward, at least not before the rise of the controlled clinical trial in the 1960s. Seldom has this handling been "fair" and "objective" according to the methodical standards called for in the eighteenth century. Rather it has been driven by implicit and explicit cultural values, medical theories, beliefs and interests.[71] Innovations have often been mixed blessings, the gains and losses as well as the standards for safety being negotiated in complex cultural processes.

The few examples presented in this chapter suggest two medical – as distinct from religious, philosophical or social – approaches to doubts about medical inventions.

Empirical innovations, without theoretical background, for instance from folk medicine (inoculation of smallpox; onions against severe burns; new methods for treating the cataract and amputating limbs) tended to be tackled medically by the "assessment" approach using explicit comparison to traditional treatments. This seemed obvious to some innovators when they set out to evaluate whether and/or where precisely they did more good than harm. If benefit was eventually agreed upon, theoretical explanations might be sought, and new ones be found, as was the case for smallpox.[72] Another case in point was the comparative, prospective testing of fruit – a folk remedy – against scurvy in the mid-eighteenth century.[73]

An innovation hardly ever gave full satisfaction from its outset. In theory-driven innovation (the examples in this chapter were the obstetric forceps and the extirpation of diseased tissues such as goitre, tuberculous foci, but the following remark also holds for tumours in nineteenth- and early twentieth-century surgery[74]), this situation primarily led to technical improvements in order to secure a new, rationally justified method that would progressively render the innovation safer. This "improvement-and-safety" approach, with its ever-changing technical standards, also included comparisons, but they were only implicit as far as traditional or competitive therapies were concerned: unilateral listings of results with the new method were deemed sufficient. Sometimes when the effectiveness of an "improvement" was to be demonstrated, there was explicit comparison, but this concerned an "innovation within the (original) innovation". The history of Theodor Kocher's total thyroidectomies, and his paper, *Vergleich älterer und neuerer Behandlungsmethoden der Knochen-und Gelenkstuberkulose* (Comparison of older to newer methods of treatment of bone and joint tuberculosis),[75] written in 1915 to legitimate his former innovation of bone and joint resections in view of the recent successes of the new non-mutilating heliotherapy, are cases in point. Sometimes convincing theories could be enemies to fairness when it came to assessing the danger (or, more generally, losses) in addition to the advantages (or, more generally, gains) of a medical innovation.

Practical doubts inevitably seem to accompany medical innovations in the long-term perspective, be it only for practitioners' psychological reasons. It may seem somewhat artificial to distinguish two ideal types of practitioners' response, since they both answered their needs in their way. But to distinguish them made it possible to conclude two points. (i) They were seen as complementary for a complete appreciation of the reliability of an innovation. While the assessment focused on the patient and/or society, the concept of safety remarkably enough lay within the medical, technical process. Both were relevant in the examples explored from the two centuries under scrutiny. (ii) Their relative implementation was historically conditioned: some examples from the eighteenth century, above all the history of inoculation, fully exhibit this complementarity of explicit comparison assessed with emerging sophisticated methodology, combined with technical safety measures and followed by legal regulation. The concurrent innovation of the forceps, by comparison, featured priority on technical safety-oriented issues, and the rules for its use continued to be set up within the profession where they remained contested. This also holds for the nineteenth- and early twentieth-century extirpations of goitre and tuberculous tissue with occasionally drastic consequences. Partly in reaction to these, today's call for fair tests of healthcare interventions focusing on the paradigm of "evidence-based medicine" again stresses sophisticated assessment, including the essential role of explicit and fair comparison, in order to "minimize harm and maximize benefit during innovation in health care".[76] This is nothing new, because these methodologies were emerging in the eighteenth century; rather it is the strengthening of a "culture of assessment" that has existed for over 200 years within medicine.[77]

Finally the long-term perspective shows that historical contingency also means that, at times, in places and situations, the approaches could converge, or that one took precedence over the other, correcting it to become the inspiration for new investigations in a continuing circle.[78,79]

Notes

1   Geneviève Miller, *The Adoption of Inoculation for Smallpox in England and France*, Philadelphia: University of Pennsylvania Press, 1957.
2   Adrian Wilson, *The Making of Man-Midwifery: Childbirth in England 1660–1770*, London: University College Press, 1995.
3   Jeffrey K. Aronson, *An Account of the Foxglove and its Medical Uses, 1785–1985*, London: Oxford University Press, 1985.
4   Ulrich Tröhler, *"To Improve the Evidence of Medicine": The 18th Century British Origins of a Critical Approach*, Edinburgh: The Royal College of Physicians of Edinburgh, 2000; pp. 59–63, pp. 95–105.
5   Ulrich Tröhler, "Die Gewissheit der Chirurgie: Grundlagen klinisch-therapeutischer Bewertung um 1750", *Praxis*, 1987, 76, pp. 958–61.
6   See the classical study by Miller, *Adoption of Inoculation*, 1957. For an updated bibliography consult Andreas-Holger Maehle, 'The Ethics of Prevention: German Philosophies of the Late Enlightenment on the Morality of Smallpox Inoculation,' in John Woodward and Robert Jütte (eds), *Coping with Sickness: Perspectives on Health Care, Past and Present*, Sheffield: European Association for the History of Medicine and Health Publications, 1996, pp. 91–114.
7   Andrea A. Rusnock, *Vital Accounts: Quantifying Health and Population in Eighteenth-Century England and France*, Cambridge: Cambridge University Press, 2002, pp. 81–6; Harry M. Marks, "When the State Counts Lives: Eighteenth Century Quarrels over Inoculation", in

Gérard Jorland, Annick Opinel and George Weisz (eds), *Body Counts: Medical Quantification in Historical and Sociological Perspective / La Quantification Médicale: Perspectives Historiques et Sociologiques*, Montréal: McGill University Press, 2005, pp. 19–50.

8 Rusnock, *Vital Accounts*, pp. 44–5; Newton Copp and Andrew Zanella, *Discovery, Innovation, and Risk*, Cambridge, MA: MIT Press, 1993, pp. 249–50.

9 Quoted in Miller, *Adoption of Inoculation*, p. 124.

10 See Thomas Schlich in Chapter 1 of this volume.

11 Miller, *Adoption of Inoculation*, pp. 121–3.

12 Andrea Rusnock, "The Weight of Evidence and the Burden of Authority: Case Histories, Medical Statistics and Smallpox Inoculation", in Roy Porter (ed.), *Medicine in the Enlightenment*, Amsterdam and Atlanta: Rodopi, 1995, pp. 198–222.

13 Miller, *Adoption of Inoculation*, p. 270.

14 Maehle, *Ethics*.

15 Rev. Edmund Massey, quoted in Miller, *Adoption of Inoculation*, pp. 103–4.

16 Miller, *Adoption of Inoculation*, p. 270.

17 Rusnock, *Vital Accounts*, pp. 92–3.

18 Miller, *Adoption of Inoculation*, p. 270.

19 Quoted in Miller, *Adoption of Inoculation*, p. 142.

20 William Smellie, *A Treatise on the Theory and Practice of Midwifery*, 2 vols, London: Wilson and Durham, 2nd edn, 1752, vol. 1, pp. 248–9.

21 Friedrich Benjamin Osiander, *Handbuch der Entbindungskunst*, 3 vols, vol. III: Johann Friedrich Osiander, *Die Ursachen und Hülfszangen der unregelmässigen und schweren Geburt*, Tübingen: C. F. Osiander, 2nd edn, 1833, p. 287.

22 See Heinrich Fasbender, *Geschichte der Geburtshilfe*, Stuttgart: Fischer, 1906; repr. Hildesheim: Olms, 1964, pp. 922–3.

23 Smellie, *Treatise*, p. 291.

24 Smellie, *Treatise*, pp. 265, 273.

25 Smellie, *Treatise*, pp. 264–5.

26 There was no discussion about long-term effects on the child.

27 Ulrich Tröhler, "Quantifying Experience and Beating Bias: A New 'Culture' within British Clinical Medicine, c. 1800", in Jorland *et al.* (eds), pp. 51–64, *Body Counts*.

28 For an illustrated description see Walther Kuhn and Ulrich Tröhler (eds), *Armamentarium obstetricium Gottingense: A Historical Collection of Perinatal Medicine*, Göttingen: Vandenhoeck and Ruprecht, 1987, pp. 157–70.

29 Jürgen Schlumbohm, " 'The Pregnant Women are here for the Sake of the Teaching Institution': The Lying-In Hospital of Göttingen University 1751 to c. 1830", *Social History of Medicine*, 2001, 14, 59–78; Hans-Christoph Seidel, *Eine neue "Kultur des Gebärens". Die Medikalisierung der Geburt im 18. und 19. Jahrhundert*, Stuttgart: Franz Steiner, 1998, pp. 232–9.

30 Ornella Moscucci, *The Science of Women: Gynecology and Gender in England 1800–1929*, Cambridge: Cambridge University Press, 1990, pp. 47–8, 50; Schlumbohm, *Pregnant Women*.

31 Moscucci, *Science of Women*, p. 48.

32 Schlumbohm, *Pregnant Women*.

33 Moscucci, *Science of Women*; Seidel, *Medikalisierung*.

34 Dale C. Smith, "Appendicitis, Appendectomy and the Surgeon", *Bulletin of the History of Medicine*, 1996, 70, pp. 414–41.

35 Thomas Schlich, "The Emergence of Modern Surgery", in Deborah Brunton (ed.), *Medicine Transformed Health, Disease and Society in Europe 1800–1930*, Manchester: The Open University, 2004.

36 Ulrich Tröhler, *Der Nobelpreisträger Theodor Kocher, 1841–1917: Auf dem Weg zur physiologischen Chirurgie*, Basle: Birkhäuser, 1984.

37 Tröhler, *Nobelpreisträger*, pp. 123–4; Theodor Kocher, "Über Krankheitserscheinungen bei Schilddrüsenerkrankungen geringen Grads", in *Les Prix Nobel en 1909*, Stockholm: Imprimerie Royale, 1910, pp. 1–59; p. 36.

38 Tröhler, *Nobelpreisträger*, pp. 125–32.

39 Quoted from Tröhler, *Nobelpreisträger*, p. 110 [author's translation].

40 This controversy had a very important social aspect: a course of heliotherapy lasted for many months. Given the then very poorly developed social security system, the therapy was practically unaffordable for the less well-to-do. See Ulrich Tröhler, " ' To Operate or Not to Operate?' Scientific and Extraneous Factors in Therapeutical Controversies within the Swiss Society of Surgery, 1913–1988", *Clio Medica*, 1991, *22*, pp. 89–113.

41 Quoted from Tröhler, *Nobelpreisträger*, p. 111.

42 Quoted from Tröhler, *Nobelpreisträger*, p. 111.

43 Tröhler, "To Operate".

44 See, for instance, the innovation of (radical) breast cancer surgery at the same time, in Barron H. Lerner, *The Breast Cancer Wars*, Oxford: Oxford University Press, 2001, pp. 17–40.

45 Iain M. L. Donaldson, "Ambroise Paré's Account in the Œuvres of 1575 of New Methods of Treating Gunshot Wounds and Burns", in Iain Chalmers *et al.* (eds), *James Lind Library* (available online at www.jameslindlibrary.org, accessed 12 September 2004).

46 Donaldson, "Ambroise Paré's Account".

47 Bernard S. Bloom, "Controlled Studies in Measuring the Efficacy of Medical Care: a Historical Perspective", *International Journal of Technology Assessment and Health Care*, 1996, *2*, pp. 299–310; a specific history of ideas of comparisons in medicine and their practical realization remains a desideratum.

48 Max Neuburger, *Die Lehre von der Heilkraft der Natur im Wandel der Zeiten*, Stuttgart: Enke, 1926.

49 Tröhler, *To Improve the Evidence*, pp. 19, 32, 116.

50 Pierre Dionis, *A Course of Chirurgical Operations, Demonstrated in the Royal Garden at Paris*, London: Jacob Tonson, 1710.

51 Tröhler, *Die Gewissheit*.

52 Anselme-Barthélémy Richerand, *Histoire des Progrès Récens de la Chirurgie*, Paris: Béchet jn., 1825, p. 27 [author's translation].

53 Michael Emmons Dean, *The Trials of Homeopathy Origins, Structure and Development*, Essen: kvc Verlag, 2004, pp. 87–153.

54 Roseline Rey, *History of Pain*, Paris: Editions la Découverte, 1993, pp. 95–7; Richard Toellner, "Die Umbewertung des Schmerzes im 17. Jahrhundert in ihren Voraussetzungen und Folgen", *Medizinhistorisches Journal*, 1971, 6, pp. 36–44.

55 Andreas-Holger Maehle, *Drugs on Trial: Experimental Pharmacology and Therapeutic Innovation in the Eighteenth Century*, Amsterdam and Atlanta, GA: Rodopi, 1999, pp. 223–45.

56 Tröhler, *To Improve the Evidence*, pp. 95, 105.

57 Quoted in Tröhler, *To Improve the Evidence*, p. 32.

58 Tröhler, *Die Gewissheit*.

59 Maehle, *Drugs on Trial*, pp. 1–54.

60 Maehle, *Drugs on Trial*, passim.

61 Erwin H. Ackerknecht, "Die therapeutische Erfahrung und ihre allmähliche Objektivierung", *Gesnerus*, 1969, *26*, pp. 26–35.

62 Tröhler, *To Improve the Evidence*, pp. 1–21.

63 Tröhler, *To Improve the Evidence*, pp. 59–81, 97–9; see also Ulrich Tröhler, "Edward Alanson 1782: Responsibility in Surgical Innovation", in Chalmers *et al.* (eds), *James Lind Library*.

64 Caleb Hillier Parry, "Experiments relative to the medical effects of Turkey Rhubarb, and of the English Rhubarbs No I and No II made on patients of the Pauper Charity", *Letters and Papers ... of the Society instituted at Bath*, 3, (1786), pp. 407–22. For more details of the experiment and biographical data on its author, see R. Rolls, "Caleb Hillier Parry, MD, FRS (1715–1822)", in Chalmers *et al.* (eds), *James Lind Library*.

65 Ted J. Kaptchuk, "Intentional Ignorance: A History of Blind Assessment and Placebo Controls in Medicine", *Bulletin of the History of Medicine*, 1998, 72, pp. 389–433; Iain

Chalmers *et al.*, "Differences in the Ways Treatment Outcomes are Assessed", in Chalmers *et al.* (eds), *James Lind Library*, where more details, original passages of the Paris trial and biographical data on its author can be seen.

66 Chalmers *et al.*, '*Differences*'.

67 Quoted in Tröhler, *To Improve the Evidence*, pp. 18–19.

68 Tröhler, "Quantifying experience", in Jorland *et al.* (eds), *Body Counts*.

69 John Harley Warner, *The Therapeutic Perspective, Medical Practice, Knowledge and Identity in America, 1820–1885*, Princeton NJ: Princeton University Press, 1997; J. Rosser Matthews, *Quantification and the Quest for Medical Certainty*, Princeton, NJ: Princeton University Press, 1995; Harry M. Marks, *The Progress of Experiment: Science and Therapeutic Reform in the United States 1900–1990*, Cambridge: Cambridge Univesrity Press, 1997; Jan P. Vandenbroucke, "Clinical Investigation in the 20th Century: The Ascendancy of Numerical Reasoning", *The Lancet*, 2001, *352*, Suppl. 2, pp. 12–16.

70 For a chronology of records see Chalmers *et al.* (eds), *James Lind Library*. Historical explanations are given by J. Rosser Matthews, *Quantification*, and Abraham Lilienfeld, "'Ceteris paribus': The Evolution of the Clinical Trial", *Bulletin of the History of Medicine*, 1982, *56*, pp. 1–18.

71 Tröhler, *To Improve the Evidence*; Harry M. Marks, "Trust and Mistrust in the Marketplace: Statistics and Clinical Research, 1945–1960", *History of Science*, 2000, *38*, pp. 343–55; Tröhler, "Quantifying Experience".

72 Miller, *Adoption of Inoculation*, pp. 241–66.

73 Tröhler, *To Improve the Evidence*, pp. 69–81.

74 Tröhler, *Nobelpreisträger*, pp. 100–4, 106–8, 112–16; Lerner, *Breast Cancer Wars*, pp. 17–40; Seija-Sisko Krudup, *Das Krebsproblem in den "Verhandlungen der Deutschen Gesellschaft für Chirurgie" von 1872 bis 1914*, MD thesis, University of Göttingen, 1990, pp. 65, 79–80.

75 *Deutsche Zeitschrift für Chirurgie*, 1915, *134*, pp. 1–53.

76 Iain Chalmers, "Minimizing Harm and Maximizing Benefit During Innovation in Health Care: Controlled or Uncontrolled Experimentation?", *Birth*, 1986, *13*, pp. 155–64.

77 Tröhler, "Quantifying experience".

78 Vandenbroucke, *Clinical Investigation*.

79 Acknowledgements: this contribution was much improved by discussions with Silke Bellanger, Nicholas Eschenbruch and Thomas Schlich. I am equally grateful to Margaret Andergassen for her valuable and unwearied language assistance.

3 Anaesthesia and the evaluation of surgical risk in mid-nineteenth-century Britain[1]

Ian Burney

Inhalation anaesthesia entered British surgical practice on a wave of enthusiasm. The use of ether in 1846, and chloroform in the following year, was greeted by contemporaries, and has since been ratified by historians, as a revolutionary innovation. It was, according to one commentator writing only a few months after ether's debut in the operating theatre, "one of the most remarkable events in the history of medicine".[2] For its admirers, anaesthesia quickly acquired a synechdotal relationship to modern, civilized treatment, a connection relentlessly pressed by its leading British advocate, James Simpson. For Simpson, the use of anaesthesia in surgery represented a liberation from unnecessary cruelty, one that coincided with the humanitarian spirit of the age. Anaesthesia joined with contemporaneous campaigns – those against slavery and corporal punishment, for example – as harbingers of a coming moral order free from subjugation and suffering.[3] Its first promise, of course, was to free patients from the "sickening horrors" of surgical pain. But anaesthesia also released surgeons from their former unnatural and invidious position of having, in Simpson's words, to "inflict present suffering upon [their] patients, with a prospective view to their own ultimate benefit and advantage".[4]

Enthusiasm, moreover, translated into a remarkably rapid practical adoption of this signal medical innovation.[5] In the weeks following the famed surgeon Robert Liston's highly publicized inauguration of British surgical anaesthesia, the medical press was, in the words of the *Medical Times and Gazette*, "literally inundated" with accounts of operations performed under these new conditions.[6] Such early reports, printed under titles like "painless operations under the influence of ether", extolled the quasi-magical qualities of the new surgical scene, often featuring accounts of patients waking from their state of induced oblivion in a state of joy mixed with disbelief at their escape from agony: "Operation? Operation? What operation?" was the gratifying response reported by the surgeon William Lawrence of his first anaesthetized patient.[7] These accounts formed the basis for more generalized expressions of gratitude for this boon to suffering mankind: "Let the chaplain of every hospital in which these wonders have been witnessed, be invited by the Medical Officers of the establishment to offer up their humble and hearty thanks for the late mercies vouchsafed to the patients under their charge," a correspondent to the *Lancet* urged. "There should be public acts of thanksgiving throughout the land, for this signal favour to man present and to come."[8]

In both form and content, then, anaesthesia was an innovation that prompted a deeply charged, visceral response, and this initial emotive quality, not surprisingly, remained characteristic of anaesthetic discussions in subsequent decades. But early enthusiasm was soon tempered. Accounts of difficulties in administration, and of failures to achieve a fully anaesthetized state in the surgical theatre, began to vie for attention with the more celebratory accounts in the medical press.[9] Theoretical objections were raised alongside these practical considerations. In some cases, objections were directed against the very principle of painlessness itself. Arguments about the physiological and diagnostic function of pain, for example, were proposed, especially in relation to obstetrical anaesthesia. More common than rejection on fundamental principle, however, were the cautionary voices raised about the need to moderate "enthusiasm", to question the individual and collective rush to insensibility, to establish what Martin Pernick has described as a "calculus of suffering".

According to Pernick, inhalation anaesthesia was the first significant medical innovation to be subjected to utilitarian risk assessment. His important study systematically lays out the component elements of this cost–benefit analytical framework, showing how a spectrum of risk positions emerged from different views on the social, moral and medical significance of pain. His primary concern is to show how this form of comparative assessment itself represented an important professional and ideological intervention in the history of American medicine. For Pernick, the calculating framework within which anaesthesia was debated represented a new, neutral pathway through a mid-century American medical world polarized between the heroic interventionism associated with Benjamin Rush and his disciples on the one hand, and a variety of naturalistic systems on the other. Utilitarian calculus provided a new professional identity legitimated not on allegiance to first principle, but on the judicious comparison of statistically generated outcomes of therapeutic alternatives. The "numerical method" associated with the work of Pierre Louis in the 1830s thus seemed to provide this new breed of medical utilitarians with a demonstrably objective means of measuring the risks and rewards of intervention without entering into ethical or sectarian disputes.[10]

Cost–benefit analysis, in Pernick's account, was the means for cutting through ideology – or perhaps better, of constructing an ideology grounded in technical, rationalistic calculation. In his analysis, the specific link between anaesthesia and risk assessment is largely a matter of historical circumstance – anaesthesia was a dramatic therapeutic innovation that coincided with the rise of this probabilistic medical thinking. There is, however, another way of interpreting the link, one that looks more closely at how the specific characteristics of anaesthesia might render it a subject in special need of rationalistic analysis. In what follows, I will be arguing that the singularly emotive frame of interpretation and action within which anaesthesia was debated led to a widespread embrace of risk assessment as a way of objectively managing the passions and anxieties provoked by anaesthesia. To be sure, any major medical innovation, by disrupting and thus disturbing existing practice, carries with it the potential to generate anxiety amongst practitioners and patients alike. But anaesthesia, with its promise to spare a vulnerable, embodied subject from suffering, was a topic that inextricably addressed the volatile realm of the passions. Into this situation, risk analysis could be seen as a means for projecting rationally bounded actors onto this unstable scene of (potentially) irrational and ungovernable nerves. Through its very calculative rationality, in other words, a more stable referent anaesthetic practice might be constructed.

I will pursue this idea through an examination of the debates over patient risk as they developed in the first decade of British surgical anaesthesia. During this period an explicit cost–benefit analysis emerged, appropriately grounded in the utilitarian language of comparative pleasure and pain, and asking a fundamental set of questions: what, if any, were the risks of anaesthesia?; how much, and what kind of suffering, justified these risks? In this period, it should be noted at the outset, two distinct anaesthetic agents were employed. Ether, the first to be introduced, lasted barely a year as Britain's principle anaesthetic, and was rapidly supplanted by chloroform following its initial use (announced to the world by Simpson himself) in November 1847. However, my discussion does not seek to make any systematic differentiation between the two agents, since in the period under consideration the focus of risk analysis in Britain was not (as it was to become in later years) the relative merits of ether and chloroform, but the relative costs and benefits of painlessness itself.[11] This was a question of fundamental importance in these early years, when the principle of anaesthetization, irrespective of agent, was very much a matter of debate.

The rational, objective assessment of risk, as I have just indicated, appealed to those arguing for and against restrictions on anaesthetic administration, but did so for different reasons. For restrictionists, it provided a means of moderating what one critic described as the "anaesthetic mania" that had seemingly taken hold of both the public and the profession.[12] The public had embraced anaesthesia "with the ardour of infatuation", according to another commentator, understandably so, since the promise of painlessness by-passed the rational faculties and spoke instead to embodied feeling. This natural desire was being inflamed by the "strenuous exertions" of its advocates, leaving the bulk of the profession powerless to resist: "the thing was too vast, the impulse too strong, and the promoters too *nimble* to be obstructed", one exasperated commentator complained.[13] A sober reckoning of costs and benefits would refocus the debate from a desperate, desiring body to a reasoning, self-protective intellect.

For Simpson and his supporters, too, reason was ultimately preferable to emotion as the basis for their practice. Practitioners and the public "swept up" in the promise of anaesthesia were equally likely to become disenchanted at the first perceived set-back, substituting an unreasoning terror for an unreasoning enthusiasm. To be free from the vicissitudes of particular experience, then, anaesthetic practice had to move from celebratory accounts of painless operations, however gratifying they might be, to the more abstracted ground of aggregate outcome. Given the "marvellous, almost supernatural" qualities with which anaesthesia had been initially invested by those who had experienced it directly, one sympathetic medical reviewer argued, it was especially important that it was considered "with the cool blood of philosophy".[14]

But if risk assessment emerged as a recognized feature of the early controversy over anaesthetic practice, there was still much room for disagreement as to how to define and measure the variables. For those advocating anaesthetic moderation – which, as Pernick shows, constituted the great majority of practitioners on both sides of the Atlantic – the analysis should be based on a comparative reckoning of the benefits of painlessness against the risks of inducing the anaesthetic state. This comparison was bounded by two stark alternatives: every surgical patient, in the words of the *Westminster Review*, had to choose between the "torture which [an operation] inflicts, and a descent into the 'valley of the shadow of death', with the possibility that he may be unable to return".[15] In justifying the "terrifying shape" of the alternative it posed, the *Westminster* invoked one of the central issues in the anaesthetic debate: the (relatively rare) incidences of patient death whilst under the influence.[16]

Against the stark threat of anaesthetic death, patient suffering took on the character of the relative variable. In this conservative analysis, the elimination of pain was predominantly viewed as a humanitarian good. Anaesthesia was grounded essentially in compassion, a laudable basis for medical practice, to be sure, but one that needed to be tempered by an assessment of countervailing dangers. Enthusiasts, from this perspective, were yielding to their own desires to relieve themselves from the dreadful responsibility of inflicting pain, or, less charitably, were simply pandering to the public's understandable but unwise desire for relief. It was the duty of the profession, however, to exercise judgement, and to refuse to engage in a practice that entailed structural elements of risk in cases where it could be avoided – that is, where the pain caused was not so intense as to interfere with surgical success.

Restrictionists did admit that in some instances pain relief was a medical, rather than a purely humanitarian measure. Certain operations, for instance, either because of their protracted nature or their complex performative requirements, could more safely be conducted on an inert, insensible body. What was needed, then, was an agreed scale of operative suffering to which surgeons might refer when deciding whether to anaesthetize. Different thresholds of tolerance were proposed: in some, toe-nail and tooth removal constituted an appropriate cut-off point, while in others simple amputations still did not meet the requisite standard of intolerable pain. Commenting on the fatal outcome of an operation to remove an ulcerated leg, the *Lancet* – despite its overall support for anaesthesia – invoked what from our vantage point seems a Spartan standard of assessment:

> Was the intensity or duration of the pain in an amputation of the leg sufficient to justify the risk in such a subject? Or can it be said that insensibility was essential to the surgeon's proceedings? Surely not. There are those who will agree with us in thinking that it were better that a thousand individuals should each bear, when necessary, the momentary pain of amputation, than that one of the thousand should die in an attempt to remove this momentary suffering.[17]

But wherever the line was drawn, and this is the point I wish to stress, this mode of assessment was predicated upon the possibility of correlating act and effect, class of operation and level of pain, of establishing a stable calculus of suffering.

As I have already indicated, anaesthetic enthusiasts, led by Simpson's tireless public advocacy and supplemented by the more methodical practical and experimental researches of the London practitioner John Snow, agreed that their actions should be justified on measured grounds. In their hands, however, the units of measurement, and the perceived threats to be weighed, were considerably more complex. Anaesthesia was, of course, a humanitarian intervention, the relief of suffering an unambiguous good. But they rejected the place that restrictionists assigned painlessness in their cost–benefit assessment, in which, because it was *merely* humane, it constituted a risk element that needed to be justified. For enthusiasts, painlessness was not a non-medical extra, justified only by virtue of low risk. It was, instead, a fundamental physiological good. Beyond the blessing of annulling pain, as Snow promised in 1847, anaesthesia would be shown to confer "the still greater advantage of saving many lives".[18]

Anaesthesia's capacity to save life was explained by the fact that pain was itself a core pathological phenomenon – that it could, in short, kill. This belief, which had been a recognized (if contested) tenet of Western medicine since classical times, was readily taken up by anaesthetic enthusiasts.[19] Simpson backed his claims about the destructive effects of pain by calling on past authorities, including the sixteenth-century French surgeon Ambrose Paré, who urged that pain should be assuaged wherever possible because "nothing so much dejects the powers of the patient".[20] Contemporary surgeons who had embraced anaesthesia agreed: in James Miller's view, pain represented "a heightened and perverted condition of the sensory functions" through which it "may in itself become a dangerous symptom".[21] By construing pain as an isolable condition with its own physiological consequences requiring proactive medical intervention, proponents of an unrestricted anaesthetic regime sought to place the fatal consequences of patient suffering as an objective feature of their risk assessment.

Pathogenic pain was thus at the heart of arguments for a differently structured calculus, with painlessness no longer a risk factor but a crucial element of safety. The key statement of this position was contained in a three-part article written by Simpson that appeared at the end of 1847 in the *Monthly Medical Journal*. These articles, representing Simpson's first sustained defence of anaesthetic practice, in fact paid less attention to anaesthesia itself than to an explicit and detailed embrace of the emergent "numerical method" as the best means of setting anaesthesia (as indeed any medical innovation) on secure, rational grounds. Simpson opened with a lengthy and seemingly irrelevant discussion of smallpox vaccination.[22] Statistical returns provided by the Registrar General's office in recent years, he claimed, proved the safety and legitimacy of Jenner's revolution. But as Jenner in his own day did not have the benefit of this form of statistical proof, he faced resistance based on prejudice and passion. The parallels to his own position as a champion of anaesthesia were patent, and Simpson drew the connections explicitly. The main point of introducing his defence of anaesthesia through the mirror of inoculation, however, was to highlight the critical role of statistical data in assessing the value of medical innovation.

Turning to anaesthesia, Simpson claimed that, despite the existence of what he considered fringe arguments about the insignificant or even beneficial nature of pain, the true debate over the proper scope of administration was a cost–benefit one. All observing and feeling individuals agreed that pain in surgery was almost unexceptionally a moral and physical evil, he ventured. Yet many still insisted that the aim of painlessness came "at the hazard or certainty of a greater and disproportionate amount of future evil".[23] Determining the truth-value of this view was a problem "that no mere reasoning or mere opinion could ever certainly and satisfactorily solve", Simpson insisted, adding: "It is one of those allegations, the accuracy or inaccuracy of which is a matter that can be fully and finally determined by one method only, – namely, by an appeal to the evidence of facts, and to the evidence of facts alone."[24]

By evidence of facts, he meant statistics, a topic to which he devoted the entirety of his second article. Here he embraced the fundamental axioms of this new and controversial approach to medical assessment. He echoed Poisson's "law of large numbers", asserting that "there is ever a mighty uncertainty as to the results, if we consider only single cases, or a small and limited number of instances; but our results approach more and more to certainty, in proportion as we deduce these results from a greater and more extended number of instances".[25] Quoting Laplace on the indeterminacy of all human knowledge, Simpson insisted that the "calculation of probabilities" represented by statistical analysis was the only realistic basis on which to build a rational medical and surgical regime.[26] He countered the

commonplace objections to medical statistics – that no two cases were sufficiently alike in their detail to be classed together, and that knowledge of the
individual cases comprising such groups was commonly inaccurate, for
instance – by claiming that classification was a core element of medical
knowledge, and that the structured nature of statistical surveys ensured
greater observational accuracy upon which to make these necessary group-
ings than *ad hoc* case reports. His proposed study, moreover, was so simple in
the facts to be adduced (was an amputation performed?; what part of the
limb was involved?; did the patient live or die?) that there was little chance
for error.[27]

In the series's concluding instalment, Simpson finally laid out the
methodology and results of the statistical survey he had undertaken. The
centrepiece of his study was the outcome of 302 major limb amputations
conducted with anaesthesia in 49 public hospitals of England, Scotland,
Ireland and France in the first half of 1847. These results were generated by
responses to a simple tabular questionnaire circulated by Simpson, in which
he had asked surgeons to break down the total number of cases and deaths
by limb involved, and by reason for amputation (accident or disease).
Finding a composite death rate of 23 in 100, he then compared this with
published figures from existing well-known investigations of amputation
mortality for a similar hospital profile in the pre-anaesthetic period, the
lowest of which reported a death rate of 29 in 100. On the basis of this
historical comparison, Simpson boldly and controversially concluded that six
patients out of every hundred had been "saved" by having their pain
annulled.[28] These figures, Simpson declared, "speak in a language much
more emphatic than any mere words that I could employ in favour of anaesthesia, not only as a means of preserving surgical patients from pain, but as a
means also of preserving them from death".[29]

Simpson provided no substantive causal explanation for the comparative
safety of surgical anaesthesia. Acknowledging this omission at the close of
his study, he rather weakly – and in some respects contradictorily – referred
the reader to his previous sampling of individual, ostensibly authoritative
statements on the pathogenic nature of pain. But Simpson's eschewal of
cause, considered from within the logic of medical statistics, was in another
respect perfectly consistent. Probabilistic inference, rather than determinant
mechanism, was what one was seeking through the power of numbers.[30]

Simpson thus claimed to have demonstrated, by the incontestable objectivity
of statistical reasoning, that the restrictionist calculus was miscalibrated. It
was not the anaesthetic agent that conferred surgical risk, but the pain
caused by surgery in the *absence* of anaesthesia. By turning the focus onto the
dangers of pain rather than onto anaesthesia, Simpson had thus fundamentally reframed the issue. His study was not about deaths under anaesthesia,
but was instead an undifferentiated comparison of two types of *surgical* death
– with and without anaesthesia. The potential risk factors in anaesthetic
administration (conditions and method of delivery, patient constitution, for

example) were therefore excluded from view as a matter of design, with surgery itself taking anaesthesia's place as the category of identified, and thus assessable, risk.[31]

Simpson's conclusions provoked a mixed response. Critics of medical statistics rejected its results on principle, while others, more sympathetic to the project overall, called attention to flaws in Simpson's methodology.[32] Admirers, on the other hand, praised Simpson's considered exposition of the still-novel principles of the numerical method, and held the study out as a key moment in the quest to secure the legitimacy and viability of the anaesthetic practice. Simpson's articles, according to James Arnott, author of more sophisticated statistical returns of anaesthetic outcomes in the 1850s, had proved "as influential with surgeons as the Northampton Life Tables have been with Assurance Companies".[33] The varied responses to Simpson's figures, however, belied a more fundamental commonality between those arguing for and those against the unrestricted use of anaesthesia. Both sides, that is, embraced the principle of calculated suffering as a means of bypassing the emotive nature of the debate.

But if pain could be made to work within a common, if contested, vision of calibrated risk evaluation, it equally presented complications that threatened to undermine this rationalistic frame of analysis. For the purposes of my analysis, the most telling of these complications was the way that pain was seen to interact with another inherently unstable element: fear. Like pain, lay and medical opinion alike regarded fear as physiologically damaging, even fatal. Andrew Combe's best-selling *Principles of Physiology* observed that "death itself is not a rare result" of the emotions of the mind; the Edinburgh physician and public health investigator William Pultney Alison maintained that "Joy, Grief, Anger, Fear, when acting in the utmost intensity, affect the circulating system just as a concussion does, and sometimes with fatal effect"; while the noted physiologist W. B. Carpenter declared "there is abundant evidence that a *sudden* and *violent* excitement of some depressing Emotion, especially Terror, may produce a severe and even a fatal disturbance of the Organic functions". Expressions like "frightened to death", C. J. B. Williams's *Principles of Medicine* warned, "are not always mere figures of speech".[34]

Release from fear, in this view, was (like relief of pain) a core physiological benefit conferred by anaesthesia. But unlike pain, which was seemingly amenable to objective risk evaluation, fear was based on an altogether different, and inherently unstable, dynamic. In the view of Benjamin Travers, surgeon to St. Thomas's Hospital and a widely quoted authority on pathogenic sensation, fear "operates with real and serious force against the best efforts of human skill, and this is excited in a degree, professionally speaking, by no means corresponding to the occasion".[35] The *Lancet* applied Travers's canonical account of the ungrounded nature of patient fear to the terms of the anaesthetic calculus: "There can be no doubt that the most terrible operations are much less painful, in reality, than they are imagined to be; that, in fact, the emotion of fear supplies a great part of the pain suffered under the operating-knife."[36] Such abstract arguments were supplemented by accounts from the surgical theatre, which highlighted patients' "unreasoning" and "distorted" sensibilities. George Wilson, in a letter to Simpson signed "An Old Patient", gave poignant testimony to the unreliability of patient self-assessment when contemplating surgery: "That the dread of pain keeps many a patient from submitting to operations, which would save life, is notorious," he observed, "but the dread of a particular mode of inflicting pain is a more dissuasive motive with many than the dread of the pain so inflicted." In Wilson's estimation, it was the purposive intentionality of surgically inflicted pain that lay at the root of disproportionate patient fear, leading many to "suffer prolonged agonies for months, rather than submit to a fraction of the same amount of pain at a surgeon's hand, because, as produced by him, it takes the form of an incision with a sharp knife".[37]

A patient-centred calculus, in short, having at its foundation a process animated not by dispassionate consideration of self-interest but by an essentially irrational (and possibly deadly) one, presented inhospitable grounds indeed for a usable model of risk evaluation. Yet since fear – however ill-judged – had real physiological consequences, it was a necessary feature of any attempt to construct such a model. This complicated both conservative and liberal regimes of risk assessment. Conservative reliance upon type of operation as the objective basis for decision-making was clearly problematic, since patients' unreasoning fears would disrupt whatever ostensibly objective correlation might be posited between surgical seriousness and projected danger. For anaesthetic liberals, the instabilities of fear presented even greater difficulties, foremost among which was the possibility that patient fear might itself be reified as a risk factor contraindicating anaesthetization.

There were well-established precedents for considering fear as a factor in assessing the proper course of medical intervention. Surgical manuals, generally citing some notion of systemic depression, had long advised against operating upon patients suffering from a state of acute nervousness, and such warnings were readily applied to debates surrounding anaesthesia. Since deaths under anaesthesia were most often related to causes "aggravated and even caused by emotional influences", one of the earliest textbooks on anaesthetic practice declared, "nothing more than this points out how necessary it is to proceed gradually and to induce confidence and calm".[38] Mental tranquillity ought to be considered an absolute prerequisite for administration, another practitioner insisted: "If [the patient] should feel any apprehension or gloomy forebodings, [anaesthesia] should be steadfastly refused."[39] This concern was underscored by reference to both contemporary physiological theory and practical experience. Marshall Hall's observation that deaths on the operating table had "frequently been foretold in the most positive terms by the patient" seemed especially apposite in the context of anaesthesia, where early reports of fatalities remarked upon pre-operative patient fear.[40]

The first reported victim of chloroform, the 15-year-old Hannah Greener, "appeared to dread the operation", according to the *London Medical Gazette*.[41] In the view of John Snow, chloroform's next reported victim, a "healthy muscular young" male, succumbed to syncope "through fear of the operation or of the inhalation, concerning which he had been led to entertain apprehensions".[42]

The combined weight of physiological theory and practical experience, in the view of one advocate of restriction, thus fully justified "withholding the administration of chloroform under the well-marked symptoms of nervous depression, and of rendering it culpable in any one using it until such a state is relieved".[43] Anaesthetic liberals, while agreeing that patient perception was an important consideration, rejected this factor as a determinant of practice. If fear proved intractable, John Snow insisted, the anaesthetist was duty bound to proceed. This was not because Snow thought it was marginal – quite the opposite: reviewing the causes of chloroform-related death in 1854, Snow concluded that "mental emotion of some kind is frequently the immediate cause of sudden death".[44] It was because fear was such a significant factor in surgical outcome, Snow argued, that it was a fatal mistake to deny chloroform on the assumption that fear increased risk beyond an acceptable level. In their anxiety about patient fear, anaesthetists would be abandoning the very class of patient – the ranks of the "nervous and feeble" – who most required their services. This was not merely a therapeutic mistake, but also a demonstrable error in logic. A patient who had agreed to be anaesthetized, Snow reasoned, had already made his or her own implicit risk analysis, and in so doing had effectively removed from the equation the imponderable dimension seemingly introduced by fear. "For whatever undefined and unreasoning fears a patient may have when the moment comes for inhaling," Snow argued, "he has only chosen to inhale it on account of a still greater fear of pain." Withholding anaesthesia in such cases contravened the patient's own embodied fear–pain ratio, and merely condemned the patient to "the still greater fear of the pain, as well as the pain itself".[45]

Snow based this syllogistic model for justifying the anaesthetization of a frightened patient on the patient's own calculus of suffering. However, by giving the avowedly unreliable economy of patient perception such an important place in the rationale for anaesthetic administration, Snow and his colleagues had to confront a discomfiting prospect: that the more anaesthesia was feared, the more problematic its use became. Rather than being an objective measure for determining practice, in other words, the very calculation of anaesthetic "risk" could itself be regarded as – and thus become – a direct factor in producing the risk being measured. This, in turn, meant that managing the *perception* of risk would be of critical importance in determining the future of anaesthetic practice. A confident public would prove a safe pool of subjects.

Anaesthetic advocates were thus acutely sensitive to what they considered the undisciplined discussions of risk which too often attracted the attention of the medical and lay press. Responding to newspaper coverage of one of the first British fatalities involving ether, a *Lancet* correspondent despaired that the reports were "calculated to strike a certain amount of terror into the minds both of the public and of the members of the medical profession", while a *Times* correspondent, writing in the wake of a later series of chloroform fatalities in London hospitals, denounced the "senseless but popular terror of chloroform which appears to be daily gaining ground".[46] Terror might equally be stoked by the ill-judged efforts of anaesthetic enthusiasts to promote faith in its safety and efficacy. When the noted chemist William Brande inadvertently smothered a guinea pig while giving a public demonstration of chloroform at the Royal Institution, a *Lancet* contributor bemoaned the event as "calculated to do much harm, by exciting an unnecessary degree of alarm. Who among that large assemblage, if the inhalation of chloroform should be at any time proposed to them," the correspondent quite plausibly continued, "would not remember the fate of that animal, and dread its application to themselves?"[47]

Concern with the management of public perception can also be discerned in a key disagreement that emerged between the leading advocates of anaesthesia, one centred on divergent national "styles" of administration. Following Simpson's teachings, most practitioners in Edinburgh, and in Scotland as a whole, administered chloroform via the "open" method – pouring an unmeasured amount onto a piece of cloth or gauze, and replenishing it as required until the patient was fully narcotized. The London school, informed by John Snow's experimental researches, held that Simpson's "slovenly" method smacked of unscientific empiricism. Snow maintained that accidents during administration were caused by the action of immoderately administered chloroform on the heart, and that careful management of the quantity and intensity of the vapour inhaled was the proper means for ensuring success. Insisting that practitioners using a cloth or sponge "have no control" over these key determinants of successful administration, Snow's research drew attention to a host of variables affecting chloroform's action (room temperature and air pressure, for example) and to the instrumental and dosimetric means of managing chloroform's effects.[48]

From Edinburgh, however, the dangers of administration lay not in any inherent properties of the drug, but in a timidity on the part of the administrator stemming from an ungrounded fear of chloroform. London's concern with the patient's circulatory system led them to place too much emphasis on signs of stress in the patient at the early stages of inhalation – gasping, delirium, spasmodic struggling, for example. These signs, though admittedly terrifying to the novice, were, Simpson explained, signs that the vapour was being given too slowly, or in too small a quantity, resulting in an excitation of the patient which could, if prolonged by further tentative administration, lead to asphyxiation. "The simple remedy, as every one properly experienced in its action knows," he declared, "is at once to increase the dose in order to pass the patient as speedily as possible into the *second*, or full narcotic stage."[49] This was precisely what practitioners south of the border failed to do: instead, regarding these signs as "very alarming, all attempts at further inhalation stops, exactly where and when the dose of the vapour should have been increased".[50] For Simpson and his Edinburgh disciples, this difference in approach directly and indirectly accounted for the higher reported death rate from chloroform in England: by withholding chloroform at the critical moment when the patient required calm perseverance with the inhalation, and by their obsession with instrumentation and measurement which suggested the existence of false dangers, English practitioners were feeding a deadly alarm. London's misplaced efforts to manage anaesthetic risk, paradoxically, tended to "give the public a dread of chloroform and to limit the advantages which it confers".[51]

Anaesthetic restrictionists were themselves fully alive to the importance of this perceptual element of the debate, identifying it as a risk factor that in itself militated against an unfettered regime of use. James Braid, a leading mesmerist and later a founding figure of British hypnosis, argued in 1848 that recent reports of anaesthetic death had themselves increased the risk of administration: "now that an alarm has been excited as to the danger ... the emotional feelings of the patients have been adding greatly to the danger of applying them". As a consequence, Braid concluded, a provisional "suspension" of all inhalation anaesthetic was necessary, leaving the way clear for the return of "safer" practices like mesmerism.[52] It was the mere existence of doubt in the public mind, independent of its actual value as a measure of risk, the obstetrician W. Tyler Smith insisted, that mitigated against widespread use of anaesthetics: "Unless the proper case for etherization can be distinguished with something approaching to certainty, patients upon whom it may be used will go under the knife influenced by previous dread rather than confidence. ... Such is the constitution of the human mind," he concluded, "that a few fatal cases, even by the side of a great number of successful ones, will be sufficient to transmute hope into fear, confidence into timidity and mistrust."[53] Smith's uncompromising insistence on absolute safety admittedly placed him at an extreme end of the risk assessment spectrum. It is noteworthy, then, that he justified this high threshold for selective anaesthesia not in terms of risk intrinsic to the agent itself, but rather on the decidedly murkier terrain of risk perception.

Anaesthetic advocates like John Snow, unsurprisingly, reacted strongly to suggestions like those made by Braid and Smith – that public perception of anaesthetic risk was itself justification for restricting practice. I want, by way of conclusion, to pay attention to the terms of his dissent, for they indicate just how much conceptual ground the two camps actually shared – how much, in fact, the early debates about anaesthetic administration had come to revolve around a self-reflexive concept of risk. To limit anaesthesia to only the most serious cases in deference to public uncertainty, Snow argued, was a strategy that missed the fatal implications of its own logic: "if the practice could only be advised for extremely painful operations", he warned, "the patient would be necessarily impressed with an idea of its essential danger, and the *greatest benefit* connected with the discovery, that of *preventing the anxiety and mental anguish arising from the anticipation of an operation*, would be altogether lost".[54] As a method for regulating anaesthetic delivery, then, risk assessment could claim no exogenous space. Instead, in the case of the early debates about British inhalation anaesthesia, risk, and more crucially the perception of risk, was itself a constitutive element of the very controversy that it purported to adjudicate.

Notes

1 Thanks to Chris Lawrence, Martin Pernick, John Pickstone and Stephanie Snow for comments on earlier drafts of this essay.

2 "On Etherization, or the Inhalation of the vapour of ether", *British and Foreign Medical Review* (hereafter *BFMR*), 23, 1847, 547–76; 547.

3 Simpson made these connections explicitly in a letter written to an American critic, cited in Martin Pernick, *A Calculus of Suffering: Pain, Professionalism and Anesthesia in Nineteenth-Century America*, New York: Columbia University Press, 1985, 78–9.

4 Simpson's own reputed sensibilities were inextricably bound up with the transformative powers of anaesthesia: according to his biographer, Simpson contemplated abandoning his medical studies in response to witnessing the terrors of surgical pain. H. Lang Gordon, *Sir James Young Simpson and Chloroform*, London: T Fisher Unwin, 1897, 91. In his writings, Simpson often praised the humanity of pre-anaesthetic surgeons like William Cheselden who endured "anxiety and sickness" before performing operations. Simpson, "Etherization in surgery, pt. I: Its effects; objections to it, etc.", *Monthly Journal of Medical Science* (hereafter *MJMS*), 8, 1848, 145–66; 161.

5 For an overview account of the introduction of anaesthesia into British surgical practice, see A. J. Youngson, *The Scientific Revolution in Victorian Medicine*, London: Croom Helm, 1979, ch. 3. Though historians like Alison Winter have drawn attention to the more complex context within which it was introduced and deployed than is recognized in accounts like Youngson's, it is none the less clear that, as Martin Pernick observes, anaesthesia was more rapidly incorporated into practice than any other pre-twentieth-century medical innovation. Alison Winter, *Mesmerized: Powers of Mind in Victorian Britain*, Chicago: University of Chicago Press, 1998; Martin Pernick, *Calculus*, 7. The only systematic study of anaesthesia in Britain is Barbara Duncum's classic *The Development of Inhalation Anaesthesia, with Special Reference to the Years 1846–1900*, London: Oxford University Press, 1947. Stephanie Snow is currently completing a book manuscript, entitled *Science, Ethics and Medical Values: John Snow and Anaesthesia in Victorian Britain*, that will provide a much-needed reconsideration of the topic.

6 "Ether", *Medical Times and Gazette* (hereafter *MTG*), 16, 1847, 24.

7 "Mr. Lawrence's case of operation performed after the inhalation of the vapour of sulphuric ether", *London Medical Gazette* (hereafter *LMG*), 4 (ns), 1847, 138–9; 138.

8 "Etherization" *Lancet*, 1, 1847, 265.

9 Liston himself reported failures in January 1847, leading him to consider giving up the practice altogether. He died soon after, however, without having made a definitive statement on the subject.

10 Pernick, *Calculus*, esp. chs 2–5. There is a large literature on the origins and growth of the "numerical method" in medicine. See, especially, Richard Shryock, "The history of quantification in medical science", *Isis*, 52(168), 1961, 215–37; Ian Hacking, *The Taming of Chance*, Cambridge: Cambridge University Press, 1990, esp. ch. 10; J. Rosser Matthews, *Quantification and the Quest for Medical Certainty*, Princeton, NJ: Princeton

University Press, 1995, and Joshua Cole, *The Power of Large Numbers*, Ithaca: Cornell University Press, 2000.

11 There were, to be sure, significant differences between the two, differences that moreover could be mapped onto a discussion of risk. Chloroform was preferred by British practitioners primarily on the grounds of its comparative ease. As experience with chloroform deepened, however, it was also recognized that its greater potency made it potentially more dangerous, and by the end of the period now under discussion the relative merits of ether and chloroform were subjects of lively debate. But in the discussions that form the subject of my analysis, ether and chloroform were for the most part conflated as agents that promised painlessness, but at a possible cost. Stephanie Snow's work (see n. 5, this chapter) develops a more systematic discussion of the ether–chloroform debates.

12 "Chloroform in Medical Practice", *Lancet*, 2, 1848, 181.

13 Liverpool Medical and Pathological Society discussion, "On the abuses of chloroform", *LMG*, 8 (ns), 563–8; 563. Emphasis original.

14 "On etherization", *BFMR*, 547, 556.

15 "Review: Snow *On Chloroform*, Simpson, *Obstetric Memoirs*", *Westminster Review*, 15 (ns), 1859, 99–146; 138.

16 The number of deaths associated with anaesthesia were not officially compiled until much later in the century, and figures collected by individuals varied according to the criteria adopted for what constituted a death under anaesthesia. Dr Crisp, a member of the Medical Society of London, put the number of chloroform deaths between 1847 and 1852 at thirteen, while John Snow counted eighteen for the same period. Crisp's figures were published in the *Lancet*, 1, 1853, 523; Snow's are cited in Youngson, *The Scientific Revolution*, 80.

17 "The Use and Abuse of Chloroform", *Lancet*, 2, 1854, 513.

18 John Snow, "A Lecture on the Inhalation of Vapour of Ether in Surgical Operations", *Lancet*, 1, 1847, 551–4; 553.

19 Pernick, *Calculus*, 81.

20 Simpson, "Etherization in surgery, pt. I", *MJMS*, 164.

21 Miller, *Principles of Surgery*, 3rd edn, 1853, 45. It should be noted that the conviction of Miller and other surgeons that minimizing pain enhanced surgical safety pre-dated the advent of inhalation anaesthesia. In the 1846 edition of his *Principles*, for example, Miller identifies the speed of operation as an important factor in surgical outcome in part because speed reduced pain: "The mere absence of protracted pain confers a most important advantage on the reparative powers of the system; and, so far, celerity is commendable." Miller, *Principles*, Edinburgh: Adam and Charles Black, 5.

22 Simpson, "Etherization in surgery, pt. I", *MJMS*, 145–53.

23 Simpson, "Etherization in surgery, pt. I", *MJMS*, 165.

24 Simpson, "Etherization in surgery, pt. I", *MJMS*, 166.

25 Simpson, "On Etherization in Surgery, Pt. II: Proper mode of investigating its effects; statistical propositions and results, etc.", *MJMS*, 8, 1848, 313–33; 314. "Truth and precision," he insisted in a discussion of his first paper, "could only be attained by generalising upon large numbers." "Discussion at the Medico-Chirurgical Society of Edinburgh", *MJMS*, 8, 1848, 302–10; 304.

26 Simpson, "Etherization in surgery, pt. II", *MJMS*, 330.

27 Simpson, "Etherization in surgery, pt. II", *MJMS*, 331.

28 Simpson, "Etherization in surgery, pt. III: Does etherisation increase or decrease the mortality attendant upon surgical operations?", *MJMS*, 8, 1848, 697–710; 707.

29 Simpson, "Etherization in surgery, pt. III", *MJMS*, 709.

30 Numbers could, however, be marshalled to explain, rather than merely empirically demonstrate, the relative safety of surgical anaesthesia. This was a task undertaken by Simpson's more experimentally minded counterpart, John Snow, who used his substantial clinical experience to inquire into the physiological workings of anaesthesia. The key to its protective effects in the surgical theatre, Snow concluded, lay in its capacity to protect

the circulatory system from the stresses incumbent upon major operations, a conclusion which he grounded in a comparative measurement of pulse rates of patients undergoing operations with and without the assistance of anaesthesia. The higher rates in the latter cases demonstrated, in his view, that patients with a weakened heart would run a greater risk from pain than from anaesthesia. See, e.g., Snow, *On Chloroform and other Anaesthetics: their Action and Administration*, London: J. Churchill, 1858, 56.

31 It is significant that the lack of differentiated mortality statistics in this study designed to demonstrate the absence of risk contrasted to those that Simpson invoked in his background discussion on statistical method, in which he cited studies (e.g. of lithotomy operations) in which patient condition was broken down by age and severity of disease. Simpson, "Etherization in surgery, pt. II", *MJMS*, 324–7.

32 See, e.g., "Discussion at the Medico-Chirurgical Society of Edinburgh", in *MJMS*, 8, 1848, 302–10.

33 James Arnott, "On the Effects of Chloroform Upon the Result of Surgical Operations", *MTG*, 34, 1856, 412–14; 412.

34 Andrew Combe, *Principles of Physiology*, 3rd edn, Edinburgh: MacLachlan, Stewart, 1835, 337; W. P. Alison, *Outlines of Physiology and Pathology*, Edinburgh: Blackwood, 1833, 334; W. B. Carpenter, *Principles of Human Physiology*, London: J. Churchill, 1855, 784; C. J. B. Williams, *Principles of Medicine*, 6th edn, 1843, 26.

35 Benjamin Travers, *An inquiry concerning that disturbed state of the vital functions usually denominated constitutional irritation*, London: Longmans, Rees, Orme, Brown and Green, 1827, 15.

36 *Lancet*, 1, 1847, "Etherization in Surgical Operations", 74.

37 Letter from Dr George Wilson, in J. Y. Simpson, *Works*, vol. 2, 264–5, 267.

38 A. E. Sansom, *Chloroform: Its Action and Administration: a Handbook*, London: J. Churchill, 132.

39 "Deaths from the administration of chloroform" *Lancet*, 2, 1853, 409.

40 Marshall Hall, *On the diseases and derangements of the nervous system*, London: H. Baillière, 359.

41 "Poisoning by Chloroform – Conflicting Medical Opinions", *LMG*, 6 (ns), 1848, 283–4; 283.

42 *Edinburgh Medical Journal* (hereafter *EMJ*), 72, 1856, 1849, 86.

43 "Deaths from chloroform in Edinburgh", *MTG*, 33, 19–20.

44 Snow, "Deaths from chloroform in Edinburgh", *MTG*, 29, 1854, 606.

45 Snow, *On Chloroform*, 76.

46 Letter from "Scrutator", *Lancet*, 1, 1847, 423; letter from "MRCS, Guy's Hospital", *The Times*, 11 October 1858.

47 "Experiment with Chloroform", *Lancet*, 2 April 1848, 163.

48 Snow, "On Narcotism by the Inhalation of Vapours, Pt. VII", *LMG*, 7 (ns), 1848, 840–4; 841. More broadly, see Snow, *On Chloroform*.

49 "Dr. Simpson's Report on the Early History and Progress of Anaesthetic Midwifery", *MJMS*, 8, 1848, 244–5. Emphasis original.

50 Medico-Chirurgical Society of Edinburgh, discussion of "Report on the Employment of Chloroform in Midwifery, etc.", *MJMS*, 9, 1849, 54–5; 54.

51 James Syme, "Lectures on Clinical Surgery", *Lancet*, 1, 1855, 56.

52 James Braid, "On the Use and Abuse of Anaesthetic Agents", *EMJ*, 70, 1848, 486.

53 W. Tyler Smith, "A Lecture on the Utility and Safety of the Inhalation of Ether in Obstetric Practice", *Lancet*, 1, 1847, 321–3; 323.

54 Snow, "Chloroform in London and Edinburgh", *Lancet*, 1, 1855, 108; emphasis added.

4 Redemption, danger and risk

The history of anti-bacterial chemotherapy and the transformation of tuberculin

Christoph Gradmann[1]

Risk, danger and medicine in the nineteenth century

"Large doses cause damage ... whereas small doses don't help."[2] At first sight, Robert Koch's tuberculin, presented as a cure for tuberculosis late in the summer of 1890, appears to be a classic example of a risky medical innovation. The passage cited above was published in late 1891 by Paul Baumgarten, a professor of pathological anatomy in Tübingen, and summed up a year of experience with the supposed remedy. Indeed, even a superficial look at the process of research, publication, application and the way in which the medicine was discussed in public reveal the features of a risky, if not a hazardous enterprise. Tuberculin was presented as a secret remedy, with only insufficient and partly misleading information supplied about its constitutive components, its preparation and the associated animal testing. Furthermore, accusations were raised about unethical human experiments and rumors concerning the grandiose commercial plans harbored by the inventor did even more damage to its reputation. After a short period of euphoria, tuberculin was considered to be therapeutically ineffective by most physicians.[3]

Indeed, injections of tuberculin could be very dangerous, as is illustrated by the example of Max Simon, a patient treated in Elberfeld in December 1890. Having just recovered from pulmonary tuberculosis, he was given what his physicians considered to be a small, diagnostic injection of 2 mg of tuberculin. What followed was a disaster:

> Only three hours after the injection high fever up to 40 degrees was observed, feeble almost undetectable pulse (about 150 per minute); on top of it vomiting, unquenchable thirst. 12 hours after the injection, death came with the symptoms of paralysis of the heart[4]

Still, it took at least three month before it became widely accepted that tuberculin was not a cure for tuberculosis and that its use was potentially dangerous. Even then, no consensus was reached concerning this remedy, and the debate lingered on for years. This chapter focuses on the debate, allowing us to address some questions around the historicity of notions of risk in medicine. How, when and by who did tuberculin come to be considered a risky medicine, on what evidence was such knowledge based, and what role did the risk of using tuberculin play in the evaluation of the medicine? Finally, some attention will be paid to the semantics of the evaluation of risk and in particular to the question of how the language used in this case is in any sense related to the language of health risks and their evaluation at the present day.

This last question is particularly thorny and so, before entering into our analysis of the short-lived career of Koch's remedy, I would like to make two preliminary remarks concerning the history of medicine in relation to the concept of risk and clinical trials in late-nineteenth-century medicine, in order to sharpen the focus of the chapter.[5] However familiar the concepts of "risk" and "clinical trial" might seem to a modern observer, they are none the less not well suited for use in a historical analysis of nineteenth-century medical practice. Thus, while recent actors in the field, as well as historical or sociological analysts, make regular use of such concepts,[6] this does not mean they can be straightforwardly projected back onto the late nineteenth century. Although the term "risk" (*Risiko* in German) was in current usage during this period, it was not used in the context of the possible outcome of a medical intervention. While everybody was well aware that the application of drugs could lead to unforeseeable events, the term was hardly ever applied in these cases. Instead contemporaries preferred to speak about dangers (*Gefahren*), thereby evoking quite a different notion, leaving the use of the term risk almost exclusively to the financial or commercial risks involved in insurance, trade or the stock market.[7] Such risk was regarded as something that could be calculated and quantified and might, for example, result in an increased insurance rate. Nineteenth-century scientists were certainly accustomed to making statistical statements about medical practices, such as claims relating to smallpox inoculations, but we have no indication that the language of risk was used to evaluate a medical intervention such as surgery, for example. The modern notion of a medical intervention being relatively safe, but carrying a few residual risks, was not yet in place. Instead, medical interventions were conceived of as being dangerous in general, implying a much broader notion of unpredictable, immeasurable events, seen to remain in the hands of fate.

Even if they did not employ the language of risk, the possible dangers associated with medical interventions were none the less quite obvious to Koch's contemporaries. However, for this analysis it is important to note that in the context of drug therapies there was no such thing as a clinical trial at that time, with the important contemporary distinction being drawn instead between human experimentation and therapy.[8] Whereas the first could be – and was indeed – seen as highly problematic, the attitude towards therapy was positive and regulation was correspondingly lax, even though the term therapy was applied to many practices that a modern observer would consider to be clinical trials if not experimentation. Against the background of the high esteem in which medical science was held at the time, such associated dangers were seen as an inherent by-product of medical activity. The side effects of drugs, which came to be an important issue for twentieth-century medicine, received little systematic attention at the time.[9] In addition to this, the widespread practice of self-experimentation by doctors lent even more legitimacy to dangerous therapies.[10]

While in the case of surgical intervention there was a tradition of discussing matters such as patient consent, the possible dangers associated with certain procedures and medical malpractice,[11] nothing of this sort existed for antibacterial chemotherapy. In reality, this type of treatment existed only in scientists' imaginations during the 1880s,[12] which meant that any unpleasant side effects were equally non-existent. The dream of finding antibacterial therapies was, however, widespread, with both scientists and the wider public convinced that the contemporary hunt for microbes, which coincidently implied a radically new conception of diseases, would result in a range of specific remedies. It should be born in mind that the very popularity acquired by bacteria rested on a peculiar balance of notions of danger and control. Thus, it was not so much the discovery of the existence of microbes as such that was sensational, but rather the revelation of the threat posed by these "smallest, but most dangerous enemies of mankind",[13] and the concomitant pledge by the scientists to fight and control these dangerous microbes.[14] For many in the late nineteenth century the discovery of bacterial pathogens carried with it the promise of mankind's redemption from the totality of infectious diseases. When in 1882 Robert Koch presented his seminal discovery of the tubercle bacillus, he pointed out to his audience that knowledge about a pathogen included the promise of a cure: "[i]n the future the fight against this horrible plague of mankind will no longer deal with an undefined something, but with a concrete parasite, whose conditions of life have been fully revealed"[15] He added the observation that measures against the disease could now be developed under what he termed "particularly favorable conditions".[16] Only a few years later, when Louis Pasteur presented his rabies vaccine, such dreams were seen to have become reality, and Gerald Geison has described the wild enthusiasm of its reception that left critics almost no space to express their doubts.[17] Furthermore, the commercial success of the vaccine quite literally laid the foundations of the Pasteur Institute.[18]

In the meantime the hopes that Robert Koch had raised both for himself and for others proved to be harder to fulfill. While preventive measures based on bacteriological hygiene such as disinfection became available in the 1880s, antibacterial therapies for infected patients were nowhere to be seen. It has to be borne in mind that, when he finally made his announcement that he had found a cure for tuberculosis,[19] Koch had already spent at least half a decade searching for such a treatment and was under no small pressure to provide one.

Euphoria

How was tuberculin presented by Koch, what was its purported effect, and what information did the inventor supply concerning the possible dangers of its use? In his address to the audience at the Tenth International Congress of Medicine held in Berlin in August 1890, Koch claimed to have discovered a substance with remarkable properties:

> I can say ... this much, that guinea pigs, which are highly susceptible to the disease, no longer react upon inoculation with the tubercle virus after having been treated with this substance and that in guinea pigs that are sick (with tuberculosis), the pathological process can be brought to a complete standstill.[20]

No information was supplied concerning the composition of the medicine or a method for preparing it. Tuberculin, when it became available in November 1890, was a secret remedy in which doctors and patients placed their trust on the sole basis of Robert Koch's prestige. In November he reported in some more detail about the method of use, described the typical symptoms of local and general reactions to tuberculin, and reported on more animal experiments and some trials on humans.[21] As we now know, testing had in fact started in a rather uncontrolled manner, with the first subjects being Koch himself and his seventeen-year-old mistress. She recalled the event in the following terms: "He called upon my readiness to make a sacrifice, by pointing out the value for mankind. I might become rather ill, but most probably not very. In any case dying was very unlikely."[22] Next in line to serve as human guinea pigs were some of Koch's assistants, and all of this testing seems to have taken place prior to the announcement at the Berlin congress.[23] The purpose of these tests seems to have been to show that the remedy posed no danger to healthy individuals.

Starting in September 1890, the remedy was tested on a small number of tuberculous patients in a few Berlin clinics.[24] However, in his second publication that appeared in November, Koch only mentioned that these trials had taken place, saying nothing about their outcome or any possible dangers associated with using tuberculin.[25] Instead, he supplied detailed instructions for its use, and described the effect it had on various sorts of tuberculosis. The inventor claimed that tuberculin affected infected tissues and not the bacteria itself, producing a necrosis of the affected tissues and thus preventing any further propagation of the bacilli in the organism by depriving them of their supply of nutrition. This process – a kind of bacteriological scorched-earth strategy – took the form of a local inflammatory process accompanied by a general reaction, including fever, shivering, pain in the limbs, and nausea. The local reaction, which was essential for the cure, could best be observed in cases of tuberculosis of the skin, or lupus.[26] Following the injection, "the parts that exhibit lupus start to turn red and they do so before shivering starts". Upon further development the tissues turn "brown-red and necrotic", the tuberculous parts are "transformed into scales, which fall off after 2–3 weeks and what remains – in some cases this is already the case following the first injection of the remedy – is a smooth red scar".[27]

Still, Koch gave no information whatsoever about the constitution of the treatment, simply insisting that the reaction could be controlled and finely tuned. In contrast to the detailed and constraining instructions for use of the treatment, the range of indications was remarkably wide. Beyond the purported therapeutic effect, Koch regarded the characteristic reaction of patients suffering from acute tuberculosis to the remedy as a diagnostic tool: whereas healthy individuals only showed general symptoms, if any at all, tuberculous individuals displayed particularly strong general and local reactions.

The introduction of tuberculin onto the market in mid-November 1890 triggered a euphoria that at least matched if not surpassed that associated with Koch's successful microbe hunt of the early 1880s (See Figure 4.1).[28] As a local newspaper put it, Berlin became "a place of pilgrimage for physicians from every country",[29] crowded with patients and doctors. Coffee houses were being turned into "wild" clinics, etc.[30] Shortly after tuberculin became available,

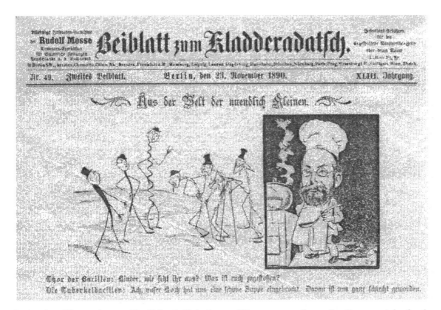

Figure 4.1 "From the world of the infinitely small", a cartoon from the German joke book *Kladderadatsch* of 23 November 1890, The tuberculosis bacteria are discussing tuberculin while facing their extermination: "*Chorus of bacilli*: Hi boys, why do you look like that? What happened to you? *The tubercle bacilli*: Our cook [Koch] has got us into a pickle. That's what made us feel sick."

Source: "Aus der Welt der unendlich Kleinen", Kladderadatsch 23.11.1890, issue 49, 1.

numerous reports were published about instant cures, fuelling the euphoric frenzy. There was scarcely any mention of the possible dangers associated with the cure, and no one seemed to realize that using tuberculin could have fatal results. The strong reaction that followed the injection was almost universally interpreted as a positive sign of its healing activity. In Hamburg an eleven-year-old girl suffering from lupus on both cheeks was well on her way to recovery after only four days.[31] If patients died while receiving tuberculin, it was assumed that it was a result of their being terminally ill before the treatment began.

Besides its use as a therapy, tuberculin was also commonly used as a diagnostic tool. In order to obtain more knowledge about the tuberculin reaction, some doctors acted rather negligently: terminally ill patients were given rapidly increasing doses to study the development of the reaction that resulted. In Berlin Frau Hermann, suffering from severe pulmonary tuberculosis, was given eight injections starting at 1 mg and rising to 4 mg between 21 November and 8 December. While she displayed almost no reaction, her state of health deteriorated and she died three days after the last injection. Presenting the pathological evidence of this case and a second similar one to the Berlin Medical Society, Ernst von Leyden, the Director of the Charité Hospital's Internal Clinic where the injections had been performed, remarked:

> Both cases were treated starting the very day we got hold of the new remedy. Therapeutic success was hardly to be expected, and the intention was rather to augment our observations and knowledge. Therapeutic success was neither intended, nor was this an issue. ... I note that these two patients have in no way experienced any damage due to the administration of the medicine and it is entirely unthinkable that exitus was accelerated in these cases.[32]

Thus, during the initial tuberculin euphoria, the issue of any possible danger associated with tuberculin simply did not exist. With the exception of one of Koch's critics, who had not succeeded in getting his share of tuberculin and subsequently warned against its use,[33] there was a general belief that the only precaution that needed to be taken was to raise the dosages slowly in order to avoid what one doctor called "evil accidents".[34] The reaction to this purported medicine, which twentieth-century scientists would come to understand as an essentially uncontrollable allergic shock, was seen at the time as predictable and perfectly controllable. Paul Gutmann, the Director of a Berlin Hospital, found that one of the advantages of the treatment was precisely that the precision of its action could be "refined to a surprising degree".[35]

The only danger that was mentioned was of rather a peculiar variety: as Koch emphasized, tuberculin was so difficult to prepare that its composition and method of preparation had to be kept secret in order to secure a reliable level of quality and ensure that only the tuberculin produced by Koch's laboratory would be put on the market.[36]

Therapy and experiment

However, as 1890 gave way to 1891, the euphoria around tuberculin was slowly fading. Several reasons can be identified for this. Rumors were spreading to the effect that Koch had imposed strict secrecy for what were not purely medical reasons, and that he was, in fact, using this means to cover up his own extensive commercial ambitions.[37] In so far as the topic of risk is concerned, however, it is more pertinent to note that the wide range of indications and uses for tuberculin was giving rise to clinical events that raised criticism.

In some cases the therapeutic and experimental uses of the medicine were hard to distinguish. Thus, for example, when a baby considered fatally ill with "tuberctoulous meningitis" was injected with tuberculin, the body could be used post-mortem to provide more information on the pathological anatomy of the tuberculin reaction.[38] In other cases, the frontier between diagnostic use and human experimentation had evidently been breached. Thus, Julius Schreiber from Königsberg, for example, was injecting tuberculin into healthy children and babies from families whose members were infected with tuberculosis, with the aim of testing current theories about the hereditary nature of tuberculosis. He reported that it was hard to find suitable subjects for this experiment:

> It has always been a problem to obtain such children and so far I have only been able to inject one boy. It was done in a casual manner supposedly to punish some petty misdemeanor. The boy comes from a worker's family, where the mother fell ill with pulmonary tuberculosis. Initially, the parents didn't want to allow the injection, later, however, when the boy had – as I mentioned – committed some petty misdemeanor the father said: "All right, now you are going to be injected ..."[39]

Events like these quickly made their way into the press, but did not immediately result in the idea of tuberculin being dangerous. Still, with reports about successful cures becoming somewhat thinner on the ground, accidents were gradually gaining more attention. The central problem at first appeared to be one of appropriate use, and the answer was seen to lie in careful dosage, although opinions on the subject were beginning to diverge. One doctor raised doubts about whether tuberculin could actually cure any sort of tuberculosis, while another questioned the efficacy of tuberculin as a remedy and a third found it impossible to make any confident judgement concerning its therapeutic effect and even doubted its diagnostic value.[40] During the winter of 1890–91, most doctors observed a multitude of atypical reactions to the medicine, but for the most part they retained their faith in it.[41] Although some ethical questions also started to be raised at that time, the dangers associated with using tuberculin were not amongst them. Issues for discussion at that time were problems around the correct indications for the use of tuberculin, as well as accusations that some doctors were conducting human experiments. Statistical evidence gathered from Prussian university clinics and published at the end of 1891 looked inconclusive, but certainly not entirely discouraging: among the 1,769 cases treated, 319 were reported to have substantially improved and 431 to have improved somewhat. However, only twenty-eight patients had been definitely cured whereas 55 had died while under treatment.[42]

It was only in the middle of January 1891 that the first major criticism was raised. In a high-profile demonstration using pathological preparations, the pathologist Rudolf Virchow showed that tubercular infection had continued in cases treated with the remedy and that fresh tubercles could be found developing on the fringes of Koch's necrotized tissues. This meant that the model of necrosis proposed by Koch, which posited that necrosis would prevent any further spreading of the disease, was inaccurate.[43] In fact, as one of Virchow's collaborators suggested, tuberculin could even accelerate the pathological process.[44] This attack and mounting pressure from the public as well as government institutions finally forced Koch to publish a general description of the preparation of tuberculin, which turned out to be an extract made from pure cultures of tubercle bacilli.[45] The inventor admitted that he had tried unsuccessfully to isolate a single component of tuberculin responsible for its pathological effect. The secrecy surrounding tuberculin, which had initially contributed to the sensation caused by the new discovery, now backfired on its inventor. Tuberculin, initially a private mystery known only to its inventor, now became a public mystery with Koch's procedure exposed to scrutiny. To make matters worse, when Koch was confronted with Virchow's evidence he was unable to produce the guinea pigs he had claimed to have cured with tuberculin.

Although it is difficult to identify a single turning point in the history of tuberculin, which continued to be used and praised by many, it was in the period between late January and early February 1891 that the euphoric atmosphere around Koch's remedy gave way to one of scandal. Up to this point, tuberculin had enjoyed unanimous confidence, and the rare critics had had to work hard to justify their objections. Now the burden of proof shifted onto those who continued to trust the medicine, most notably Koch and his collaborators. Koch, however, failed to provide any substantially new evidence, choosing instead to quit the scene by setting off for Egypt on a long holiday (See Figure 4.2).

Still, the potential dangers played only a minor role in the general swing of opinion away from tuberculin that took place starting in January 1891. The crucial arguments were the mounting evidence for the ineffectiveness of tuberculin as a treatment, suspicions that it was being used for human experimentation, and the findings based on pathological anatomy that

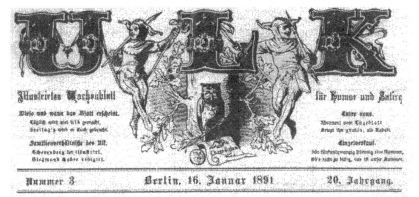

Musteirtes Wochenblatt

Wie und wann das Blatt erscheint.
Täglich oder vier Ulk gemacht,
Freitag's wird er Euch gebracht.

Famulienverhältnisse des Ulk.
Scherenberg der illustiert,
Sigismund Haber redigirt.

für Humor und Satire

Entre nous.
Abonnent vom Tageblatt
kriegt ihn gratis, als Rabatt.

Einzelverkauf.
Für Fünfundzwanzig Pfennig eine Nummer,
Ist's nicht zu billig, das ist unser Kummer.

Nummer 3   Berlin, 16. Januar 1891   20. Jahrgang.

Damit es noch mehr fluscht.

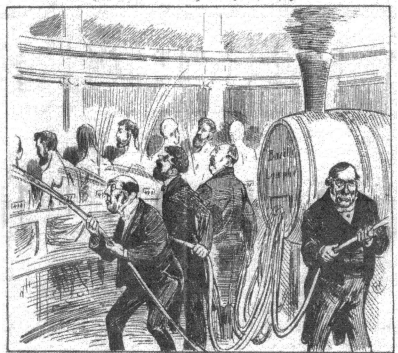

Einzelne Heilkünstler, denen das Geschäft über Alles geht, haben zu Gunsten ihres Geldschranks beschlossen,
die Einspritzungen künftig mit Hülfe der Feuerwehr zu besorgen.

Figure 4.2 "Make it work more swimmingly", cartoon from 16 January 1891. "A few remarkable therapists, to whom business means everything, have made a decision in favor of their safe. In future, injections shall be applied aided by the fire-brigade." The barrel in the centre is labeled "Bacillen Lymphe", a common name for tuberculin at this time.

Source: "Damit es noch mehr fluscht", Ulk, Beilage der Vossischen Zeitung, 16.1.1891.

contradicted Koch's theory of how it was supposed to act on infected tissues. Up until this time, accidents had mostly been blamed on irresponsible doctors, profiteers, or improper use of the medicine. Thus, tuberculin fell into disrepute not because it was considered dangerous, but because it simply did not seem to work. What had been regarded as a wonder cure started to turn into something quite unknown. The most common way that the issue of any danger associated with tuberculin had been raised was that some doctors claimed to feel uneasy about using a powerful medicine of unknown composition.[46] This feeling, coupled with the "accidents" mentioned above, resulted in doctors receiving the advice to augment the doses only slowly when administering the drug.

In spring 1891, Ottomar Rosenbach, a Breslau clinician and well-known critic of laboratory medicine, presented a critique that raised the issue of possible danger. He had taken the opportunity of a series of treatments to investigate the occurrence of fever reactions following the injection. This proved to be a good method for highlighting the dangers of tuberculin and – more importantly – the various types of fever reactions that emerged from this study seemed to be incompatible with Koch's ideas concerning the curative and diagnostic value of his remedy. It turned out that factors such as the patient's disposition or prior exposure were better predictors for the type of fever reaction than the dosage used. Rosenbach proceeded to take another step in the argument and proposed that these bouts of fever should be considered as dangerous side effects rather than as diagnostic symptoms.[47]

This critique turned out to be particularly devastating for two reasons. First, it integrated the numerous anomalies and bewildering phenomena that blurred the clinical picture of tuberculin into a new and different understanding of the bodily reaction to the substance. It transformed the fever reaction, which had been seen as a valuable diagnostic tool, into a complete mystery. Second, Rosenbach had posed the question whether a strong reaction – which was certainly what happened when tuberculin was administered – was necessarily curative. It was at about the same time that the first accusations concerning the morally questionable and experimental use of tuberculin were raised. Ernst von Leyden, a prominent Berlin clinician, complained that it was "hard to judge the effect of a medicine without actually having any knowledge about it. Moreover, we doctors were urged to experiment on sick people."[48]

With the inventor away on vacation in Egypt, tuberculin rapidly fell out of favor. While Virchow's attack in January 1891 had been restricted to the presentation of unfavorable pathological evidence, some speakers at the Tenth Congress of Internal Medicine held in Wiesbaden in early April went as far as openly to question whether tuberculin constituted a remedy or a diagnostic tool at all. The dangers associated with the administration of tuberculin were now almost universally acknowledged, while its curative and diagnostic value appeared to be in doubt, even though some speakers supported one or both uses. Friedrich Schulze, a clinician from Bonn, who had made some cautionary remarks earlier on, now declared that in light of the worsening state of some of his patients and the publication of Virchow's findings, he no longer dared to pick up his syringe and had not given any injections since February.[49] More fatalities resulting from the treatment were presented to the congress and Koch was repeatedly urged to provide more complete information on his animal experiments.

Bernhard Naunyn, a highly reputed doctor from Strasbourg, delivered a very harsh statement in his capacity as president of the assembly, coming to the conclusion that applying tuberculin was more or less useless, that it was dangerous, and that the occurrence of accidents was unpredictable.[50] While the opening speaker had already criticised the "unprecedented enthusiasm" around the reception of tuberculin, which he literally termed an "orgasm",[51] Naunyn denounced any purported cures by tuberculin and went on critically to assess the fabulous successes of late 1890. He surmised that these had been artifacts, resulting from a greatly increased cohort of patients that included many minor cases. This seems a reasonable conjecture, since the administration of tuberculin was usually preceded by a bacteriological diagnosis and successful cures were mostly observed in cases of so-called "early phthisis".[52] In the case of a lightning cure that was not followed by a relapse the best hypothesis seemed to be that they had not been infected with tuberculosis in the first place, or that they experienced a spontaneous cure.

Following the Wiesbaden congress, the dangers of tuberculin became more and more widely known. This knowledge was mobilized during a heated debate over the newly built Institute for Infectious Diseases in Berlin that took place on 9 May in the Prussian parliament. A decision had been made in November to found such an institute, giving *carte blanche* to its director, Robert Koch, and six months later the parliament had to vote on a large annual budget. It was during this session that the issue of the dangerous medicine was given a more detailed examination. Speakers now made the connection with the issue of the responsibilities and dangers faced by doctors and patients. In the fall of 1890 everybody had been enthusiastic about the new institute, but since then the euphoria had passed and the term "experimental medicine" had acquired a somewhat sinister connotation. The plans for the institute had included the founding of a department of "experimental studies", an idea that rang alarm bells for at least one representative:

> Gentlemen, you will admit that the expression "experimental studies" is not a happy choice in this case. ... [T]o my knowledge there has – up until now – never been a direct connection between an experimental department and a hospital. In the present case, there seems to be an attempt to establish an immediate link between a hospital and a research institute and it would be natural for many to assume that the result of experimental studies and scientific research could immediately be tried out on the bodies of the patients."[53]

While the advocates of tuberculin resorted to the argument that "experience needed to be obtained" even if the cases constituting this experience were miserable ones, another delegate came closer to the mark when he pointed out that the scandal around tuberculin had in fact confronted everyone with questions concerning the development and testing of a medicine on an unprecedented scale. Doctors had been applying a "highly toxic medicine" in an "unhesitant and inconsiderate way". It was precisely when they were being endangered or even violated that the rights and duties of doctors and patients became clearer than ever before. As Broemel, another member of the Prussian parliament, put it, "doctors need to stand trial before the public, the principal constituency concerned in any such matter that involves everyone's individual health".[54]

Of course, the notion that medical treatment could be experimental and dangerous was not entirely new at this time, although, as mentioned on p. 55, it had been more or less restricted to discussions of surgical treatment. In the context of bacteriological research, experimental procedures had not up to this point been considered a serious issue.[55] Now, with the rise of anti-bacterial chemotherapy and in light of the failure of tuberculin, these notions were expanded to include the administration of drugs.[56]

Dangerous medicine

Even though the dangers associated with tuberculin became common knowledge in the course of the 1890s they were mobilized in a rather particular way in the campaign against the treatment. The dangers were usually alluded to in quite general terms and never became a decisive argument in themselves. Danger played a supporting role, with the most significant accusations concerning attempts at profit-making, clinical inefficacy, negative pathological evidence and the violation of contemporary ethical standards by allegedly crossing the frontier between therapy and human experimentation. Thus it comes as no surprise that in the summer of 1891, when more severe critiques of tuberculin appeared, the dangers associated with the remedy had once again left the scene, ceding their place to two different issues.

A group of authors attempted to conduct a chemical analysis of tuberculin, and some of them even proposed their own theories concerning its mode of operation. One of these scientists, Edwin Klebs, came out with his own version of tuberculin in late 1891.[57] The aim of Klebs and other researchers was not to eliminate tuberculin from clinical use but to improve it, and it continued to be used in therapy for decades.[58] Another group of authors, however, seized the chance to launch a frontal assault on the bacteriological model of infectious diseases itself. Some of these authors were prominent mainstream clinicians like Ottomar Rosenbach, while others, like Heinrich Lahmann, were proponents of what was known as alternative medicine. However, neither group took up the issue of the dangers associated with using tuberculin as a central theme.[59]

Those who looked back to the times of the euphoria around tuberculin saw it as a period when German doctors had fallen into a collective illusion. Their main problem was that of reconciling the celebrity and standing of the inventor with the failure of the invention. The author of one of the rare critical reviews from late 1891 came to the conclusion that those who still remained faithful to tuberculin were "guided more by the indubitable authority of the discoverer than by the observations that are beyond any doubt".[60] In this context, it is worth noting that outside Germany the excitement around tuberculin seems to have been somewhat less pronounced and also that the phase of disillusionment came significantly earlier than it did in Germany.[61]

The medical community did not indulge in a great deal of self-criticism over the episode, but that was to be expected. What is more surprising is that the tuberculin scandal generated almost no explicit discussion over the dangers of antibacterial drugs. Indeed, as I have already mentioned, tuberculin continued to be used as a remedy for decades and a number of researchers even presented improved versions of the same treatment. Even when, in 1907, Clemens von Pirquet proposed a totally different explanation of the tuberculin reaction as an example of delayed hypersensitivity – which from a present-day perspective seems more accurate – some continued to remain faithful to tuberculin as a remedy.[62] As Elias Metchnikov noted during a visit to Berlin, Koch was still among them:

> Koch and I met for the last time in summer 1909. I found him in his laboratory, immersed in his researches on tuberculosis which he attempted to cure by new preparations of tuberculin.[63]

In his pioneer treatise on medical ethics from 1902, Albert Moll noted a conspicuous absence of critical questions that could and should have been asked in the case of tuberculin. He compared the case of tuberculin with the much-debated scandal of the Breslau dermatologist Albert Neisser, who had performed experiments using cell-free syphilitic serum on non-syphilitic patients, including prostitutes and children, without obtaining consent from the subjects or their parents. The revelation of these experiments caused a scandal in 1899, and not only was Neisser sued, but the case resulted in the first legal regulations concerning therapeutic experiments in Prussia.[64] Moll wrote the following concerning this case:

> It is really not my intention to defend Neisser's experiments, but it is unjust to pick out one single author and attack him repeatedly on a daily basis in the press. In this case, I'd like to recall once again the tuberculin inoculations. How could doctors justify injecting children who had been admitted to the clinic for entirely different reasons? Is a private physician entitled to treat a child suffering, for example, from some skin disease or something similar, for no other reason than to gain evidence concerning the reaction?[65]

However, even if the tuberculin scandal evinced very little systematic discussion in its aftermath, and it rather appears that nobody wanted to be reminded of the event once it was over, it could still be argued that it left some long-term traces and is a significant event in the history of risk conceptions in medicine: when new drugs were introduced in subsequent years, the atmosphere of euphoria seen in the case of tuberculin was never recreated. When Behring launched his diphtheria antitoxin only a few months later, he carefully undertook lengthy clinical trials and, even after this, the serum was not hurried into medical use, but was introduced slowly over a long period.[66] Paul Ehrlich's quest for the magic bullet which finally resulted in Salvarsan as a treatment for syphilis was accompanied by a continuous chorus of critical discussion, and the medicine itself was tested extensively before being made generally available.[67] In the second edition of his textbook from 1893 on the side effects of drugs, Leo Lewin devoted an entire chapter to Koch's wonder cure.[68]

Overall, the tuberculin scandal resulted in a grand disillusionment. Although it certainly did not result in the generalized idea that drug therapies might be risky, it can be argued that it triggered a number of changes in the evaluation of such therapies that came to assume particular importance in the twentieth century. Even though few of the arguments were made explicit at the time, the tuberculin scandal nevertheless cleared the way for future discussions on the possible dangers and risks associated with antibacterial therapies. The most important lesson to be learned was that the therapeutic promise of laboratory medicine carried with it certain specific novel forms of serious, inherent danger. Dangers of this nature were almost inconceivable prior to 1890, but would nevertheless become a distinctive feature of twentieth century medicine.

Notes

1   Ruprecht-Karls-Universität Heidelberg, Institut für Geschichte der Medizin, Im Neuenheimer Feld 327, 69120 Heidelberg, Germany: christoph.gradmann@urz. uni-heidelberg.de

2   P. Baumgarten, "Neuere experimentell-pathologische Arbeiten über Tuberculinwirkung", *Berliner klinische Wochenschrift* 28, 51, 52, 53, 1891, 1206–8, 1218–19, 1233–4. Quote from p. 1208.

3   On tuberculin and its reception in Germany: C. Gradmann, "Money and Microbes: Robert Koch, Tuberculin and the Foundation of the Institute for Infectious Diseases in Berlin in 1891", *History and Philosophy of the Life Sciences* 22, 2000, 51–71. *Idem*, "Robert Koch and the Pressures of Scientific Research: Tuberculosis and Tuberculin", *Medical History* 45, 2001, 1–32; on the international reception: M. Chauvet, "Une Cenetaire qui n'a pas tenu toutes ses promesses", *Revue médicale de la suisse romande* 110, 1990, 1067–70; M. Worboys, "The Sanatory Treatment for Consumption in Britain 1890–1914", in J. V. Pickstone (ed.), *Medical Innovations in Historical Perspective*, Houndsmills, Basingstoke: Macmillan, 1992, 47–71.

4   "Bereits drei Stunden nach der Injektion stellte sich hohes Fieber ein, bis zu 400, kleiner kaum fühlbarer Puls (: etwa 150 in der Minute:); dazu kam Erbrechen unstillbarer Durst. 12 Stunden nach der Injektion trat der Tod unter den Erscheinungen der Herzlähmung

ein ...",Geheimes Staatsarchiv Preußischer Kulturbesitz/Berlin, I HA, Rep. 76 VIII A, Nr. 2955.

5 On human experiments in the late nineteenth century see: B. Elkeles, *Der moralische Diskurs über das medizinische Menschenexperiment im 19. Jahrhundert*, Stuttgart, Jena, NY: Gustav Fischer, 1996; S. E. Lederer, *Subjected to Science: Human Experimentation in America before the Second World War*, Baltimore and London: Johns Hopkins University Press, 1995; L. Sauerteig, "*Ethische Richtlinien, Patientenrechte und ärztliches Verhalten bei der Arzneimittelerprobung 1892–1931*", *Medizinhistorisches Journal* 35, 2000, 303–34.

6 For an introduction see: J. Gabe (ed.), *Medicine, Health and Risk. Sociological Approaches*, Oxford: Blackwell, 1995.

7 See: Brockhaus's *Konversations-Lexikon*, 14th edn, 1898, Vol.13, 890, where risk is defined as "danger, venture: in particular in the economic sense the as the danger of failing of an enterprise". Cf. O. Rammstedt, "Risiko", in *Historisches Wörterbuch der Philosopie*, J. Ritter and K. Gründer (eds), Basel: Schwalbe, 1992, 1045–50.

8 From analyses of B. Elkeles, 1996; fn 4 and L. Sauerteig, 2000; fn 4 it can be gained that a certain awareness with regard to human experimentation on hospital inmates was rising in the 1890s.

9 A first treatment of the issue of drug side-effects came out in 1881: L. Lewin, *Die Nebenwirkungen der Arzneimittel. Pharmakologisch-klinisches Handbuch*, Berlin: August Hirschwald, 1899 (1881, 1893).

10 L. K. Altman, *Who Goes First? The Story of Self-Experimentation in Medicine*, Berkeley, Los Angeles; London: University of California Press, 1987.

11 The contemporary discussion is revisited in: A.-H. Maehle, "Assault and Battery, or Legitimate Treatment", *Gesnerus* 57, 2000, 206–21; U. Tröhler and A.-H. Maehle, "Anti-vivisection in Nineteenth-Century Germany and Switzerland: Motives and Models", in N. Rupke (ed.), *Vivisection in Historical Perspective*, London, New York: Routledge, 1987, pp. 149–87; R. Winau, "Medizin und Menschenversuch: Zur Geschichte des 'informed consent' ", in C. Wiesemann and A. Frewer (eds), *Medizin und Ethik im Zeichen von Auschwitz*, Erlangen und Jena: Palm & Enke, 1996, pp. 13–29.

12 For an introduction see L. Sauerteig, 2000, fn 4; W. Wimmer, "*Wir haben fast immer was Neues": Gesundheitswesen und Innovation der Pharma-Industrie in Deutschland 1880–1935*, Berlin: Duncker & Humboldt, 1994.

13 R. Koch, "Über bakteriologische Forschung', in J. Schwalbe (ed.), *Gesammelte Werke von Robert Koch*, Leipzig: Verlag von Georg Thieme, 1912 (1890), pp. 650–60; 660.

14 Cf. T. Schlich, "Repräsentationen von Krankheitserregern. Wie Robert Koch Bakterien als Krankheitserreger dargestellt hat", in H.-J. Rheinberger, M. Hagner and B. Wahrig-Schmidt (eds), *Räume des Wissens: Repräsentation, Codierung, Spur*, Berlin: Akademie Verlag, 1997, 165–90, on bacteria as functional representations of diseases.

15 R. Koch, "Die Ätiologie der Tuberkulose", in J. Schwalbe (ed.), *Gesammelte Werke von Robert Koch*, Leipzig: Verlag von Georg Thieme, 1912 (1882), pp. 428–45; 444. Cf. K. Faber, *Nosography: The Evolution of Clinical Medicine in Modern Times*, New York: Paul B. Hoeber, 1930, 110–11, on the expectations of specific remedies being raised by the discovery of bacteria.

16 R. Koch, 1912 (1882), fn 14: 445.

17 G. Geison, *The Private Science of Louis Pasteur*, Princeton, NJ: Princeton University Press, 1995.

18 I. Löwy, "On Hybridizations, Networks and New Disciplines: The Pasteur-Institute and the Development of Microbiology in France', *Studies in the History and Philosophy of Science* 25, 1994, 655–88.

19 R. Koch, 1912 (1890), fn 12. On the pompous surroundings of the 10th International Medical Congress: R. Winau, "Bakteriologie und Immunologie im Berlin des 19. Jahrhunderts", *Naturwissenschaftliche Rundschau* 43, 1990, 369–77.

20 "ich kann ... soviel mitteilen, daß Meerschweinchen, welche bekanntlich für Tuberkulose außerordentlich empfänglich sind, wenn man sie der Einwirkung einer solchen Substanz aussetzt, auf eine Impfung mit tuberkulösem Virus nicht mehr reagieren, und daß bei Meerschweinchen, welche ... erkrankt sind, der Krankheitsprozeß vollständig zum Stillstand gebracht werden kann." R. Koch, 1912 (1890), fn 12: 659.

21 R. Koch, "Weitere Mitteilungen über ein Heilmittel gegen Tuberkulose', in J. Schwalbe (ed.), *Gesammelte Werke von Robert Koch*, Leipzig: Verlag von Georg Thieme, 1912 (1890), pp. 661–8.

22 H. Schadewaldt, "Die Entdeckung des Tuberkulins", *Deutsche Medizinische Wochenschrift* 100, 1975, 1925–32.

23 August Wassermann and Shibasaburo Kitasoto. R. Koch, "Weitere Mitteilung", 673–82; 679. The testing of Koch's assistants was done in June and July. Koch's and Hedwig Freiberg's (self-)experiments are undated, but unlikely to have taken place much later.

24 With a single exception the reports of these were published in a special issue of the *Deutsche Medizinische Wochenschrift* (issue 47, 20 November 1890), i.e. one week after Koch's release of the medicine. The numbers of treated patients can be estimated at less than fifty.

25 Since testing had started with terminally ill patients it was hard to decide whether the death of a patient could be blamed on the medicine.

26 In more detail, see C. Gradmann, 2001, fn 2.

27 R. Koch, 1912 (1890), fn 20: 663.

28 For an overview see: T. D. Brock, *Robert Koch: A Life in Medicine and Bacteriology*, Madison, Wisconsin: Science Tech Publishers, 1988: chaps 14–15.

29 *Vossische Zeitung* 21.11.1890

30 T. Gorsboth and B. Wagner, "Die Unmöglichkeit der Therapie. Am Beispiel der Tuberkulose', *Kursbuch* 94 (Die Seuche), 1988, 123–45. In his memoirs, the clinician Theodor Brugsch gave a vivid account of atmosphere of these days (T. Brugsch, *Arzt seit fünf Jahrzehnten*, Berlin: Rütten und Loening, 1957, 47–8).

31 Schriftleitung der Deutschen Medizinischen Wochenschrift (ed.) 'Robert Koch's Heilmittel gegen die Tuberkulose', Berlin und Leipzig: Thieme, 1890–1, 12 Issues, Issue 2, 73–4.

32 "Beide Fälle sind vom ersten Tage an, wo wir über das neue Heilmittel geboten, in Behandlung gezogen worden, zwar nicht eigentlich mit der Aussicht auf therapeutischen Erfolg, sondern vielmehr in der Intention, Beobachtungen und Kenntnisse zu sammeln. Ein therapeutischer Erfolg hat hier weder erreicht werden sollen, noch konnte er überhaupt in Frage kommen.... Ich bemerke, dass beide Patienten von der Anwendung des Mittels in keiner Weise einen Schaden gehabt haben, dass also auch nicht im entferntesten daran gedacht werden kann, der Exitus sei hier beschleunigt worden." D. Jürgens, E. v. Leyden and D. Goldscheider, "Aus dem Verein für innere Medicin. Mittheilung über das Koch'sche Heilverfahren', in *Robert Koch's Heilmittel gegen die Tuberkulose*, S. d. DMW (ed.), Berlin und Leipzig: Thieme, Issue 3, 1890, pp. 122–29; 128. A more detailed description of both cases is to found in "Die Wirksamkeit des Koch'schen Heilmittels gegen Tuberkulose. Amtliche Berichte der Klinken, Polikliniken und pathologisch-anatomischen Institute der preussischen Universitäten", *Klinisches Jahrbuch*, Sonderheft, Berlin: Julius Springer, 1891: 15 and 53.

33 F. Hueppe, "Ueber die Heilung der Tuberculose mit specieller Beruecksichtigung der neuen Methode von R. Koch", *Wiener Medizinische Presse* , 31, 48, 1890, 1888–92.

34 "Robert Koch's Heilmittel gegen die Tuberkulose" 1890/1891, fn 30, issue 2, 16

35 "Die Wirksamkeit des Koch'schen Heilmittels gegen Tuberkulose", 1891, fn 31, 795.

36 C. Gradmann, "Ein Fehlschlag und seine Folgen: Robert Kochs Tuberkulin und die Gründung des Instituts für Infektionskrankheiten in Berlin 1891", in C. Gradmann and T. Schlich (eds.), *Strategien der Kausalität. Konzepte der Krankheitsverursachung im 19. und 20. Jahrhundert*, Pfaffenweiler: Centaurus, 1999, pp. 29–52.

37 C. Gradmann 1999, fn 35.

38 E. Hennoch, 'Mittheilungen über das Koch'sche Heilverfahren gegen Tuberkulose', *Berliner Klinische Wochenschrift* , 27, 51, 1890, 1169–71.

39 "Es ist schwer geblieben, solche Kinder zu bekommen und so konnte ich bisher nur einen solchen Knaben injizieren, beiläufig als Strafe für irgend eine Untat im Hause. Der Knabe stammte aus einer Arbeiterfamilie, deren Mutter an Lungentuberkulose erkrankt war. Anfangs wollten die Eltern die Injektion nicht zulassen, dann aber, weil der Junge, wie gesagt, etwas begangen hatte, sagte der Vater: 'So, jetzt sollst Du auch eingespritzt werden'." J. Schreiber, "Ueber das Koch'sche Heilverfahren", in *Robert Koch's Heilmittel gegen die Tuberkulose* 1890–1, fn 30, issue 8, 11–21; 18.

40 V. Czerny, "Erster Bericht über die Koch'schen Impfungen", in Robert Koch's *Heilmittel gegen die Tuberkulose* 1890–1, fn 30, issue 3, 61–8; B. Fränkel, "Ueber die Anwendung des Koch'schen Mittels bei Tuberculose", in "Robert Koch's Heilmittel gegen die Tuberkulose" 1890–1, fn 30, issue 3, 81–95; F. Schultze, "Aus der medicinischen Universitätsklinik in Bonn: Bericht über Wirkung der Einspritzung mit Koch'scher Flüssigkeit', in "Robert Koch's Heilmittel gegen die Tuberkulose' 1890–1, issue 4, 21–9.

41 E.g. P. Fürbringer, "Vierwöchige Koch'sche Behandlung in ihrer Bedeutung für die Abweichung vom Schema", in 'Robert Koch's Heilmittel gegen die Tuberkulose' 1890–1, fn 30, issue 3, 96–109.

42 "Die Wirksamkeit des Koch'schen Heilmittels gegen Tuberkulose" 1891, fn 31, 904–5.

43 R. Virchow, "Ueber die Wirkung des Koch'schen Mittels auf innere Organe Tuberkulöser", *Berliner klinische Wochenschrift*, 28, 1891, 49–52.

44 D. Hansemann, "Pathologisch-anatomische und historlogische Erfahrungen über die Koch'sche Injectionsmethode", *Therapeutische Monatshefte* 5, 1891, 77–80.

45 R. Koch, "Fortsetzung der Mitteilungen über ein Heilmittel gegen Tuberkulose", in J. Schwalbe (ed.), *Gesammelte Werke von Robert Koch*, Leipzig: Verlag von Georg Thieme, 1912 (1891), pp. 669–72; F. Hueppe, 1890, fn 32.

46 V. Czerny, 1891, fn 39: 68; "Die Wirksamkeit des Koch'schen Heilmittels gegen Tuberkulose", 1891, fn 31: 6–7.

47 O. Rosenbach, "Über das Verhalten der Körpertemperatur bei Anwendung des Kochschen Verfahrens", in "Robert Koch's Heilmittel gegen die Tuberkulose" 1890–1, fn 30, issue 4, pp. 12–30. Cf. *Idem, Grundlagen, Aufgaben und Grenzen der Therapie: nebst einem Anhange: Kritik des Koch'schen Verfahrens*, Wien: Urban und Schwarzenberg, 1891. On Rosenbach: R. Maulitz, " 'Physician versus Bacteriolgist': The Ideology of Science in Clinical Medicine", in M. J. Vogel and C. E. Rosenberg (eds), *The Therapeutic Revolution: Essays in the Social History of American Medicine*, Philadelphia: University of Pennsylvania Press, 1979, 91–107.

48 "Die Wirksamkeit des Koch'schen Heilmittels gegen Tuberkulose" 1891, fn 31, 6–7.

49 "Robert Koch's Heilmittel gegen die Tuberkulose" 1890–1, fn 30, issue 11, 51.

50 "Robert Koch's Heilmittel gegen die Tuberkulose" 1890–1, fn 30, issue 11, 48–9.

51 "Robert Koch's Heilmittel gegen die Tuberkulose" 1890–1, fn 30, issue 11, 23.

52 "Die Wirksamkeit des Koch'schen Heilmittels gegen Tuberkulose" 1891, fn 31, 904.

53 "Sie werden mir zugeben, meine Herren, daß der Ausdruck 'experimentelle Arbeiten' in dieser Verbindung nicht sehr glücklich gewählt ist. ... soweit mir bekannt, hat bisher eine direkte Verbindung zwischen einer experimentellen Abtheilung und einem Krankenhause nicht bestanden. Und wenn hier eine Krankenanstalt mit einer Versuchsanstalt in unmittelbare Verbindung gebracht wird, so ist es ganz natürlich, daß so Mancher glaubt, man könne das Ergebnis experimenteller Versuche und wissenschaftlicher Forschungen sofort an dem Körper des Kranken vornehmen und probieren," "Stenographische Berichte über die Verhandlungen ... beider Häuser des Landtages. Haus der Abgeordneten", Berlin: W. Moeser Hofbuchdruckerei, Vol. 189, 2258.

54 "Stenographische Berichte ... Haus der Abgeordneten", 1891, fn 52, 2260 and 2263.

55 B. Elkeles, 1996, fn 4: 112; S. E. Lederer, 1995, fn 4, 3.

56 Cf. L. Sauerteig 2000, fn 4, 307, who states that in the 1890s human experimentation on hospital inmates became an issue.

57 E. Klebs, *Die Behandlung der Tuberkulose mit Tuberkulocidin: Vorläufige Mittheilung*, Hamburg und Leipzig: Leopold Voss, 1892.

58 See e.g. a widely-used handbook of internal medicine form the interwar period: H. Hetsch, "Tuberkulose", in F. Kraus and T. Brugsch (eds), *Spezielle Pathologie und Therapie innerer Krankheiten*, Berlin: Urban & Schwarzenberg, 1919, 777–857, 843–6. Cf. J. M. Schmidt, "Geschichte der Tuberkulin-Therapie – Ihre Begründung durch Robert Koch, ihre Vorläufer und ihre weitere Entwicklung", *Pneumologie* 45, 1991, 776–84.

59 H. Lahmann, *Koch und die Kochianer. Eine Kritik der Koch'schen Entdeckung und der Koch'schen Richtung in der Heilkunde*, Stuttgart: Zimmer, 1890; O. Rosenbach, *Grundlagen*, 1891, fn 46.

60 G. Siegmund, "Die Stellung des Arztes zur Tuberculinbehandlung", *Therapeutische Monatshefte*, 5, 1891, 415–21; 415.

61 F. B. Smith, *The retreat of tuberculosis 1850–1950*, London: Croom Helm, 1987: 59–62; D. S. Burke, "Of Postulates and Peccadilloes: Robert Koch and Vaccine (Tuberculin) Therapy for Tuberculosis", *Vaccine*, 11, 1993, 795–804; M. Chauvet, 1990, fn 2; B. Hansen, "New Images of a New Medicine: Visual Evidence for the Widespread Popularity of Therapeutic Discoveries in America after 1885", *Bulletin of the History of Medicine*, 73, 1999, 629–78; D. Leibowitz, "Scientific Failure in an Age of Optimism: Public Reaction to Robert Koch's Tuberculin Cure", *New York state journal of medicine*, 93, 1993, 41–8.

62 A. Silverstein, *A History of Immunology*, San Diego: Academic Press, 1989, 230–2.

63 Quoted in T. D. Brock ,1988, fn 27, 302.

64 B. Elkeles, "Medizinische Menschenversuche gegen Ende des 19. Jahrhunderts und der Fall Neisser: Rechtfertigung und Kritik einer wissenschaftlichen Methode", *Medizinhistorisches Journal*, 20, 1985, 135–48.

65 "Es liegt mir durchaus fern, die Neisserschen Experimente zu verteidigen, aber einen Autor immer herauszunehmen und Tag für Tag in der Presse anzugreifen, alle analogen Vorgänge aber zu verschweigen, ist ungerecht. Ich will auch hier wieder an die Tuberkulinimpfungen erinnern. Mit welchem Recht wurden Kinder, die wegen ganz anderer Affektionen in Krankenhäuser kamen, von Krankenhausärzten mit Tuberkulin behandelt? Hat ein Privatarzt etwa das Recht, ein Kind, das vielleicht eine Hautkrankheit oder etwas Aehnliches hat, einfach mit Tuberkulin zu spritzen, um zu sehen, ob es darauf reagiert?" A. Moll, *Ärztliche Ethik. Die Pflichten des Arztes in allen Beziehungen seiner Tätigkeit*, Stuttgart: Enke, 1902, 562.

66 P. Weindling, "From Medical Research to Clinical Practice: Serum Therapy for Diphtheria in 1890s", in J. V. Pickstone (ed.), *Medical Innovations in Historical Perspective*, Houndmills, Basingstoke: Macmillan, 1992, 72–83.

67 L. Sauerteig, 2000, fn 4.

68 L. Lewin, 1899 (1881, 1893), fn 8.

5 "As safe as milk or sugar water"

Perceptions of the risks and benefits
of the BCG vaccine in the 1920s and
1930s in France and Germany

Christian Bonah

Introduction

A lesson to be learned from recent science studies is that scientific facts are
not discovered but produced and their production can rarely be tied down to
a single, precise moment but rather needs to be understood as a long and
subtle sequence of changes remodelling the network in which they are
constituted. From this perspective, the risks and benefits associated with
new therapies are not precise fixed measures that serve to evaluate any
potential harm or to aid in the prevention of random health accidents or
sickness. Rather, risks and benefits are part of the contextual network for the
genesis and development of therapeutic or preventive remedies.[1] Just like
the scientific facts they are linked to, risks and benefits are perpetually being
redefined and so there is no single risk or benefit, but many varying over
time in accordance with the varying contexts of discovery and production.
The following contribution offers a detailed analysis of the shifting meaning
of risk and benefit for various protagonists who participated in the development and evaluation of the BCG vaccination against tuberculosis.

The events analysed here should be understood against the background of
tuberculosis as a historical entity: a peculiar and frightening disease that was
common, if not ubiquitous, in the "civilized world"[2] at the beginning of the
twentieth century.[3] The story here concerns a preventive therapeutic agent,
the BCG vaccine (an acronym for Bacillus Calmette-Guérin),[4] which was
considered safe and effective by its inventors. The vaccine has been in
constant medical use since the 1920s, and has remained controversial right
up to the present. The history of the introduction of the BCG vaccine provides
an insight into how risk, safety and effectiveness were assessed and transformed
between 1918 and 1940, and I want to illustrate this point with four different
perceptions corresponding to four constellations of the vaccine's network of
invention. First, I will analyse risks and effectiveness from the perspective of
the inventor-producers, Calmette and Guérin; second and third, from two
view points of their scientific peers who criticised the vaccine; and finally,
from the perspective of a court in Germany presiding over what has become
known as the "Lübeck vaccination catastrophe".[5]

The 1920s and 1930s were a time of rationalization in the construction of the scientific evidence for new medical treatments, characterized by the rise in importance of the field of statistics. Yet clinical and laboratory evidence remained central for researchers and physicians evaluating the BCG vaccine's safety and effectiveness. Laboratory risks, clinical risks and statistical risks could converge, but they could also be quite contradictory. By bringing together the four perspectives analysed in this paper, I aim to address the following questions: what was the respective significance and weight of laboratory, clinical and statistical risk assessments in this process? How were they translated into an overall judgement of the risk and effectiveness of the vaccine that justified medical action and determined what information would be conveyed to the public? And finally, how did this final judgement concerning the risk and effectiveness of the BCG vaccine change as the BCG's network of invention progressively modified itself?

Calmette's construction and evaluation of risk; the safety and effectiveness of the BCG vaccine, 1921–27

Between 1905 and 1921, Albert Calmette (1863–1933) and Camille Guérin (1872–1961) developed an oral vaccination against tuberculosis. The BCG vaccine consists of an attenuated living bacterial strain derived from the virulent bovine Koch bacillus (BK) responsible for tuberculosis. Attenuation was obtained by growing the initial bacteria on specific culture media that, after 230 uninterrupted passages (that took 13 years),[6] appeared to produce a specific "race of a-virulent bovine bacillus".[7] Between 1921 and 1927 the scientific evaluation of safety and effectiveness of the BCG vaccine was based on laboratory, clinical and statistical evidence gathered by Calmette that led to extensive publications in 1927 and 1928.[8]

The first line of argument for evaluating the safety and effectiveness of the BCG as a new preventive agent mobilized laboratory and animal evidence. By the early 1920s, Calmette and Guérin, having tested guinea pigs, rabbits and cattle, were convinced that "the bacillus had become completely deprived of its virulence and this for any animal species"[9]. From their perspective, the risks of the vaccination were defined as the possibility that the BCG vaccine might cause tuberculosis during the months following its administration, and effectiveness was defined as the prevention of infection with the usual BK after vaccination.[10]

If we turn now to statistical arguments we see that gross morbidity and mortality rates of tuberculosis established at the turn of the century indicated two facts: there existed an "everyday-life risk" of infection and/or sickness; and certain groups within the population in general had a higher risk of infection than others. This was particularly true for infants born to mothers suffering from open tuberculosis. The rather approximate mortality rates were combined with the perception of laboratory risk to provide an assessment of Calmette and Guérin's first human trials in 1921. Despite the very positive laboratory data accumulated at the beginning of the 1920s, the initiation of experiments with humans required more justification than just animal data indicating the relative safety and effectiveness of the vaccine in these hosts. Acknowledging the inevitable risks associated with the first human administrations of the vaccine, Calmette employed a twofold strategy to further justify his action. On one hand he highlighted that the first administration resulted from medical demand and was not undertaken by the scientific investigator of the BCG vaccine. Two entirely independent physcians asked for the vaccination to be employed. On the other hand, he developed a "statistical" argument based on the construction of the notion of the "inevitable encounter" with the microbe, which transformed infants with "tuberculous mothers" into "irremediably condemned" subjects. The approximate evaluation of this somewhat exaggerated everyday-life risk defined a hopeless medical situation that invited acts of "heroic treatment".[11] Thus, under these particular circumstances any action that had some chance of improving the subject's fate was seen as worth taking. Accordingly, very limited human trials were initiated at the *Hôpital de la Charité* in Paris by Benjamin Weill-Hallé (1875–1958) and his young intern Raymond Turpin between July 1921 and June 1922 in close collaboration with Calmette.[12] Despite the official "heroic therapeutic" justification of the trial (amongst other objectives, this shielded the authors against the accusation of illegal human experimentation), Calmette was later to clearly state that this first "experiment was essentially designed to ensure the harmlessness of the ingestion of the vaccine".[13] For this safety evaluation, purely clinical parameters were analysed, such as weight curves, body temperature, clinical case reports, general observations of pathologies as well as the standard diagnostic tool, the von Pirquet's tuberculin skin test. Eighty of the 120 vaccinated children were followed up during the next four years, with only twenty-four living in a contaminated family environment. Apparently no major complications appeared in this first cohort, establishing (for Calmette and his collaborators) that there was no clinical risk. Nevertheless forty vaccinated infants disappeared from sight. After a temporary interruption due to reorganizations in the hospital, a second series of hospital vaccinations was carried out between July 1924 and January 1927. This time the overall mortality among the 469 vaccinated children amounted to thirty-three, or 7.1 per cent.[14] Out of these deaths, however, only one was attributed to tuberculosis. This led Calmette to conclude that in contaminated family environments (this was the case for 67 of the 469 vaccinated infants), the mortality rate with the BCG vaccine could be precisely calculated, and that it was 1.5 per cent.[15] In order to contextualize this result, and help progressively to transform clinical risk into statistical risk, Calmette needed to compare the rate achieved to gross mortality rates. Official sources for estimates of child mortality under the age of one were rather slim and unreliable. In order to have an estimate of the "real" mortality of children born to mothers suffering from tuberculosis, Calmette conducted an inquiry of his own in 1925.

Questionnaires were sent to physicians directing tuberculosis dispensaries in 80 French administrative regions. The responses revealed that 1,362 mothers afflicted with tuberculosis gave birth to 1,364 babies in 1922. Only 623 babies were still alive on 1 January 1925. Of the original cohort, 327 babies had died, presumably of tuberculosis, which amounts to 24 per cent.

The protagonists translated the clinical and statistical results of these hospital trials into common sense language, concluding that the vaccination was "probably effective and that its harmlessness was beyond doubt".[16] The emerging perception of statistical risk in the context of these first human trials of the vaccine compared a purported "natural risk" of contracting tuberculosis against the risk of contamination from the BCG vaccine itself. As the latter risk was unknown, Calmette and his collaborators adopted the case of a somewhat artificial therapeutically hopeless situation where "heroic experimental treatment" was "demanded and authorized", echoing Claude Bernard's version of medical duty from the 1860s.[17] If the risk of infection was almost certain (in fact the 1925 inquiry indicates that it was 24 per cent at most), then the use of the BCG vaccine could not possibly carry a greater risk. At the same time, the construction of social risk factors and risk groups (infants born to "tuberculous mothers") was being used to justify the unknown risk that was being taken with the BCG vaccine. Once this first perilous experiment had been undertaken, every further vaccination that took place without any obvious adverse effects reinforced the conclusion that the new therapeutic agent was safe. From an initial reliance on individual cases, the definition of risk was increasingly transferred to statistical aggregations. Laboratory risk, clinical risk and the emerging statistical risk progressively converged to define the overall concept that we can term the "1924-BCG-vaccine risk".

At the Pasteur Institute in Paris in 1924, while Weill-Hallé was beginning his second series of hospital trials, Calmette and Guérin considered that the safety of the BCG vaccine had been sufficiently established in young animals and young children for them to offer it to the medical profession at large. The distribution of the BCG vaccine officially started on 1 July 1924, with physicians willing to "experiment"[18] with the vaccine being able to obtain it by simply writing to the Pasteur Institute. The decisions concerning the vaccination and any follow-ups were made by the individual physicians concerned, who also performed the vaccination themselves. In turn, they were to report the results of the vaccinations and any other observations to Calmette in Paris, who established a central BCG card file precisely to collect this information. These centralized files would eventually lead to the first large-scale statistical analysis of the safety and effectiveness of the vaccine in human beings, as the number of vaccinations steadily progressed from over 4,000 in December 1924 to 21,200 in December 1926. In January 1927, two batches of figures were examined independently by two professional statisticians, to give what Calmette qualified as an "objective" analysis of the observations. First M. Moine, the statistician of the *Comité National de Défense contre la Tuberculose*, went through Calmette's centralized card files in Paris,[19] and reported on 882 infants who had been vaccinated between one and two years previously and had been brought up in tubercular environments. Of these, seven died of what were presumably tubercular lesions and 72 died of non-tubercular lesions during the first two years of life. The mortality rate was, therefore, 0.8 per cent from tuberculosis, and 8.9 per cent from all the causes taken together. A second statistics professional, Dr Y. Biraud, head of the statistics department of the hygiene institute of the medical faculty in Paris, confirmed the results of the first expert.[20]

Drawing on these two independent evaluations, Calmette claimed that the results established the safety of the vaccination beyond any doubt and proved "the effectiveness of protection with BCG against the effects of family contagion".[21] In May 1927, Calmette presented a complete manual on preventive vaccination against tuberculosis with the BCG to the tribune of the French Academy of Medicine in Paris, where the procedure gained official endorsement. Two months later, sufficient support had been gained from the French *Ministry of Labor, Hygiene and Social Assistance and Prevention* for the vaccination to be officially promoted in a circular from this body. A. Fallières, at the time in charge of the ministry responsible for public health, informed the *Préfets* of his administrative regions that:

> [a] large trial with the new BCG vaccine for the immunization of infants against tuberculosis has been conducted over the last three years in different countries. In France, more than 30,000 infants have been vaccinated and the resulting statistics tend to show that the method is not only inoffensive, but furthermore that it is effective because mortality from tuberculosis between zero and one year for vaccinated infants in permanently exposed family environments does not even reach one per cent. For unvaccinated children living in the same circumstances tuberculosis mortality is approximately 24 per cent. ... This authorization is based on the reports of the Academy of Medicine and the *Conseil Supérieur d'Hygiène Publique*.[22]

With reassuring animal and human data, a growing number of clinical trials, a user's manual and an official endorsement from the French state, the BCG vaccine was well on its way to becoming what could be called a routine preventive treatment with clearly established "absolute safety" and absence of any risk. We can call this stage of perception the "1927-Calmette-BCG-vaccine risk".

"Every medical procedure has its opponents ..." debates at the French Academy of Medicine

Starting in July 1927, the laboratory evidence and the available clinical data were reviewed by José Lignières, a veterinarian and bacteriologist trained at the Pasteur Institute, who was also a member of the Academy of Medicine and on leave in Argentina at this time. His critical questioning as to whether or not the vaccine was really completely inoffensive led to a sometimes bitter conflict at the Academy of Medicine in Paris.[23] Lignières did not straightforwardly object to the use of the vaccine; rather, he called for greater caution in its use. His argument was based on rare and variable laboratory results that, while not invalidating Calmette's results, nevertheless put in doubt the overly-perfect 1927-Calmette-BCG-vaccine risk perception.[24]

Yet, the cautious objections formulated by Lignières were presented precisely at the moment when Calmette was starting a major publicity campaign intended to convince hesitant physicians and public opinion of the total safety of his preventive treatment. Now that he would have to answer to more than 30,000 vaccinated infants, their families, state officials and international colleagues, Calmette realized that the time had passed when such a reappraisal would be possible. The network of invention had been stabilized and alliances had been sealed. Calmette's response consisted in shifting the grounds of the argument from laboratory to statistical evidence, a field where Lignières could not so easily follow. Statistics were available that proved the safety and effectiveness of the procedure, with the results of massive human trials easily overruling the findings of an isolated laboratory worker based in Argentina. In this strategy, laboratory, clinical and statistical evidence were no longer seen as being complementary; instead, they could be used independently to cover up any perceived inadequacies in one of the others.

In January 1928, Calmette answered Lignières's challenge by publishing further positive results of human vaccinations in a lengthy article that appeared in the *Annales de l'Institut Pasteur*. By then, he could rely on the results of the vaccination of more than 50,000 infants in France. The translation of the latest statistical figures into common sense language indicated that "the vaccine-bacillus remains in the human organism for a very long time without disturbing its health and only manifesting its presence by the acquired resistance against infection. This fact is of a nature as to disqualify any anxiety concerning the purported danger."[25] Thus, according to Calmette's vision, objective statistical risk assessment could be opposed to the emotional and sensationalist fears of a biased bacteriologist. In this context, laboratory risk was opposed by statistical risk.

Despite the dismissive attitude of Calmette, Lignières was not immediately reduced to silence, and returned to the tribune of the Academy in May 1928 correctly reasserting that "it has not been demonstrated that the BCG is always inoffensive".[26] The core of the controversy was the question of how it could be proved scientifically that the vaccine was "sufficiently safe". Calmette considered that as long as laboratory experiments did not show that the vaccine bacillus could recover its virulence there was no room for doubt. What is more, thousands of vaccinated children were sufficient proof of its harmlessness. Lignières objected that, because of their rarity and the difficulty in establishing stringent proof of causality, the occurrence of accidents could not be totally ruled out. What to Lignières seemed to be reasonable doubt appeared to Calmette to be extravagant hypothesizing.

Subsequently, the dispute became increasingly technical. According to Calmette, "the harmlessness and effectiveness of prevention by BCG is so evident, in France as well as in other countries, that the public health services of several cities have been able to realize the vaccination of 80 to 89 percent of infants of all families for over a year".[27] Public institutions that had been convinced by Calmette's arguments were now becoming his direct allies in the battle against recalcitrant critics who dared to question the absolute safety of the vaccine. Hoping to settle the disruptive controversy once and for all, Calmette declared that Lignières was simply arousing unjustified anxiety and panic in families that had agreed to the vaccination, and he challenged his critic in the following terms: "I am still waiting for someone to furnish me with an observation showing that an infant vaccinated with the BCG and growing up in a healthy environment has succumbed from tuberculosis caused by the BCG vaccine."[28]

This argument is of the utmost importance, as it clearly implies that the burden of proof had been reversed by 1928. It was now up to opponents of the vaccination to supply evidence to prove that the BCG vaccine was not safe. Nevertheless, rather than closing off all further debate, Calmette's statements further inflamed the controversy. In July 1928 Lignières returned once more to the Academy of Medicine. He directly answered Calmette's challenge that someone needed to show that the BCG could cause complications in humans. This time he left his usual terrain of laboratory bacteriology and presented two case histories to the assembly. Lignières had been contacted by two local physicians in Brittany about the case of two sisters, Denise and Marie D., one of whom, Denise, had been born in August 1926 and had been vaccinated with the BCG. The family environment was completely healthy and in particular exempt from tuberculosis. The family's cattle were also declared exempt from tubercular contamination. In March 1927, the infant presented a tumefaction of the neck that could not be healed with the usual treatments available at the time. At the age of one year the huge infected lymph-node was still abundantly producing pus and the girl was in a state of advanced consumption. Denise died in November 1927. Her sister Marie was born in August 1927. By February 1928, at the age of six months, the infant presented a lesion similar to that of her sister. Local treatment of the neck led to rapid improvement and Marie was doing well when Lignières reported her case history to his colleagues.[29]

Lignières went to Brittany in order to collect pus from the two vaccinated children and immediately initiated a series of inoculation experiments in guinea pigs. By July 1928, when he was presenting his first observations concerning these cases to the Parisian Academy, no definite laboratory results could be communicated since the observation of control animals required several months. Nevertheless, he assured the Academy that the preliminary observations up to this point clearly established that the bacillus identified in the extracts examined displayed characteristics that were neither those of the human nor the bovine Koch bacillus but closely resembled those of the BCG strain. The sequence of events and the total absence of a source of contamination by tuberculosis seemed sufficient to Lignières for blaming the lethal events on the BCG vaccine. Accordingly, he concluded:

> 'We have here irrefutable proof of the fact that under special circumstances of sensitivity to BCG, the vaccine can manifest a pathogenic power in children that was hardly imaginable beforehand. ... Guinea

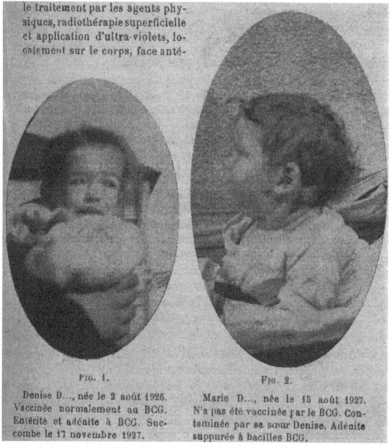

Figure 5.1 Photographic material presented by J. Lignières at the Academy of Medicine illustrating the case histories of Denise and Marie D.

Source: J. Lignières, "Le vaccin BCG, bien que très atténué et sans action tuberculigène, reste encore trop pathogène pour l'espèce humaine", *Bulletin de l'Académie de Médecine*, 1928, p. 875.

pigs support the administration of BCG well, without any problems, whereas the human species is far more sensitive.[30]

In October 1928, Lignières returned to the Academy. This time he not only presented his experiments verbally, but he also brought with him stained microscope slides of extracts of pus and stool taken from the two girls that he showed to the gathered physicians. These slides, along with results from control animals inoculated with the extracts, indicated that the bacillus responsible for the complications was not a typical Koch bacillus but, according to Lignières, could be attributed to the intrinsic pathogenic qualities of the BCG.[31] At the same meeting of 23 October 1928, Calmette made a final attempt to reduce his opponent to silence. In a polemical attack he denied that "this person with a degree as a veterinary" had any competency in such a delicate affair concerning expert clinical knowledge.[32] Furthermore the centralized BCG files proved that "Lignières is raising an alarm for no reason. There is no evidence of the evil effects of which M. Lignières has pleased himself to accuse the BCG."[33]

Isolated individual physicians or scientists such as Lignières could hardly contradict the interpretations and evaluations of the central producer-coordinator of the BCG vaccine. Laboratory risk was still being opposed to clinical risk, but the Calmette network was also effectively staging an opposition between collective expertise and the individual bacteriologist. These were the final exchanges in a scientific controversy that remained unsettled, although medical practice demanded that an overall judgement be made concerning "the" risk and "the" effectiveness of the vaccine.

By this stage, Calmette had changed his approach to advocating his vaccine. He turned to national and international commissions that would evaluate the risks and benefits of the preventive remedy and partially endorse the further extension of the vaccination campaign in France and throughout the Western world. This strategy was precisely what was at stake when the French Academy of Medicine discussed the vaccination and when the hygiene commission of the League of Nations gathered in Paris from 15 to 19 October 1928 for an international conference on the BCG vaccine. Lignières was not invited to this forum, and when Calmette spoke his final word concerning their dispute over the safety of BCG at the Academy of Medicine, he was already certain about the positive outcome of the international conference.

Statistics betrayed: Greenwood versus Calmette, 1927–28

The articles in the *Annales de l'Institut Pasteur* also attracted attention and criticism from the international scientific community working in the field of tuberculosis. In May 1927, the *British Medical Journal* published a critical editorial[34] indicating that British physicians were less eager than their French counterparts to accept the 1927-Calmette-BCG-vaccine risk and the purported effectiveness as they had been presented in France. At the end of May 1927 Major Greenwood, professor of epidemiology and vital statistics at the University of London, lent his voice to the chorus of British criticism.[35] On closer scrutiny, the initial figure of 1,877 vaccinated infants included in Biraud's statistical analysis dwindled to 367 infants, if one took into consideration only those who had been closely observed and were definitely "exposed to risk" in their first year of life.[36] As Greenwood remarked, within a few months after birth the statistical basis for discussion became rather scanty. In June 1927, Major Greenwood published a second article in the *BMJ* expanding on his criticism of Calmette's statistics.[37]

Initially, in the face of persistent criticism of his statistics, Calmette tried to adapt his figures and interpretations accordingly. But as the criticism continued and went deeper, Calmette eventually changed his strategy again to what might be called the dialectics of the clinic and statistics: whenever the statistical criticism became too difficult to answer, Calmette argued that the positive results were so obvious to clinicians that statistical difficulties could be ignored. This stand indicates at least two things. First, in the 1930s, statistics was considered an important argument in evaluating the safety and effectiveness of a new treatment. Large numbers and supposedly objective statistical figures seemed to produce evidence with mathematical precision. Yet, when Calmette's figures were criticised or interpreted in a different manner by other members of the still very small group of professional statisticians capable of unravelling the delicate construction of statistical proof, the whole statistical argument could be put aside, since clinical experience proved beyond a doubt the self-evidently positive results.[38] This argumentation amounted to what might be described as a game of "hide and seek" between statistics and clinical evidence of individual case histories (casuistry).

Table 5.1 Synthesis of statistical results produced by Calmette's statisticians by 1927, and Major Greenwood's criticism of their significance

Authors of statistics	Number of vaccinated infants included	General mortality of vaccinated infants	TB mortality of vaccinated infants	TB mortality in the same risk group without vaccination (controls)
	Greenwood: Number insufficient Not all in contaminated families		Greenwood: No autopsies. Possible local variations of TB mortality	Greenwood: Overestimated mortality rate. Realistic mortality rate: 5–10%
Moine	882	8.9%	0.8%	24%
Biraud	1,537	7.29%	1.84%	24%

Source: M. Greenwood, "Professor Calmette's statistical study of BCG vaccination", *British Medical Journal* 12.5.1928, pp. 793–5.

Calmette's reassuring tone, as well as his superficial treatment of the criticism that had been raised, exasperated commentators like Major Greenwood. Another full article in the *BMJ*[39] presented his criticism of Calmette's statistical work, concluding that statistical evidence from foreign authors had been misrepresented and that the alleged "natural" mortality rate used as a reference by Calmette (24 per cent of infants born to tubercular mothers die during the first year of life) was based on erroneous data (a realistic estimation according to Greenwood was between 5 and 10 per cent, providing a less favorable background rate against which to evaluate the effectiveness of the BCG vaccine). He also argued that the number of infants with complete records of follow-up examinations was too small to be statistically significant, that many of the vaccinated infants had not been raised in contaminated family environments, and furthermore that in the case of many of the infants who had died, no post-mortem examination had been carried out. Greenwood's final pair of grievances were of a strictly statistical nature, consisting in the complaint that the statistical samples analysed were not characterized by a circumscribed geographic locality, and that Calmette had neither used control groups nor randomized his samples. Greenwood's conclusion was clear: "Calmette has deliberately appealed to the statistical method, and, in my submission, his use of that method has been so gravely defective that no confidence can be placed either in his statistical inferences or in the reliability of the data which he has assembled. I see no hope of obtaining statistically valid data from France."[40]

This 1928 paper was not simply a stinging criticism of Calmette's work, Greenwood had served up a veritable lesson on medical statistics and how a proper clinical trial should be organized from a statistician's point of view.[41] The major change in perspective consisted in the fact that statistical methods should not be applied only once the clinical work was done, but that they should prepare and direct the collection and evaluation of data from the beginning to the end.

Although confident of the scientific validity of an ideal, statistically significant enterprise, the British observer remained pessimistic concerning the possibility of successfully putting such a method into practice in 1928:

> Whether it would be practically possible to use this method, here or in America, it is hard to say. The number of instances of births in families with one or more cases of open tuberculosis which come to the notice of the public health authorities within any one area and within a limited period of time is small, and the difficulty of strict random sampling is great. We are concerned, not with guinea-pigs, but with human beings, and it is not easy to induce those who have the medical charge of human beings to administer to any of them a treatment which they regard as worthless, or to abstain from administering to any of them a treatment which they regard as valuable. ... I do not expect that the value of BCG

will be determined on these lines. Like most methods of treatment, its use or neglect will be determined by psychological considerations.[42]

The objections presented here indicate not only that some observers were sceptical about the laboratory and clinical evidence for the 1927-Calmette-BCG-vaccine risk and effectiveness, but that some others were equally sceptical about the statistical assessments of risk and effectiveness. But how could the right note be drawn out of this chorus of dissonant voices? Who could establish whether the BCG should be used in practice, and what was the right way to arrive at such a decision? How were the medical and public health authorities to escape from what must have seemed like an endless series of scientific controversies?

On the national level, the French Academy of Medicine was an advisory body to the state and its endorsement generally carried with it full political and legal support. On the international level, Calmette demanded evaluation of the therapeutic agent in the fall of 1928 in the form of a public statement from the hygiene commission of the League of Nations mentioned above. The commission endorsed the favourable conclusions presented by Calmette almost as strongly as the Academy of Medicine, publishing an official resolution certifying that the vaccination could be extended to all infants, whether they lived in contaminated family environments or not. The assembly of eighteen experts declared: "Unanimously the bacteriologists present in the commission estimate that the experimental results authorize the conclusion that the BCG is an innocuous vaccine. ... Concerning the preventive action of the BCG against tuberculosis, the BCG vaccine produces a certain degree of immunity. But further research on the vaccinated children, carried out over a longer period and in a uniform manner is needed."[43] The international expert commission transformed the 1927-Calmette-BCG-vaccine risk and effectiveness into the 1928-Society-of-Nations risk and effectiveness. This statement provided a solid basis for the decision made by the Lübeck physicians to administer the vaccine in this city in northern Germany barely one year later. The differences expressed in the scientific controversies were transformed into a univocal overall judgement of "the" risk and "the" effectiveness of the vaccine that justified the medical action of vaccination and also determined the public information that was given.

The Lübeck BCG (monster) trial, 1931–32

The apparent consensus discussed above formed the basis for a BCG vaccination campaign undertaken in 1930 in the small town of Lübeck in Germany, which would turn into a major catastrophe with 76 new-born babies dying in the course of the following year.[44] Analysis of the subsequent public outcry and a major lawsuit that took place in 1931–1932 offer varying, often contradictory, perspectives on the scientific evaluation of risk, safety and effectiveness, and the public information provided about them. The Lübeck trial not only triggered public discussion of medical ethics in Europe, but also catalysed the introduction of the German regulations for medical research on human beings, the *Richtlinien* of 1931.[45]

The Lübeck vaccination scandal and the subsequent trial allow us to study two particular aspects of risks and safety in the 1930s. First, the trial paid considerable attention to the way Lübeck health officials had presented the vaccination to the public.[46] The process of translating specialized laboratory, clinical and statistical evidence into simpler, general information to be presented to the public allows us to analyse in some detail the issue of risk communication in relation to medical innovation in 1930. The second point concerns how risks and safety were perceived and identified by the medical actors as well as legal judges in Lübeck once what had been only a potential danger had turned into a real catastrophe with its 76 "little victims".

Before turning to the issue of public information in Lübeck, it will be helpful briefly to analyse how Calmette and his collaborators presented the BCG vaccine to the French public once its use had received ministerial support. A rare surviving information leaflet from the city of Béziers, dated 1926, can be taken as representative of this kind of literature:

City of Béziers. Office of charity.
Read immediately and carefully.

Future mothers, Young couples, tuberculosis kills 25 per cent of children born to tubercular parents or growing up in an environment with an individual with tuberculosis.

Sooner or later tuberculosis also kills many children of healthy parents or growing up in a healthy environment....

Young couples, mothers of tomorrow, think about it!

You should also know that now you can save your children and prevent them from succumbing to tuberculosis.

You can have them vaccinated.

Two French scientists: Professor Calmette, member of the French Academy of Medicine, assistant-director of the Pasteur Institute in Paris and Mr Guérin, his collaborator at the Pasteur Institute, after 15 years of studies and numerous experiments, all very encouraging, have recently discovered a product they have named the BCG vaccine (Calmette-Guérin bacillus). "The vaccine is inoffensive; it has not caused the slightest accident, neither fever reactions, nor any kind of physiological disturbances" (Professor Calmette).

This is not a commercial specialty. The vaccine is prepared at the Pasteur Institute and its exclusive distribution is assured by the Institute free of any charge. ...

During the last four years over 10,000 children have been vaccinated. Not a single incident or accident has occurred. All the children born into and growing up in tuberculosis-contaminated families are today perfectly healthy. ...

The administrative commission of the Office of charity.[47]

The leaflet presented the usual scientific evidence claimed by Calmette, including the controversial mortality rate of 24 per cent for children growing up in contaminated family environments. At the same time, the leaflet's authors suggested that the same risk of death more or less applied to the general population as well. Although, as we have seen, this figure was dubious, even for exposed children, it nevertheless served the purpose of obtaining a maximal vaccinal coverage of the population. Furthermore, the emotionally charged presentation of the supposed omnipresent danger fitted well with the public perception of tuberculosis as a huge national scourge.[48] Everyday life presented a known, clearly calculated and almost unavoidable risk of disease, death and destruction due to tuberculosis. The leaflet went on to reassure the public that now, in 1926, this risk was no longer inevitable, as the disease could be prevented.

The names of scientists and institutions were cited in support of the view that the new preventive treatment was totally safe. The statistical evidence of "more than 10,000 vaccinated children who had remained in perfect health since their treatment" was mobilized to counter any fears the public may have had about vaccination. Thus, the value of the procedure was guaranteed not only by 15 years of hard scientific work, but also by the nation's most reputable scientific institution, universally known for its humanitarian commitment. Furthermore, the disinterestedness of those involved was reinforced by the mention of the non-commercial nature of the product, which was distributed solely in the interests of public health. Most significantly, this information leaflet shifted the burden of responsibility for any possible risk away from the inventors and producers of the new vaccine and onto its recipients. The risks portrayed were no longer those associated with the administration of the vaccine, but rather those taken by the parents who refused this inoffensive life-saving prophylactic measure that would protect their children against the unavoidable risk of infection. No sign remained of any scientific controversy, as even the slightest doubt over the procedure had been removed from the information provided to the general public in France. As presented, this information was perfectly in tune with the profound conviction of Calmette and his collaborators concerning the safety and effectiveness of the vaccine. Thus, we can see that the views made available to the public were those of the vaccine's main protagonist. If we assume that Calmette was truly convinced of his case, then the information leaflet, although perhaps tendentious, was not blatantly misleading or deceitful. In contrast, from the perspective of the vaccine's critics, many of the specific details of the leaflet were half-truths if not lies. Its authors needed to simplify evidence that remained to a large degree complex and controversial, but at the risk of sometimes oversimplifying. Thus, taking

VILLE DE BEZIERS

LUTTE CONTRE LA TUBERCULOSE

Lire d'extrême urgence et attentivement

Futures Mères, Jeunes Ménages,

La **TUBERCULOSE** tue 25 pour cent des enfants nés de parents tuberculeux ou élevés dans un milieu où il y a un tuberculeux.

Elle tue aussi, un peu plus tôt ou un peu plus tard, beaucoup d'enfants nés de parents sains et élevés dans un milieu sain.

Car cette maladie est si répandue et si contagieuse, qu'il ne faut pas songer, malgré toutes les précautions et la vigilance la plus attentive, à les soustraire à son emprise. Les plus forts résistent, et encore pas toujours ; les autres succombent ou restent infirmes (tumeurs blanches, coxalgies, mal de Pott, etc.) et sont condamnés à une existence misérable. La méningite, la broncho-pneumonie, *manifestations terribles de la tuberculose,* les guettent à tout instant et peuvent en quelques jours vider votre foyer.

Jeunes Ménages, mères de demain, songez-y !

Mais sachez aussi que vous pouvez, désormais, conserver vos enfants et les empêcher de succomber à la tuberculose.

Vous pouvez les faire **VACCINER.**

Deux savants français : M. le Professeur Calmette, *membre de l'Académie de Médecine et sous-directeur de l'Institut Pasteur de Paris, et* M. Guérin, *son collaborateur à l'Institut Pasteur, viennent, en effet, après 15 années d'études et de nombreuses expériences,* toutes concluantes, *de découvrir un produit qu'ils ont appelé* **VACCIN BCG** (bacille Calmette-Guérin).

« Ce vaccin est inoffensif : il n'entraine ni accident d'aucune sorte, ni réaction fébrile, ni troubles physiologiques quelconques.» (Professeur Calmette.)

Ce n'est pas une spécialité commerciale. *Il est préparé à l'Institut Pasteur et fourni* **EXCLUSIVEMENT** *et* **GRATUITEMENT** *par cet établissement.*

Il doit être administré au nouveau-né comme une simple tisane. dans les 10 premiers jours de sa naissance.

Depuis quatre ans, plus de **10.000** *enfants ont été ainsi vaccinés. Il n'y a eu aucun incident, ni aucun accident. Tous ces enfants, nés et élevés dans des milieux contaminés,* sont aujourd'hui bien portants.

Mais il faut que le nouveau-né soit vacciné le plus tôt possible après sa naissance, en tous cas dans les **10** premiers jours, *pas plus tard*

Jeunes Ménages, Mères de demain, ne l'oubliez pas !

Dès la naissance de votre enfant, *prévenez le Bureau de bienfaisance, rue Boïeldieu, n° 54, où un service spécial,* gratuit *est organisé ; par télégramme, il demandera à l'Institut Pasteur le vaccin préventif que, dès réception, une infirmière viendra administrer à votre nouveau-né.*

Comme tout oubli de votre part serait regrettable et irréparable, *nous enverrons chez vous, dès que nous connaitrons la naissance de votre enfant, une infirmière vous offrir le vaccin sauveur.*

Accueillez-la en amie, *nous vous aiderons,* mais aidez-nous.

N'OUBLIEZ PAS qu'il s'agit de la santé et de la vie de votre enfant, du bonheur et de l'avenir de votre foyer.

La Commission Administrative du Bureau de Bienfaisance : F. Suchon, Maire, Président; J. Fabre, Vice Président; A. Desplats, Ordonnateur; Ch. Vinnet, P. Pancol, Chanet et Bru, Administrateurs.

Figure 5.2 Béziers information leaflet for the promotion of BCG vaccination, 1927.

Source: A. Calmette, *La vaccination préventive contre la tuberculose par le BCG*, Paris: Masson, 1927, p. 243.

into account the convictions of the researchers, and the exigencies of the public authorities concerned, no simple line could, or can be, drawn dividing true or honest from false or dishonest information.

As we shall see, the physicians and public health officials of the city of Lübeck went to quite some lengths to discuss and evaluate the BCG vaccination before its administration to the infant population. The city possessed a fairly advanced and well-organized public health system, and, prior to the introduction of a public vaccination campaign, the physicians in charge had to inform and convince the representatives of the local council of public health of the project's safety and efficacy.[49] Furthermore, these physicians organized meetings with the members of the town's medical profession and midwives, during which they presented information concerning the vaccine's effectiveness and safety based on Calmette's French statistics and the official approval granted by the League of Nations. Nevertheless, during the whole procedure, there was no mention of the prior disapproval of the vaccination published in 1927 by the Reich Health Office (Reichsgesundheitsamt), which was still in force in 1929.[50]

In January 1930, the two local authorities declared themselves in favour of public vaccination. At the beginning of February 1930, E. Altstaedt, the physician in charge of the campaign, and H. Jannasch, the director of the town's tuberculosis dispensary, drew up a public information notice to be distributed to the population. Starting with its title and ending with its conclusion, the so-called "yellow flyer" reproduced the information that was circulated by Calmette and his collaborators in France:

Fighting tuberculosis

25 per cent of children growing up in a family environment with tubercular parents or with an individual with tuberculosis die of tuberculosis.

Sooner or later, many children of healthy parents, growing up in healthy environments, but occasionally exposed to infection by strangers, die of tuberculosis as well.

Therefore you should take every possible precaution to protect your children from the disease. Most importantly, children should be educated in a healthy way and should be strictly isolated from infectious individuals with tuberculosis. Furthermore, you are in the situation to assure that even an unfortunate accidental infection might bring with it reduced dangers by administering the Calmette agent during the first days of your child's life. It can be obtained free of charge from your physician or your wet-nurse.

This protective agent is totally harmless; it does not produce any disturbances in health. ... Do everything for the health and the protection of the life of your children; take advantage of the Calmette agent regardless of whether your child is growing up in a tubercular environment or not.

The Public Health Office, The Dispensary for the Prevention of Tuberculosis.[51]

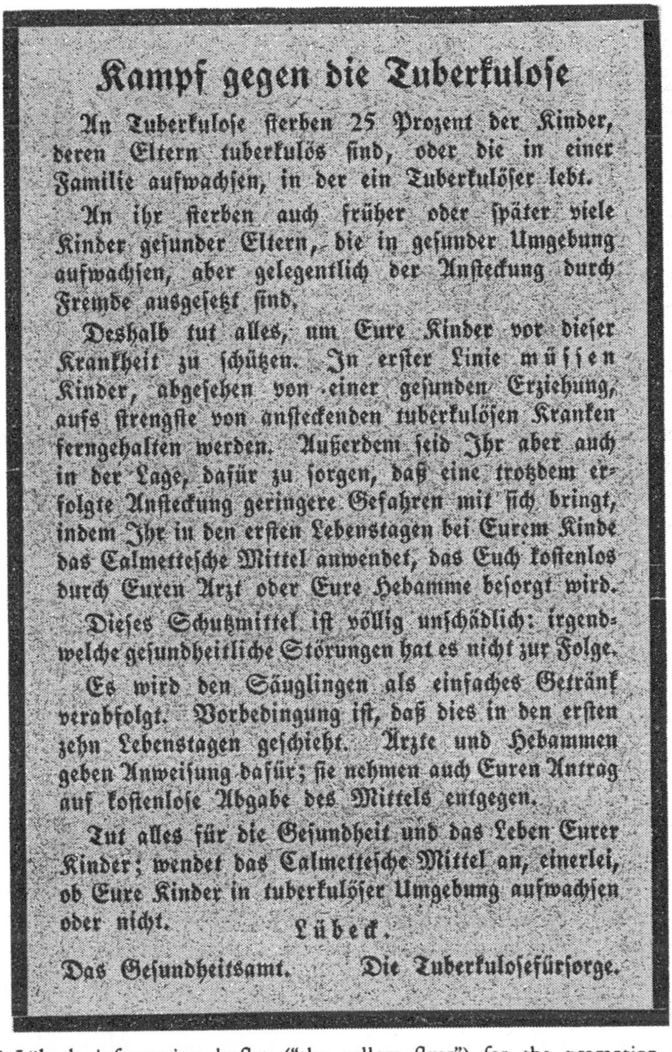

Kampf gegen die Tuberkulose

An Tuberkulose sterben 25 Prozent der Kinder, deren Eltern tuberkulös sind, oder die in einer Familie aufwachsen, in der ein Tuberkulöser lebt.

An ihr sterben auch früher oder später viele Kinder gesunder Eltern, die in gesunder Umgebung aufwachsen, aber gelegentlich der Ansteckung durch Fremde ausgesetzt sind,

Deshalb tut alles, um Eure Kinder vor dieser Krankheit zu schützen. In erster Linie müssen Kinder, abgesehen von einer gesunden Erziehung, aufs strengste von ansteckenden tuberkulösen Kranken ferngehalten werden. Außerdem seid Ihr aber auch in der Lage, dafür zu sorgen, daß eine trotzdem erfolgte Ansteckung geringere Gefahren mit sich bringt, indem Ihr in den ersten Lebenstagen bei Eurem Kinde das Calmettesche Mittel anwendet, das Euch kostenlos durch Euren Arzt oder Eure Hebamme besorgt wird.

Dieses Schutzmittel ist völlig unschädlich: irgendwelche gesundheitliche Störungen hat es nicht zur Folge.

Es wird den Säuglingen als einfaches Getränk verabfolgt. Vorbedingung ist, daß dies in den ersten zehn Lebenstagen geschieht. Ärzte und Hebammen geben Anweisung dafür; sie nehmen auch Euren Antrag auf kostenlose Abgabe des Mittels entgegen.

Tut alles für die Gesundheit und das Leben Eurer Kinder; wendet das Calmettesche Mittel an, einerlei, ob Eure Kinder in tuberkulöser Umgebung aufwachsen oder nicht.   Lübeck.

Das Gesundheitsamt.   Die Tuberkulosefürsorge.

Figure 5.3 Lübeck information leaflet ("the yellow flyer") for the promotion of BCG vaccination, 1930.

Source: Landesarchiv Schleswig-Holstein, Abt. 352, Nr. 297, *Urteil der II. Grossen Strafkammer*, 6.2.1931, p. 36.

From Calmette's 24 per cent mortality rate to his invitation to parents to do everything possible for the health of their children, the yellow flyer faithfully represented Calmette's own data. The flyer also faithfully preserved the omissions made by Calmette and his collaborators. As in the Béziers leaflet, the safety and harmlessness of the BCG vaccine were guaranteed, while any controversies or precautionary statements from health officials were omitted altogether. As in Béziers, the vaccine was to be distributed free of charge under the control of physicians and midwives. The most salient difference between the two information leaflets consisted in the fact that the Lübeck version insisted more on "healthy education" and the protection of children through isolation from contaminated individuals as a fundamental means of fighting the disease. Thus, while advocated and even recommended, the BCG vaccine appeared as a supplementary, although important, means of protection. As in France, the risks and responsibilities associated with contamination lay with non-compliant parents rather than with the vaccine itself.

The public vaccination campaign was initiated on 24 February 1930.[52] Over the following two months, 84 per cent of newborn babies in the city, a total of over 250 babies, were vaccinated. The first complications appeared in late April, and in May the vaccination campaign was stopped and a murder trial was instigated in the criminal courts. What had been only abstract and hypothetical risks had become a tangible and painful reality. In the public's view, the BCG vaccine was no longer seen as a safe and harmless protective agent, but rather seemed to be a risky enterprise that had caused more harm than it could ever have prevented. As to the question of the public information about the vaccine, in retrospect judgements concerning its quality seemed ultimately to depend to quite some extent on the eventual outcome of the vaccination programs themselves. At least, this is what the Lübeck catastrophe and the subsequent trial suggest. In the immediate aftermath, the public health scandal required an explanation and the victims were seeking not only justice but also information concerning the issue of who was responsible.

Lawyers, prosecutors and public critics of the BCG vaccine accused the two physicians in charge of having deliberately withheld information from the public.[53] When the physicians responsible for the introduction of the BCG in Lübeck were asked by the court whether they knew of the controversies around Lignières and Greenwood and why they chose to ignore them, one of them, Altstaedt, declared "that he had been aware of critics of the BCG, but that every medical procedure had its opponents".[54] The second Lübeck physician, Georg Deycke, declared that despite the controversies it was his firm conviction that the BCG was harmless. Although he would later concede that this was a scientific mistake,[55] Alstaedt instead continued to declare publicly that he considered the BCG to be "as safe as milk and sugar water"[56] and publicly vaccinated his young daughter with the BCG during the trial. The official proceedings of the court trial as well as the verdict signalled that the physicians had deliberately withheld information from the local Senate, the council of public health, and the general public, because they considered, just like Calmette, that the criticism was unjustified. But the legal argumentation had its own rationale. The starting point for the litigation and the eventual judgement was the act that led to the fatal contamination, in other words the administration of the BCG vaccine. According to this argument, any decision prior to that act, such as the decision-making process concerning the introduction of the vaccination in the first place, as well as the provision to the public with information about risks, safety and effectiveness, were not legally relevant despite their bearing on the justification of the actions. Nevertheless, as far as the public was concerned, they remained a crucial element in the dysfunction of the health system in Lübeck. The accusation of providing misleading and dishonest information remained unanswered.

The fundamental issue for the court was to establish an explanation for the deaths of 76 babies. What had happened? Even during the trial, expert evidence and opinions still diverged widely over not only the evaluation of the risks and safety associated with the BCG, but also the causes of the Lübeck accident. Three possible scenarios were under consideration: immoral human experimentation; bacterial variability indicating the uncertainty of a fundamental scientific fact; and an accident involving poor laboratory practice during the production of the vaccine.[57] The third hypothesis was the interpretation that was finally adopted by the court, designating a laboratory accident due to sloppy practice as responsible for an exchange or contamination of vaccination cultures during the production process of the BCG vaccine in the Lübeck laboratory.[58] Most interesting for our analysis here, the judgement identified a new risk that did not explicitly exist before the Lübeck catastrophe. The cause determining the tragic events in Lübeck was not a potential harm inherent to the vaccine itself (the BCG was not responsible for the deaths of the children), but a failure that appeared during its large-scale production in Lübeck. Calmette's BCG in France, even after Lübeck, was still considered as a harmless and safe preventive vaccine, whereas local production could destroy these supposedly fixed characteristics. Invention and production were dissociated in this procedure, and separate, yet related risks now existed for each of the two elements, research and production. The Lübeck tragedy was considered only to be related to the production side of the vaccine. In the French view, BCG produced by the Pasteur Institute had nothing to do with this scandal, and so BCG vaccination was pursued without any restrictions during the following decade west of the Rhine.

Conclusion

This presentation seems to call for three concluding remarks. First, the risks and safety of the BCG vaccination were conceived and identified in multiple and varying ways. There was not one permanent and universal risk associated with the vaccination but manifold and divergent ways of defining and assessing such risks. The development of the preventive treatment involved several steps that progressively modified and adjusted the vaccine throughout the period from 1921 to 1934. Perceptions and definitions of risk varied accordingly. In the courtroom, too, the scientific evaluation of risks and safety remained controversial. But practicing doctors and judges had to draw conclusions that they could then use as the basis for their actions, and in such a situation, some uncertainty inevitably remained.[59] Scientific controversies can be open-ended and remain unsettled for a long time, but medical decision-making and legal judgements need to reach conclusions within a limited period of time. The Lübeck physicians had concluded that the BCG was safe, and the judges concluded that the BCG had been accidentally contaminated by virulent bacteria during its production. Both conclusions were reached at a given moment, based on what seemed most probable from a practical point of view, but, in the end, they were not necessarily true in an absolute sense.

Second, risks and their definition changed, along with the perspectives of specific actors and users of the vaccination. Such assessments changed substantially in light of the possibility that risk could become reality so clearly highlighted by the Lübeck case. Under these circumstances, information about risks was not simply a question of truth versus deceit. In his 1935 monograph *Genesis and development of a scientific fact*, Ludwik Fleck asserts that information is not simply communicated, but rather it is inter-subjectively and unconsciously shared and transformed. This also holds for the risks and safety associated with the introduction of the BCG vaccine. According to Fleck, the evaluation of and information about scientific facts are partial and biased by the very essence of their existence and their exchange. He underlines that every piece of information or "didactic intro-duction" is therefore literally a "leading into" or a "gentle constraint".[60] This contribution argues that the same relativist conclusion applies to the notions of risk, safety and effectiveness since they directly depend on "scien-tific facts".

Last but not least, the BCG story shows that the inherent risks of medical inventions change over time and are not necessarily tied to the inventive networks that produce them. Public information about these risks needs to be situated in their local contexts of production and meaning. Yet this contextual nature is squarely opposed to the imperatives of clear and simple information to be communicated to the profane. The question that remains for our present society is whether bioethical review boards and courtroom responses can effectively mediate the essential tension between complex and contextual medical innovation and comprehensible public information about them, mediate between the worlds of science, technology and society.

Notes

1 L. Fleck, *Genesis and development of a scientific fact*, Chicago: University of Chicago Press, 1979. (German original, 1935)
2 A. Calmette, *L'infection bacillaire et la tuberculose chez l'homme et chez les animaux*, Paris: Masson, 1922 (2nd edition), p. 538.
3 O. Faure and D. Dessertine, *Combattre la tuberculose, 1900–1940*, Lyon: Presses Universitaires de Lyon, 1988; D. Barnes, *The making of a social disease. Tuberculosis in nine-teenth-century France*, Berkeley: University of California Press, 1995; G. Feldberg, *Disease and class. Tuberculosis and the shaping of modern north American society*, New Brunswick:

Rutgers University Press, 1995; S. Haehner-Rombach, *Sozialgeschichte der Tuberkulose*, Stuttgart: Steiner, 2000.

4 S. R. Rosenthal, *BCG vaccination against tuberculosis*, Boston: Little, Brown and Company, 1957; L. Bryder, " 'We shall not find salvation in inoculation': BCG vaccination in Scandinavia, Britain and the USA, 1921–1960", *Social science & medicine* 49, 1999, 1157–67. P. Menut, "Ethique et ethos de la recherche biomédicale en France: l'introduction de la vaccination par le BCG, 1921–1933", in C. Bonah, E. Lepicard and V. Roelcke (eds), *La Médecine expérimentale au tribunal: Implications éthiques de quelques procès médicaux du XXe siècle européen*, Paris: Editions des Archives Contemporaines, 2003, 95–124. C. Bonah, *Histoire de l'expérimentation humaine en France : discours et pratiques, 1900–1940*, Strasbourg: Habilitation, 2003.

5 S. Hahn, " 'Der Lübecker Totentanz'. Zur rechtlichen und ethischen Problematik der Katastrophe bei der Erprobung der Tuberkuloseimpfung 1930 in Deutschland", *Medizinhistorisches Journal* 30, 1995, 61–79; P. Menut, "The Lübeck catastrophe and its consequences for anti-tuberculosis BCG vaccination", in A. M. Moulin and A. Cambrosio (eds), *Singular Selves: Historical issues and contemporary debates in immunology*, Amsterdam: Elsevier, 2001, 202–10; C. Bonah, "Le drame de Lübeck: la vaccination BCG, le 'procès Calmette' et les Richtlinien de 1931", in Bonah *et al.*, *La Médecine expérimentale au tribunal*, 2003, 65–94.

6 A. Calmette, "Sur la vaccination préventive des enfants nouveau-nés contre la tuberculose par le BCG", *Annales de l'Institut Pasteur* (hereafter AIP), 1927(a), 201–32; here pp. 204–5.

7 A. Calmette and C. Guérin, "Vaccination des bovidés contre la tuberculose et méthode nouvelle de prophylaxie de la tuberculose bovine", *AIP*, 1924, p. 373.

8 Bonah, *Histoire de l'expérimentation humaine*, 2003, pp. 92–143.

9 Calmette and Guérin, "Vaccination des bovidés", 1924, p. 373.

10 A. Calmette, *La vaccination préventive contre la tuberculose par le BCG*, Paris: Masson, 1927(b), p. 74.

11 E. Ackerknecht, "Aspects of the history of therapeutics", in *Bulletin of the History of Medicine 36*, 1962, 389–419; A. Berman, "The heroic approach in 19th Century therapeutics", in J. Leavitt and R. Numbers, *Sickness and health in America. Readings in the hitory of medicine and public health*, Madison: University of Wisconsin Press, 1978.

12 A. Calmette, C. Guérin and B. Weill-Hallé, "Essais d'immunisation contre l'infection tuberculeuse", *Bulletin de l'Académie de Médecine* (hereafter BAM), 24.06.1924, pp. 787–96; Calmette, *Vaccination préventive*, 1927(b), p. 186; Menut, "Ethique et ethos", pp. 99–103.

13 Calmette, *Vaccination préventive*, 1927(b), p. 187.

14 B. Weill-Halléand R. Turpin, "Sur la vaccination antituberculeuse de l'enfant par le BCG", *AIP*, 1927, 254–70.

15 Weill-Hallé and Turpin, "Vaccination antituberculeuse", 1927, p. 261. Calmette, *Vaccination préventive*, 1927(b), p. 187.

16 Calmette *et al.*, "Essais d'immunisation", 1924, pp. 795–6.

17 C. Bernard, *Introduction à l'étude de la médecine expérimentale*, Paris: Baillière, 1865, pp. 172–82.

18 Calmette, "Sur la vaccination préventive", 1927(a), p. 213.

19 Calmette, "Sur la vaccination préventive", 1927(a), pp. 213–18.

20 Calmette, "Sur la vaccination préventive", 1927(a), p. 218.

21 Calmette, "Sur la vaccination préventive", 1927(a), p. 218.

22 A. Calmette, "La prémunition ou vaccination préventive des nouveau-nés contre la tuberculose par le BCG. Statistiques et résultats du 1er juillet 1924 au 1er décembre 1927", *AIP*, 1928, 1–34; citation p. 18.

23 J. Lignières, "Contribution à l'étude des qualités pathogènes du vaccin BCG contre la tuberculose", *BAM*, 1927(a), 127–45.

24 Lignières, "Contribution à l'étude des qualités pathogènes", 1927(a), p. 144.

25   A. Calmette, "La vaccination préventive des nouveau-nés contre la tuberculose par le BCG: statistiques et résultats du 1er juillet 1924 au 1er décembre 1927", *BAM*, 1928(a), p. 59.

26   J. Lignières, "A propos de la prémunition dans les milieux non infectés de tuberculose", *BAM*, 1928(a), p. 470.

27   A. Calmette, "A propos de la communication de M. Lignières sur la prémunition dans les milieux non infectés de tuberculose", *BAM*, 1928 (b), p. 495.

28   Calmette, "A propos de la communication de M. Lignières",1928 (b), p. 495.

29   J. Lignières, "Le vaccin BCG, bien que très atténué et sans action tuberculigène, reste encore trop pathogène pour l'espèce humaine", *BAM*, 1928(b), 865–78; here p. 876.

30   Lignières, "Le vaccin BCG, bien que très atténué", *BAM*, 1928(b), pp. 877–8.

31   J. Lignières, "Résultats expérimentaux obtenus avec les bacilles des petites Denise et Marie D* pour la recherche de leur identité avec le BCG", *BAM*, 1928(c), 1027–37.

32   A. Calmette, "Réponse à M. Lignières", *BAM*, 1928(c), 1038–48; here pp. 1038–9.

33   Calmette, "Réponse à M. Lignières",1928(c), p. 1042.

34   Anonymous, "Prophylactic vaccination of the newly born against tuberculosis", *British Medical Journal* (hereafter BMJ), 1927, 845–6.

35   M. Greenwood, "Prophylactic vaccination of the newly born against tuberculosis", *BMJ*, 1927(a), 896–7.

36   Greenwood, "Prophylactic vaccination", 1927(a), p. 897.

37   M. Greenwood, "Prophylactic vaccination of the newly born against tuberculosis", *BMJ*, 1927(b), 1082–3.

38   Anonymous, "A criticism of 'BCG' ", *BMJ*, 1928, p. 364.

39   M. Greenwood, "Professor Calmette's statistical study of BCG vaccination", *BMJ*, 1928, pp. 793–5.

40   Greenwood, "Professor Calmette's statistical study of BCG vaccination", 1928, p. 795.

41   Bonah, *Histoire de l'expérimentation humaine*, 2003, pp. 92–143.

42   Greenwood, "Professor Calmette's statistical study of BCG vaccination", 1928, p. 795.

43   Société des Nations, Organisation d'Hygiène, Rapport de la conférence technique pour l'étude de la vaccination antituberculeuse par le BCG. Tenue à l'Institut Pasteur de Paris du 15 au 18 octobre 1928, Genève: Société des Nations, 1928, pp. 7–9.

44   Landesarchiv Schleswig-Holstein (hereafter LASH), Abt. 352, Nr. 297, *Urteil der II. Grossen Strafkammer*, 06.02.1931, pp. 59–60.

45   Bonah, "Le drame de Lübeck", 2003, pp. 65–94.

46   J. Moses, J., *Der Totentanz von Lübeck*, Radebeul/Dresden: Madaus, 1930. W. Kröner, W. and V. Noack, *Anti-Calmette*, Berlin, 1931. W. Kröner, W., *Unsere Kinder = Versuchskaninchen? Die Sachverständigenkomödie von Lübeck*, Berlin, 1930.

47   Calmette, *Vaccination préventive*, 1927(b), p. 243.

48   Barnes, 1995.

49   LASH, *Urteil*, pp. 13–36.

50   LASH, *Urteil*, pp. 19–20.

51   LASH, *Urteil*, p. 36.

52   LASH, *Urteil*, p. 38.

53   LASH, *Urteil*, pp. 91–2.

54   LASH, *Urteil*, p. 29.

55   LASH, *Urteil*, pp. 103.

56   LASH, *Urteil*, pp. 167.

57   LASH, *Urteil*, pp. 122–56.

58   LASH, *Urteil*, pp. 92–121.

59   M. Callon, P. Lascoumes and Y. Barthe, *Agir dans un monde incertain: Essai sur la démocratie technique*, Paris: Seuil, 2001.

60   L. Fleck, *Genesis and development of a scientific fact*, Chicago: University of Chicago Press, 1979, p. 104.

6 From danger to risk

The perception and regulation of X-rays in Switzerland, 1896–1970[1]

Monika Dommann

Perhaps the time will soon be here when every barber sports a "focus tube" to accompany his razor.[2]

Schweizerische Blätter für Elektrotechnik, 1897

A human being today in the first 30 years of his or her life is exposed to 3400 milliroentgens of natural radiation; in addition to this, artificial radiation accounts for: 700 milliroentgens from X-ray exams, 3 milliroentgens from shoe-fitting machines, 60 milliroentgens from luminous dials, 30 milliroentgens from the television, and 30 milliroentgens from nuclear explosions (as of 1956).[3]

Hans Rudolf Schinz, 1958

The first side effects

At the end of December 1895, the physicist Wilhelm Conrad Röntgen informed the public about his discovery of the baffling entity that could render the interior of the human body visible on a light-sensitive photographic plate, which he called "X-rays".[4] Although they had remained unknown for so long, these rays were produced using apparatus that could be found in any physics laboratory by this time, such as the Rühmkoff inducer and a Crooke's tube. In the following months, physicists, photographers, technicians, and medical doctors would test possible procedures for using X-rays as a diagnostic tool, constantly manipulating this recently discovered radiation. The fact that the rays were invisible to the human eye, while being able to affect a photographic plate and being easily detectable after having passed through the human body, simultaneously fascinated and confused the scientists concerned. Confusion reigned even amongst the physicists right up until 1912 when Max von Laue furnished the experimental proof that X-rays consisted of electromagnetic radiation of extremely short wavelength, well outside the range of the visible spectrum.

The first reports of the depilatory effects of X-rays appeared in the *Lancet* as early as 1896,[5] and reports were published in Switzerland soon after about "sunburn" resulting from contact with X-rays.[6] In January 1896, Aimé Forster, a physics professor at the University of Berne, started to work with

Röntgen's procedure, and, in collaboration with his assistant Hans Schenkel, succeeded in producing 506 X-ray photographs for the *Inselspital* in the period before February 1897,[7] with the exposure times for these photographs varying between half a minute and a full hour. After the procedure, each patient was asked whether he or she had experienced any special sensation. Only two or three of the "*Geixten*" ("X-ed") answered affirmatively, although they were unable to put into words what kind of feeling it actually was.[8] Forster also conducted experiments on himself. Thus, he irradiated his hand every day for approximately 10 minutes from a distance of 5 centimeters for 10 days without observing any changes in the skin. A patient did finally present himself to Forster in a state of great excitement over his hair loss, having been treated with X-rays twice in Forster's physics laboratory during the preceding three weeks. The symptoms became worse, developing into a round, completely hairless patch about the size of a five franc coin. The hair had become so loose in the region close to the bald spot that it could be removed using the fingers, and without applying any force.[9] This discovery appears to have been no cause for concern for Forster, indeed quite the opposite. In 1897 he published an essay in the trade journal for Swiss electrical engineers, which culminated in the euphoric hope that X-rays represented a practical new depilatory tool.[10]

Through the quite typical example of the University of Berne we can see how, in the months following the discovery of X-rays, physics laboratories were already busy working with these entities. We can also see how the daily papers and technical journals were reporting on this work. Of course, electricity and any related phenomena had all been hyped in the futuristic medical discourses of the fin-du-siècle, with utopian predictions concerning the future being loudly proclaimed in the most public arenas. Each new phenomenon was immediately tested therapeutically, and X-rays were no exception.[11] If physicists and medical doctors did take any interest in the physiological effects of X-rays in the euphoric decade of experimentation that followed their discovery, then it was with respect to the possibilities of their therapeutic use, not their potential hazards. Thus, when a scientist reported "some effects of X-rays on his hands" in *Nature* in 1896, he did not ask whether the production of X-rays marked the introduction of a dangerous new material into the laboratory, even though he noted that the effects were "most unpleasant and inconvenient to myself".[12]

In line with the theme of this volume, I want to focus on risk in relation to medical innovation, but to do this requires addressing fundamental problems associated with the history of X-rays. Initially, Röntgen's procedure was not itself a medical innovation, but was an accidental discovery made in a physics laboratory. Its subsequent development over the next twenty years took place in the context of an extended phase of experimentation in which the technology had to be fine-tuned to generate a visual representation of differences in density. Only once this had been achieved could X-rays be introduced as a standardized medical diagnostic tool. During this phase, the

X-ray equipment had to be adapted and modified for medical use as well as being invested with appropriate symbolic meaning.

Furthermore, in this context the notion of risk itself, a topic that has become very fashionable in the social sciences over the last twenty years, is a treacherous one. The term "risk" was never used by any of the participants in relation to the deleterious effects of the X-rays, as they preferred to use the word "damage", a term that at the end of the nineteenth century was associated with "injury or impairment of one's life and health or of one's possessions irrespective of the author or cause".[13] Nevertheless, we can ask whether the concept of risk is a useful analytical category from a historical perspective. The sociologist Ulrich Beck has promoted the emergence of the risk associated with modernity (the irreversible endangering of animal and plant species as well as the human race, and the generalized danger that such global problems represent as they affect all classes indiscriminately) into a feature that defines an epoch.[14] Did X-ray technology pose this kind of risk associated with modernity at the end of the nineteenth century, or was it just another occupational hazard associated with industrial society? After all, this hazard was not limited to the working class but also threatened high-ranking members of the science and technology community. Adopting a historical perspective, it is insufficient just to attribute only to either the industrial or modern society. One has to focus on the relevant historical and social context. That means to analyse local laboratory practices in connection with the history of professionalization and projects for national health regulation. From this perspective, we can explain why it was that X-rays only became subject to national control and regulation relatively late (the end of the 1950s), even though the rays' harmful effects had been widely observed within the scientific community as early as 1905, and already by the 1920s a number of compensation suits had been launched, alerting the public to the danger outside the confines of the X-ray laboratories themselves.

In order to understand the stages by which the perception of X-rays changed, it is not enough just to analyse the associated technoscientific practices. We also need to study the communication about these rays. Adopting this approach, it becomes clear that the question of who was using X-rays as a diagnostic tool, and who later acquired control over them, represent crucial factors in explaining the transformation of the phenomenon from the object of diagnostic euphoria to the subject of national legislation.[15] Although the actors themselves never mentioned the term risk in connection with X-rays, I want to use the term myself as an analytic category, thereby mobilizing Niklas Luhmann's distinction between danger and risk.[16]

As X-ray radiation had been discovered in the physics laboratory, it was initially predominantly physicists who had control over the all-important knowledge needed to handle the apparatus and thus managed entry into the field. At the same time, there was a great deal of interest expressed by the medical community in the new procedure, which argued for the integration of X-ray laboratories into hospitals and other medical settings. In Berne, the installation that had been improvised at the University's physics laboratory was replaced by a new X-ray institute at the *Inselspital* in December 1897, with Hans Schenkel, Aimé Forster's former assistant, appointed as its director. In May 1899, Schenkel made the first report concerning the appearance of "fissures and marks" on his hands to the director of the hospital. Despite intensive treatment by physicians, he suffered from severe pain that seriously impaired his ability to work.[17] The hands were particularly exposed to the danger, as they were used to measure the intensity of the rays in the course of these experiments. While Hans Schenkel experienced the damaging effects of X-rays himself, he nevertheless spoke out against starting any public debate on the topic, adopting the view that discussions in the daily press were to be avoided. In this context, he had this to say as a result of the news that had been reported in both the daily papers and the specialist medical press concerning the severe damage caused by X-rays: "Such reports, particularly in the daily papers, are likely to render the public suspicious of this new diagnosis aid, which is practically indispensable in many cases".[18] He advised his colleagues strictly to limit their discussion of the harmful effects of X-rays to a small circle of experts. In 1901, Hans Schenkel resigned his post at the X-ray laboratory, but the unhealthy nature of the work was probably just one factor in this decision. He must have realized that the discipline of radiology was emerging in the context of medicine, and that consequently the promotion opportunities for a physicist like himself were severely limited, and this may well have contributed to his decision to resign.

The threat begins to be perceived by the scientific community: from danger to risk

Hans Schenkel's resignation from the X-ray laboratory coincided not only with a new phase in relation to the professionalization of radiology but also with a reassessment of the potential hazards associated with the rays themselves. The question remains as to which events contributed to the paradigm shift that took place in the years that followed with respect to the perception of X-rays. Indeed, the development of the situation in Switzerland can only be understood in the context of the international debate over the issue. Between 1900 and 1910 the heterogeneous, but constantly professionalizing, scientific community that had formed around X-rays effected a slow but marked about-face in terms of the perception of this phenomenon. In his outstanding study of the early history of the protection measures adopted against radiation, Daniel Paul Serwer has suggested several different causes that might explain this change in attitude.[19]

Although the scientific community was shaken up by the first trials demanding compensation for radiation damage that were launched in

Germany in 1898, the scientists were still able to fend off the accusations at this early stage. In 1902, however, the first physician was found guilty of having caused bodily harm through negligence.[20] In the same year, it became known that Thomas Edison's assistant in the U.S.A. had contracted an X-ray induced cancer that would end by taking his life in October 1904. The specialist journals immediately characterized this death as a case of scientific "martyrdom", with the *Lancet* announcing the death of Clarence M. Dally under the title "A Martyr to science".[21] It had now become clear that X-rays did not just simply cause "dermatitis", but also had carcinogenic effects.

Moreover, the scientific community, which had up until this time been characterized by its pluralism and openness, was now assuming a more formal structure, which allowed it to be more exclusive. Thus, it reacted to the dramatic turn of events not only by introducing the first technical preventive measures, but also by demanding that procedures for granting formal permission be put in place for those wishing to work with X-rays. This marks the beginning of a process that, following Niklas Luhmann's terminology, one could term a transformation of X-rays from a "danger" to a "risk". Luhmann characterizes a danger as "any damage that is due to causes that lie outside of our own control", such as natural phenomena.[22] Risk is characterized as the damage that is the consequence of a conscious decision and that could have been prevented by the use of technology or by other means. In this context, technology is not understood just as a collection of instruments, but as something that reduces the complexity of a situation. Thus, the change in the perception of X-rays can be regarded as a shift from seeing them as representing a vague danger to seeing them as a risk that could at least be influenced or attenuated, even if not entirely eliminated.

The first technical preventive measures concerned the architecture of the institutes. Thus, in the 1906 extension to the X-ray institute at the *Inselspital* in Berne, the patient would be separated from the X-ray apparatus by a newly introduced lead wall during the process of irradiation.[23] These structural innovations were complemented by the introduction of lead gloves, lead aprons, and lead screens, aimed at containing the rays in order to prevent dangerous secondary radiation.[24] General hygiene measures were also introduced, such as regular washing of the hands, putting grease on them, going for walks, or opening the windows. In 1912, an X-ray specialist reported that the "noticeable tingling of the skin" disappeared when he thoroughly washed himself.[25]

Beyond the structural changes in buildings and the improvement in the X-ray apparatus itself, there were also demands for other measures of control associated with professional politics. Those medical doctors who had specialized in X-ray technology now aligned themselves against their non-specialist colleagues, and speaking as experts in the use of X-rays demanded the regulation of X-ray diagnostics. Thus in 1903, even before the death of Clarence M. Dally, and so at a time when the harmful effects of

X-rays on the internal organs were still not proven, the radiologist H. E. Albers-Schönberg wrote in an article about preventive measures that "only competent physicians should be allowed to use X-rays on patients".[26] This statement merits particular attention, as the cases that were starting to be brought before the courts concerned almost exclusively physicians.

It is reasonable, therefore, to suppose that the X-ray specialists, who in 1905 had formed their own society in Germany, were turning these lawsuits for radiation damage to their own professional ends. Thus, when the German X-ray Society announced in 1907 that the deliberate use of X-rays by an "unapproved" person constituted an illegal act, we can ask whether this was an attack aimed at the numerous non-physicians who were still active and often held important positions in the X-ray laboratories.[27]

The pioneers of radiation research, who had worked for years with X-rays, practiced another way of reducing the associated risk by withdrawing from the practical activities of the laboratory. Wilhelm Mayer-Lienhard, for example, who had been responsible for radiography in the X-ray institute of the Basel *Bürgerspital* since 1896 became so seriously ill in 1905 that the administration hired a female assistant worker for the first time. This woman took over all the practical tasks, while Mayer-Lienhard's role was limited to directing the laboratory. One might describe this measure as the delegation of the risk to a subordinate female assistant.[28]

The scientific study of the effects of radiation and the efforts to measure doses were still in their infancy at this time.[29] It was only in the mid-1920s that agreement was reached over standards for dosimetry and what was to be considered the Tolerance Dose. The concept of the Tolerance Dose was based on a procedure that one could describe as risk negotiation, balancing the risk that physicians, scientists and their employees were exposed to against the practical demands of the use of X-rays.[30] Based on investigations conducted in different X-ray laboratories, the American physicist Arthur Mutscheller determined the maximal dose that elicited no complaints from the laboratory workers. The skin erythema dose was finally agreed upon as an international standard, and consisted of 0.2 roentgens per day.

Insurance against the risk

Using Niklas Luhmann's distinction between danger and risk, we have described how in this case danger was transformed into risk. The damage was identified as being a consequence of the use of X-rays and attempts were made to bring the problem under control using architectural and technical measures, as well as amending work practices and establishing international agreements. So far, our analysis has been focused on the scientists, physicians and autodidacts who were exposed to the radiation during the course of their professional lives, but we can also ask how the process was perceived by the patients who were brought into contact with X-rays in the course of a diagnosis or treatment. Following decisions made by other people, they were exposed to dangers that they neither chose nor controlled (doses of radiation, distance from the X-ray tube, etc.). This reminds us of what Niklas Luhmann has to say about one person's risk becoming another person's danger.[31] If we turn our attention to the liability claims made by injured patients, we could argue a variation of Luhmann's position as other people's danger becoming one man's risk, as radiologists faced a financial risk associated with their medical diagnoses and treatments. In 1927, a case involving serious physical injury connected with X-ray therapy attracted widespread public interest and sympathy. The case eventually made it to a federal court where the patient was awarded 110,000 francs in damages.[32] During the 1920s, when the demands for compensation following injuries received from radiotherapy were rising sharply, both independent physicians and hospitals took out insurance against potential liability. The *Inselspital* in Berne concluded an insurance deal in 1924 to cover itself against damages related to accidents and injuries suffered by their patients. It seems likely that this insurance was taken out because of the risk associated with the X-ray institute, as this institute was explicitly referred to by name in the policy.[33]

Zürich's *Kantonsspital* also took out liability insurance at this time covering both the head of the institute and his female assistants.[34] The policy explicitly noted that the head of the institute was responsible for the activity of the institute, and that the female assistants were not to take radiographs on their own initiative. In practice, however, a large part of the responsibility of the day-to-day operation of the institute before 1920 fell to the female assistants. This situation continued unchanged until well into the 1920s, when large, rationalized X-ray institutes that operated according to a hierarchic structured division of labour with an academically trained radiologist at the top replaced the original structures. Of course, the introduction of insurance policies that assigned the ultimate responsibility for any injuries to the chief radiologist helped this transformation towards a hierarchic organization of labour. On the other side of the picture, however, professional liability insurance for doctors was never a profitable business for the *Zürich Unfall- und Haftpflicht-Versicherungs AG*, and in 1930 the area was classified as a "bad" risk by one of its staff, as nearly every year it generated heavy losses due to the risk of irradiation.[35]

Radiation damage to the female assistants who were the most widely exposed to the X-rays led to frequent sickness leave as well as a large number of resignations. The head of surgery at the *Kantonsspital* in Zürich, Ernst Ferdinand Sauerbruch, made the following comment on the large number of leave requests and resignations: "the second sister is also beginning to ail and will shortly be requesting leave. Work with the X-ray service is no doubt implicated because of the harmful nature of the work due to the use of X-rays, meaning that anemia and other damage is readily brought about."[36] While the insurance companies had experience in dealing with cases of liability involving patients, the occupational health problems experienced by the personnel did not fit into any of the insurers' existing categories.

In November 1922, Hans Rudolf Schinz, the director of the X-ray institute at the *Kantonsspital* in Zürich, made enquiries at the *Zürich Unfall- und Haftpflicht-Versicherungs AG* concerning the possibility of insuring himself and the other personnel at the institute against "bodily injury". The insurance company rejected the request on the grounds that the only case in which it would take responsibility for bodily injury was if it was accidentally inflicted by an external agent, and manifested itself immediately and concomitantly with the accident. Swiss federal insurance law stated that such an accident had to be the "sudden unintended damaging result of the action of a more or less unusual cause external to the human body".[37] The criterion of the "suddenness" of the effect disqualified much of the "chronic" damage caused by the X-rays such as anemia, peripheral neuropathy in the fingers, "X-ray nervous excitation", or "X-ray cachexia", that were often seen as a delayed consequence of long-term exposure to the radiation. Only the severe injuries experienced while exposed to the X-rays were clearly recognized as accidents and so could be covered by the insurance.

Thus, X-ray injuries did not fit into the normal definition of occupational illnesses. One of the main problems was that, unlike all other industrial enterprises, neither the hospitals nor the X-ray institutes were covered by the mandatory national Swiss institution for accident insurance (SUVA). Furthermore, because X-rays were categorized as "energy" and not as a classic "poison" they were not included in the list of "materials the production and use of which cause dangerous diseases".[38] The legislators had only envisaged "chemicals" as constituting this kind of "poison", which only exacerbated the problem. Thus a state of ambiguity and disagreement existed both for the insurance industry and for the Swiss government right up until the beginning of the 1960s, leading to the eventual technical and legal regulation of X-ray use in the laboratory.

Scientific research

The second wave of lawsuits demanding compensation for X-ray injury (predominantly as a consequence of radiotherapy) in Switzerland came at the same time as radiology was seeking recognition as a discipline and integration into the university curriculum. The emerging group of radiologists and other physicians specializing in X-rays reacted skillfully to this development by launching an investigation into the issue of "radiation damage" in collaboration with the wider medical profession. These specialists not only presented themselves as experts on questions of such radiation damage in their dealings with government institutions but also petitioned for self regulation in order to fend off any possible interference from the state.

These cases of X-ray damage lent additional weight to the demands for specialist technical training for radiologists, and, starting in the mid-1930s, the Swiss specialist community not only obtained chairs at the universities dedicated to radiology, but also saw the introduction of large X-ray institutes organized along the lines of rational management outlined on pp. 98–99. Thus, the community of radiologists managed to combine the exigency of minimizing the risk associated with X-rays with their own interest in professionalizing their discipline.

The issue of X-ray damage was raised for the first time at the Swiss X-Ray Society in 1916, when Max Steiger and Hermann Hopf asked the group whether it "was concerned by the recent very frequent cases of X-ray damage and what position it would like to adopt".[39] Nevertheless, it took nine years before a scientific study was undertaken in 1925 concerning this issue.

Thus, at precisely the time when X-ray damage compensation suits were being pursued in many different places at once, the Swiss X-Ray Society, in collaboration with the most important Swiss medical associations, launched a systematic data collection project concerning "accidents" and "injury" occurring in Swiss institutions using X-rays.[40] This survey was conducted by Hans Rudolf Schinz, Professor of Radiology in Zürich, assisted by two other radiologists, Adolf Liechti, Professor of Radiology in Berne, and Adolf Zuppinger, a young radiologist who would later be appointed as full professor in Berne.

From its launch in 1925 to its conclusion in 1928 and the final publication of a report in 1930, the study was taken in hand by the radiologists. Right at the beginning of the report the authors presented the goals of the study, which were that X-ray injuries should be "damned" while at the same time any prejudices against the X-ray or radium therapy should be eliminated. Another goal set out in the report was to create a body of expert knowledge and make it available to the courts and insurance companies in the form of a set of guidelines.[41] The authors deliberately stressed that the study was not comprehensive, and that the true number of X-ray-related injuries that had occurred was probably much higher than that reported.[42] Altogether there were 103 cases, 77 involving radiotherapy and five due to the large electrical currents involved; these were mainly burns from coming into contact with the power supply in the X-ray laboratory. Nearly all the compensation claims, which were mostly settled out of court, were for injuries due to radiotherapy. Nine cases involved damage caused by the diagnostic use of X-rays, mainly following fluoroscopy, in particular of the stomach, which involved passing X-rays through the body. The authors attributed the injuries following this procedure to the fact that the patients had been exposed for a long time (over five minutes). These injuries were severe: one patient died, and four had to have cancers surgically removed. The authors nevertheless stressed that all these cases had originated in the "old days" and would have been avoidable in the present state of practice.[43] Thus, X-ray injuries due to diagnostic techniques would completely disappear in the future as a consequence of new precautionary measures that had been introduced. Casting this in Luhmann's terms: from the perspective of the radiologists, the X-rays were no longer a danger, but had become a risk that they believed could be eliminated by instituting appropriate measures.

The study also looked at twelve cases of "X-ray injury" suffered by the personnel of X-ray laboratories, and in this context the authors suggested several prophylactic measures: "a lunch break of two hours, 1 half day off work per week", and the suggestion to the staff that "if possible they spend their free time in the fresh air and engaging in sporting activities".[44]

The conclusions of the study sought to convey a clear message; that the use of X-rays did not itself represent any danger, and it was only their unregulated use that posed a threat. "The list of radiation injury that we have presented is not a small one. Only a minority of these, however, were unforeseeable and inevitable. Only a small number were the result of chance or force majeure. The majority were the result of ignorance, negligence or malpractice."[45] This claim was supported by statistics: out of approximately 90 cases involving patients, 20 were put down to an oversight, 37 to ignorance, 5 were considered predictable, while 28 were considered unforeseeable.

On 4 April 1936 a memorial was inaugurated in Hamburg, dedicated to the memory of all those who had died following their exposure to X-rays and radium in the course of their professional lives.[46] Thus, the scientific community found a way to bury its dead while contributing to its own development as a profession. By declaring these former colleagues "martyrs", the community hoped to be able to bury not only its own inglorious past along with the hundreds of victims, but also the specter of the dangers associated with the technique.

The creation of this monument should also be understood against the background of a second wave of compensation claims in the 1920s, as the negative publicity that accompanied them threatened to undermine the status of the still-emerging discipline of radiology. Thus, the international scientific community was seeking to mark the end of the pioneering phase of radiology, both by introducing internal regulation into the profession, including the establishment of international standards through the "X-Ray and Radium Protection Commission" created in 1928, and by the symbolic act of inaugurating the monument in Hamburg.[47]

Professionalization

The report made two principle suggestions; first, the institutionalization of training, and second, the introduction of voluntary guidelines. These demands coincided with the radiologists' efforts to integrate radiology into the existing academic institutions and to advance the professional standing of their specialty. Another measure that was considered by the radiologists in their report was the regulation of the "use of the energy of X-rays and radium" by means of legislation, such as placing all the institutions that used X-rays under state control. However, the medical profession strongly opposed the extension of "any regulation". Future radiation injuries could only be avoided by "good initial training, good professional training, and continual advanced training"[48] and not by any laws or the introduction of national or private regulation. This opposition reflects a fundamental reluctance on the part of the medical profession to accept any government interference, but it probably also reflects the fear of non-radiologists that they would lose access to the procedure, and see it assigned exclusively to the radiologists in their capacity as experts. In the end, only two Swiss cantons introduced clauses into the medical legislation making the use of X-ray apparatus subject to official government approval: Geneva in 1926, and Waadt in 1928.[49]

Moreover, in 1928 the Swiss X-Ray Society introduced the very first set of "Guidelines for the Foundation and Running of X-Ray Institutes". These were voluntary guidelines internal to the profession that the members of the society pledged they would follow.[50] The guidelines contained recommendations concerning the technicalities of X-ray use, security measures, and the procedures for measuring radiation exposure according to international standards for dosimetry. The society recommended that its members noted all the radiographs they took and all their fluoroscopies, which they were also advised to limit to precise times, bearing in mind the possibility of compensation claims.

In the study's conclusion, X-ray use was explicitly referred to as a medical activity, heralding the coming battle against the "physics teachers", "X-ray engineers", "retired locksmiths", "metal workers" and "subaltern mechanics" who regularly made use of X-rays as a diagnostic tool.[51] One practice that was severely criticised was the use of fluoroscopy in shoe stores. Thus, the aim at the end of the 1920s was to define the X-ray apparatus as a medical instrument making its use the exclusive domain of the physicians responsible for medical practice in Switzerland.[52] The "pedoscope", which started to be introduced into Swiss shoe shops at the end of the 1920s, would develop into the central issue in X-ray regulation in the following decades. This instrument became the main symbol in the battle fought by the medical profession for exclusive control over X-ray technology, and in the beginning of the 1960s it would also become the symbol for the acceptance of legislative protection measures against radiation damage.

The pedoscope: an X-ray machine for fitting shoes

A shoe dealers' fair held in Boston in 1920 was the occasion for the launch of an X-ray instrument that promised to revolutionize the practice of fitting shoes.[53] The new machine was the expression of a scientific approach to the body that had already adopted the use of modern machines as early as the end of the nineteenth century. During the 1920s the Swiss shoe industry underwent a structural change, moving away from a tradition of made-to-measure shoes and towards mass-manufactured ones, which also contributed to the rise of the pedoscope. Furthermore, the new large-scale shoe businesses like Bata and Bally had their own distribution networks and outlets that successively replaced the traditional shoemakers.[54] At the beginning of the 1930s, the Swiss shoe manufacturer Bally introduced its first "hygienic shoes" onto the market, under the brand names of *Vasano* and *Sanoform*. These new models were intended to combat "modern ills" such as flat feet, skewed feet and splayed feet.[55] These shoes were manufactured according to "scientific principles" and were claimed to "conform to the foot", even though they had not been produced following any individual measurements made on the customer's feet. Bally, nevertheless, stressed the importance of the professional fitting of mass-manufactured items, particularly children's shoes: "The only help in this case is the reliable assessment of the shop assistant by palpation supported by the X-ray apparatus, which is available to the public free of charge in every modern children's department."[56]

Importing the pedoscope from Great Britain constituted an important element in the campaign for the new range of hygienic shoes. The shoe industry thus took advantage of the meaning associated with the use of X-rays, which had already been presented to the public as an objective, modern, scientific diagnostic tool. Bally recruited retailers to use the "X-ray – Shoe-fitting – Pedoscope" that would be "at the service of the customer in every efficient, forward looking shoe retailer" and would furthermore guarantee increased sales.[57] The medical specialists in X-ray technology greeted this development negatively, pointing out the harmful nature of irradiating the foot for several minutes.[58] Such arguments were, however, insufficient to arrest the triumphant march of the pedoscope, with around 1,500 being installed in Swiss shoe shops by the beginning of the 1960s.[59] The popularity of the pedoscope in these shoe shops reflected the continuing fascination that X-rays held for the public, despite the disturbing reports on the harmful effects of the radiation in the newspapers that had been published since the mid-1920s.

The accidents that cost the lives of a number of doctors, scientists, technicians and physicists, their assistants and their patients were seen by the groups representing the medical profession as so many regrettable incidents, but were not considered to constitute an obstacle to the path they were already pursuing. According to the scientific community the professionalization of the discipline in tandem with technological and scientific progress would put things right, a view that was not challenged by the public. Thus, the accidents in the X-ray laboratories did not trigger any society-wide debate over the safety of the apparatus in question. In 1940, the Swiss X-Ray Society collaborated with the federal Ministry of Health in measuring doses of radiation generated by these X-ray machines, but such investigations remained sporadic and were not mandatory.[60] Discussion of the issue was mostly limited to a small circle of doctors, radiologists and selected lawyers.[61] At this point, the utopian image of the radiation age still remained intact.

New radiation contamination

The positive image of the radiation age could not, however, remain unchallenged after 6 August 1945, the day the USA dropped the first atomic bomb on Hiroshima. The severe physiological effects of ionizing radiation –

a term taken from physics that was adopted by physicians in the 1920s – were analysed by the researchers who comprised the "Atomic Bomb Casualty Commission" sent to Japan to examine the site of the bomb. It now became clear that ionizing radiation caused mutations in living organisms, a phenomenon that geneticists had first observed in the late 1920s.[62]

World War Two turned into the Cold War, and the destructive potential of radiation became associated with the most powerful weapons known to man. This confirmed the place of nuclear physics as the new "leading science" that it had achieved during this war, supported by heavy financial investment from the military. The mid-1950s witnessed the first public debates over atomic energy in Switzerland. The origin of these debates lay in the US-sponsored international conference "Atoms for Peace" that was held in Geneva in August 1955, which sought to advance the cause of "the peaceful use of atomic energy".[63] In the wake of this conference, Paul Scherrer, a professor of physics at the ETH in Zürich, and the entrepreneur Paul Bovery acquired the Geneva experimental atomic reactor, which was put into service as a test reactor in Würenlingen in 1957 by the Reactor Company. At the same time, groups of Swiss officers launched a public discussion about the possibility of providing the Swiss army with nuclear weapons. Paul Scherrer had already been involved in secret discussions with army officers over the possibility of Switzerland developing its own nuclear arsenal. After the parliament announced on 11 July 1958 that it had agreed in principle to supply the army with nuclear weapons, the issue had a much broader public impact. This change in the domestic context, combined with the reports of the numerous nuclear tests carried out abroad, explains why in the 1950s people started thinking about radiation differently from how they had thought about it in the 1930s and 1940s. This change in perspective started with the small circle of experts and eventually spread to the general public. The inauguration by the parliament of a "Commission for Monitoring Radioactivity" under the direction of the physicist Professor Paul Huber from Basel in 1955 bears witness to the development of social awareness concerning the dangers of nuclear radiation. The commission set up measurement stations throughout the country to measure radioactivity in the air, soil, food and the human body, indicating that the state had assumed the role of providing protection against radiation.

In 1955, the Swiss federal public health authority published the first guidelines covering radiation in medical use in laboratories, trade and manufacturing industry, the latter being directed at the radium dial paint industry.[64] Although these guidelines were not legally binding, they nevertheless represent the first initiative undertaken by the medical profession in partnership with research laboratories and industry, and furthermore, they were published by a government body rather than by the private X-Ray Society. The guidelines were drawn up by a technical committee consisting of medical professionals, physicists, chemists, as well as representatives of insurance companies and lawyers.

On 25 November 1957, following a referendum, the Swiss changed their constitution, granting the federal government exclusive authority to legislate on issues of atomic energy, thereby enabling the parliament to issue regulations concerning protection against ionizing radiation. Thus, a "Federal law on the peaceful use of atomic energy and protection against ionizing radiation" came into effect on 1 July 1960.[65] This formed the legal basis for the elaboration of further Swiss federal regulations dealing with protection against radiation, and the creation of a "Department for Protection Against Radiation" as part of the public health authority.

The negotiation of the regulations concerning protection against radiation

The 1950s witnessed the introduction of radioactive emissions and X-rays as a topic of discussion in the political arena. The politicization of this issue, which for over half a century had been a topic of discussion almost exclusively confined to scientific circles, was in part due to the fact that many of the participants who were concerned with the topic of protection against radiation for professional reasons were also involved in the much more public debates over the nuclear armament of Switzerland.

The man who was chosen to direct the newly-created "Department for Protection Against Radiation" on 1 October 1958 was the 38-year-old biologist and schoolteacher Gerhart Wagner.[66] This biologist had already become actively engaged in the struggle against the introduction of atomic weapons into Switzerland even before the parliament's public announcement on 11 July 1958 in support of this initiative. To this end, he had collected a lot of material concerning radioactivity and gave public lectures on the subject.[67] Thus, the motivations of Wagner as he coordinated the elaboration of the regulations concerning protection against radiation over the next five years were always allied with his politically marked anti-nuclear stance with respect to the Swiss army. Although he endorsed the civilian use of nuclear energy, the dangers connected with its military deployment seemed more alarming. Gerhart Wagner, was not, however, the only scientist to present himself as a radiation expert in the public debate over nuclear weapons in Switzerland. On the other side of the debate there were Paul Huber, physics professor at the University of Basel, and Hans Rudolf Schinz, Professor of Radiology at the University of Zürich, who gave talks in favour of the Swiss having nuclear weapons. In 1959, both these professors contributed to a brochure produced by the Swiss Education Service (*Schweizerischen Aufklärungs-Dienst* or SAD).[68] The brochure built up both military and scientific arguments for the introduction of nuclear weapons into Switzerland. The text written by the radiologist Hans Rudolf Schinz was about "radiation damage to the body and genetic material" and ended with the claim that Switzerland needed atomic weapons. Schinz, who willingly presented himself to the public as an expert in protection against radiation, and who in 1958 voted to outlaw the pedoscope due to the additional radiation exposure it caused, did not think that equipping Switzerland with atomic weapons would pose the same danger.[69] The communist "East", in the eyes of this radiologist at least, represented a greater danger than this kind of radiation. Schinz not only took this stance in the political arena. In 1962 he wrote the following in a widely read medical periodical:

> Thus it follows that as our soldiers want and have to defend our homeland against foreign attack only the best weapons are good enough. We cannot use rifles to fight against nuclear weapons. Western pacifist groups do not realize that by means of their propaganda they are working hand in hand with communism at the very moment when the free West is engaged in a life and death ideological struggle against the communist East.[70]

Gerhard Wagner's interest in protection against radiation was initially aroused by his concern about the dangers that nuclear weapons posed to living organisms. In the subsequent years he spent as a civil servant working on this area, he was concerned with the question of how the state could control and regulate the use of radioactive material in medicine, industry and scientific research. Establishing the regulations for protection against radiation followed a typical form of negotiation in which agreement had to be reached between various different disciplines and institutions. The thirty-strong technical committee consisted of chemists, physicists, physicians, lawyers, representatives of insurance companies, the SUVA and factory inspectors. The guidelines from 1955 as well as the international agreements such as that established by the United Nations' Scientific Committee on the Effects of Radiation served as a basis for negotiation. In October 1961, a first draft of the main proposal was presented to the public. Around 250 federal or cantonal representatives, societies, companies, parties, trade unions and private individuals expressed their views on the proposal in a public hearing.[71] The revised version was finally approved by parliament on 19 April 1963, and passed into law on 1 May of the same year. This process represents a highly differentiated procedure issuing in a "socially robust" form of regulation.[72] Possible conflicts were identified and defused through compromise during the initial process. Two topics proved particularly controversial: first the question of the professional competence of the chiropractor in the field of radiography; and second the demand for a ban on the pedoscope.

A conflict between the physicians and the chiropractors concerning the use of X-ray apparatus arose early on in the negotiations.[73] Chiropractors were part of a relatively young profession at this time, being recognised by only thirteen Swiss cantons in 1962.[74] Nevertheless, the question of recognizing chiropractors in Switzerland had already given rise to violent confrontations during the 1930s.[75] These conflicts resurfaced in the 1960s, with the physicians demanding that the chiropractors only be allowed to treat one of their patients at the physician's explicit request.[76] When it came to drawing up the regulations for protection against radiation, the physicians, and in particular the radiologists, demanded that the chiropractors should only be permitted to perform radiography on the upper part of the spinal column. They justified this restriction by suggesting that preparing X-rays of a wider area brought the beam of radiation too close to the gonads. The chiropractors for their part stressed the necessity of evaluating the position of the whole of the spinal column as well as the pelvic girdle for their work. Thus they needed to be able to obtain radiographs of the whole area.[77] In turn, the chiropractors accused the physicians of trying to use the regulations for protection against radiation to foil them, undermining their position just because the physicians perceived them as unwanted intruders in the Swiss medical market. The technical committee responsible for putting together the proposal on protection against radiation was reluctant to stop chiropractors from using radiography for legal reasons, as such a ban would have "represented a singular infringement of the freedom of medical professional practice" as specified in the medical legislation. Thus, chiropractors would be allowed to take radiographs, but only after they had passed an examination administered by the Swiss state, and so the radiologists failed in their attempt to use these guidelines to marginalize their opponents.[78] Most of the members of the technical committee, like the federal authorities themselves, did not see a great difference between the established and the new medical professions, and so accepted that chiropractors obtain their X-ray licenses. The mandatory examination to obtain this license represented a compromise between the different camps, as a physician who had a regular Swiss federal diploma did not need to sit the examination.

A second controversial point for the committee was the question of whether or not to ban the pedoscope. This device, which had proved so popular in Swiss shoe shops, had been the target of criticism in the medical literature as early as 1957. Following a report of a case of dermatitis of the feet attributed to the use of a pedoscope that was published in the December 1957 issue of the *British Medical Journal* the instrument was immediately criticised by both the radiologists and the Cantonal health authorities.[79] Although no case of cancer caused by the pedoscope was ever reported in Switzerland, a child did lose his life after being electrocuted by a faulty pedoscope.[80] In October 1958, the public health authority of the Canton of Waadt banned the use of the pedoscope for children under 12, on the grounds that the reproductive organs of small children were particularly exposed to radiation by these machines.[81] At the end of May 1959, chemists working for the city and the canton conducted measurements of the X-ray apparatus in a Zürich shoe shop and came up with disturbing results. At a distance of one meter, the measured dose was fifteen times greater than the maximum recommended dose proposed in the 1955 guidelines. These results also alarmed the technical committee working on the regulations for protection against radiation, and on 4 June 1959 they decided permanently to outlaw the approximately 1,500 pedoscopes in Switzerland. Assuming that each pedoscope was used ten times a day, the committee arrived at the estimate of four and a half million irradiations per year, the same figure as all the medical radiological investigations conducted in Switzerland. The ban was not, however, based on the high dose of radiation used, but was seen as a measure to prevent the effects of all "unnecessary" radiation, as the population was already being exposed to much higher doses of radiation due to the existence of atomic reactors and nuclear weapons testing.[82] By outlawing what was seen as unnecessary radiation, the committee introduced a central concept that would guide the preparation of these regulations aimed at protecting the population from such radiation.[83] The goal was not only the reduction of individuals' exposure to radiation, but also the protection of the genetic material of the whole population. Arguments that combined considerations of politics and population ("protection of the family taking the future into account"[84]) were combined with an estimate of the utility of the different uses of radiation to form the basis for the justification of any such ban. The decision to accept a risk should depend on a concomitant estimation of the utility associated with it.

Members of the shoe industry and the importers of the apparatus rejected this ban, and for the next few months fought vehemently against what they considered to be a disproportionate reaction. They questioned the legal basis of such a ban, arguing that the use of this apparatus was well-established and contributed to the reduction of foot damage due to badly-fitting shoes.[85] The commission was now faced with a dilemma; should they push the ban through, and possibly see it challenged in the courts, or should they try to make a deal with the shoe industry? Furthermore, the physicians and physicists did not have a long-term interest in imposing on the use of X-rays national limitations that were too strict, as these could serve to provoke wider public fears and debates over the risk of ionizing radiation, and they also had little interest in seeing the state assume too extensive a range of authority over the regulation of the use of X-rays. In October 1959, Gustave Joyet, the director of a betatron and isotope laboratory at the University Hospital at Zürich, argued against a ban, favouring instead the introduction of strict norms and controls: "In my opinion we should not use the ephemeral fear of radiation to justify taking totalitarian measures, but rather we should try skillfully to protect and encourage the useful applications of this radiation."[86] Instead of a prohibition, which threatened to endanger research by its capacity to alarm the public, the pedoscope needed to be subjected to standards concerning the doses of radiation delivered, just like any other piece of X-ray apparatus.

The result of the controversy over the pedoscope, which dragged on for five years, was the introduction of regulations that radically limited their use.[87] The shoe industry could only use machines that had been examined by the Swiss Electrical Engineering Society and had received a license from the Swiss public health authority, and they had to be clearly labelled as X-ray machines. Finally, their use on children under ten years old was strictly forbidden. These measures were aimed at eliminating the pedoscope, as these machines were publicized by the shoe industry precisely for the purpose of fitting children's shoes. Nevertheless, in November 1963 the industry reluctantly communicated these new regulations to their members.[88]

In 1963, Bally introduced a new model for the X-ray apparatus for fitting shoes (the Ultra Model Orthoscope), that was guaranteed to be safe and "corresponded to the strict standards of the public health authority".[89] All the same, through the report made by the Swiss Electrical Engineering Society and the public health authority in 1969 on the number of licenses granted for these machines, it became clear that they were gradually dying out. Where at the beginning of the 1960s there had been approximately 1,500 pedoscopes in the shoe stores, by the time of the report there were only 110 such machines in use, and in 1970 the number was down to 106.[90] A sales gimmick from a period where people still believed in the positive image of the radiation age now found its place among other hazardous waste.[91] The pedoscope, which had been the pride of the shoe industry in the 1920s, providing the industry with a modern, scientific image as well as a competitive edge, was finished. The disappearance of this machine was a victory for the medical profession and marked the wider introduction of measures aimed at protecting the public against radiation.

In the regulations for protection against radiation that came into force on 1 May 1963, permission to use an X-ray machine for diagnostic purposes was only granted to those in possession of a medical diploma recognized by the Swiss federal government – with the exception of the chiropractors mentioned above, who had to pass a special examination. The state now had the power to enforce the regulations and could seize X-ray machines in case of contravention. The rules also made it a legal requirement that those exposed to radiation in their work receive regular blood check-ups. The regulations also recommended that physicians limit the number of radiographs and irradiations "as far as possible".[92] Thus the responsibility for regulating the use of ionizing radiation was taken out of the hands of physicians and scientists for the first time and placed under national control, under the auspices of the newly created Office for Protection against Radiation (*Amt für Strahlenschutz*). The 1963 regulations for protection against radiation should be understood in terms of the need to impose a national system of control over radioactive material and nuclear energy, which became of particular importance to the state in the 1950s in connection with the new issues of nuclear energy and nuclear weapons. Thus, the use of radiation in science, medicine and industry needed to be brought into line with the regulatory requirements in these other areas. The medical profession did manage to retain the right to train the staff who would work in medical X-ray departments, and the profession was also meant to handle the risks associated with the technique internally. Starting in the 1950s, the radiologists had asked for the introduction of laws "which would strictly limit the human application of X-rays and radioactive isotopes to specially trained physicians" to avoid the procedure slipping "into laymen's hands".[93] Thus, the regulations were in line with this group's professional politics, as they granted a monopoly over the therapeutic and diagnostic use of radiation to radiologists and dermatologists.

Thus, X-rays, which at the beginning of the century had served as the object of utopian futuristic fantasies, had now become the subject of national regulations. A decade after the initial discovery of X-ray radiation, scientists started to acknowledge the dangers associated with this phenomenon, and the first protective measures were introduced. Thus, at least for scientists and doctors in this case, the initial danger was transformed into a risk. Research into the causes of radiation damage, the definition of standards and the reduction of the risk lent legitimacy to the new discipline of radiology that was fighting for its own recognition and the exclusion of non-physicians from the domain. This process initially took place without any intervention from state authorities, with the medical profession left free to regulate its own affairs in the matter. Thus, it was only at the end of the 1950s, when public awareness of ionizing radiation was raised by debates over atomic energy and nuclear weapons, that the issue became a political one and national legislation was drawn up specifically to deal with such radiation.

Notes

1 The following text is based on Monika Dommann, *Durchsicht, Einsicht, Vorsicht. Eine Geschichte der Röntgenstrahlen, 1896–1963*, (Interferenzen; 5), Zürich: 2003.

2 "Ueber die physiologische Wirkung der X-Strahlen", *Schweizerische Blätter für Elektrotechnik und das gesamte Beleuchtungswesen*, 2 (1897), p. 29.

3 "Strahlenschutz bei Schuhdurchleuchtungsapparaten", *Neue Zürcher Zeitung*, 22 Juni 1961.

4 W. C. Röntgen, "Ueber eine neue Art von Strahlen (Vorläufige Mitteilung)". Sitzungsberichte der physikalisch-medicinischen Gesellschaft Würzburg, Würzburg, 1896 (reproduced in George Sarton, 'The Discovery of X-rays', *ISIS*, 26 (1936), pp. 349–64.

5 " 'X' Rays as a Depilatory", in *Lancet*, 9 May 1896, p. 1297.

6 William Rushton, "Sunburn by the Röntgen Rays", *Lancet*, 15 August 1896, p. 492.

7 StAB (Staatsarchiv Bern) BB III b Hochschule Philosophische Fakultät II: Physikalisches Institut 1891–1900. Brief von Aimé Forster an den Erziehungsrat, 15 February 1897.

8 Röntgen, "Ueber die physiologische Wirkung der X-Strahlen", p. 28.

9 Röntgen, "Ueber die physiologische Wirkung der X-Strahlen", p. 28.

10 In the USA, X-rays were introduced as depilatory agents in beauty salons soon after World War Two. Rebecca Herzig, "Removing Roots. 'North American Hiroshima Maidens' and the X Ray", *Technology and Culture*, 40.4 (1999), pp. 723–45.

11 For more on X-ray therapy, see Arne Hessenbruch, "Calibration and Work in the X-Ray Economy, 1896–1928", *Social Studies of Science*, 30.3 (2000), pp. 397–420.

12 "Some Effects of the X-Rays on the Hands", *Nature*, 20 October 1896.

13 *Deutsches Wörterbuch von Jacob und Wilhelm Grimm*, Achter Band, Leipzig: 1893, p. 1970–82.

14 Ulrich Beck, *Risikogesellschaft. Auf dem Weg in eine andere Moderne*, Frankfurt a. M.: 1980.

15 Andrew Abbott, *The System of Professions. An Essay on the Division of Expert Labor*, Chicago: 1988.

16 Niklas Luhmann, *Soziologie des Risikos*, Berlin/New York: 1991.

17 StAB Insel-Akten, Verwaltungsrat, Verwaltungsausschuss 42, 1898–1900. Briefe von Dr. Schenkel an Direktor Surbek, 2 March 1899 and 25 May 1999.

18 Hans Schenkel, "Zur Wirkung der Röntgenstrahlen", in *Correspondenzblatt für Schweizer Ärzte*, 23 (1899), p. 109. "Solche Publikationen, besonders in Tagesblättern, sind sehr geeignet, das Publicum diesem nunmehr für viele Fälle fast unentbehrlichen Hülfsmittel der Diagnose gegenüber misstrauisch zu machen." Compare this with another article on Schenkel: G. Felder, "Redaction des Correspondenzblattes für Schweizer Aerzte", *Correspondenzblatt für Schweizer Ärzte*, 23 (1899), pp. 727–8.

19 Daniel Paul Serwer, *The Rise of Radiation Protection {Mikroform}. Science, Medicine and Technology in Society, 1896–1935. Informal Report*. Brookhaven National Laboratory, Upton, N.Y. Prep.: Biomedical and Environmental Assessment Division; National Center for Analysis of Energy Systems, Washington 1976, pp. 27–107.

20 See Bruno Schürmayer, "Röntgentechnik und fahrlässige Körperverletzung", *Fortschritte auf dem Gebiete der Röntgenstrahlen*, 6 (1902–3), pp. 24–43. Guido Holzknecht, "Die forensische Beurteilung der sogenannten Röntgenverbrennungen", *Fortschritte auf dem Gebiete der Röntgenstrahlen*, 6 (1902–3), pp. 145–52.

21 "A Martyr to Science", *Lancet*, 22 October 1904, p. 1172.

22 Niklas Luhmann, *Soziologie des Risikos*, pp. 30–1.

23 Jahresbericht der Insel- und Aussenkrankenhauskorporation pro 1904, pp. 42–43. Jahresbericht der Insel- und Aussenkrankenhauskorporation pro 1906, p. 52.

24 Ernst Sommer, "Über Blenden und Schutzvorrichtungen im Röntgenverfahren", *Röntgentaschenbuch*, 1 (1908), pp. 70–9.

25 Bruno C. Schürmayer, "Selbstschutz des Röntgenologen gegen Schädigungen durch Röntgenstrahlen", *Röntgentaschenbuch*, 4 (1912), pp. 151–2.

26 H. Albers-Schönberg, "Schutzvorkehrungen für Patienten, Ärzte und Fabrikanten gegen Schädigungen durch Röntgenstrahlen", *Fortschritte auf dem Gebiete der Röntgenstrahlen*, 6 (1902–3), pp. 235–8.

27 *Verhandlungen der Deutschen Röntgen-Gesellschaft*, 3 (1907), p. 26.

28 See Otto Hesse, *Symptomatologie, Pathogene und Therapie des Röntgenkarzinoms*. (Zwanglose Abhandlungen aus dem Gebiete der medizinischen Elektrologie und Röntgenkunde), Leipzig: 1911, pp. 57–9. StaBS (Staatsarchiv Basel-Stadt) Bürgergemeinde Basel E 3,1 Bürgerspital Mitglieder des Pflegeamtes Beamte und Angestellte 1875–1941, Brief Pflegeamt an Bürgerrat Basel, 16 January 1930.

29 In 1910 there were two instruments for measuring doses of radiation that were used in the context of radiation therapy. The Chromoradiometer had been developed by Guido Holzknecht in 1902, and the Sabourat-Noiré patch introduced in 1904, whose use was generalized after World War One. Subsequently, ionizing chambers became the generally accepted measurement technique.

30 Daniel Paul Serwer, *The Rise of Radiation Protection {Mikroform}*, pp. 195–264.

31 Niklas Luhmann, *Soziologie des Risikos*, p. 171.

32 See Hans Rudolf Schinz and F. Zollinger, "Materialsammlung von Unfällen und Schäden in Schweizerischen Röntgenbetrieben", Sonderdruck aus: *Röntgenpraxis*, 2 (1930), p. 1. Compare E. Steiner, "Die zivilrechtliche Haftbarkeit des Röntgenarztes nach schweizerischem Recht", *Schweizerische Ärztezeitung*, 15.29 (1934), pp. 381–4. StAZH (Staatsarchiv Zürich) S 226 b 2: Akten Lina Mächler Gysling und Anna Umbricht.

33 Jahresbericht der Insel- und Aussenkrankenhauskorporation 1925, p. 40.

34 StAZH, S 226 b 1, Röntgeninstitut des Kantonsspitals 1897–1922. Brief der Verwaltung des Kantonsspitals an die Direktion des kantonalen Gesundheitsamtes, betr. neuer Unfallversicherungsvertrag, 10 November 1922.

35 Zürich Financial Services Unternehmensarchiv, A 101 203 589 Typoskript eines Angestellten über die Geschichte der einzelnen Versicherungsarten in der Schweiz (ca. 1930).

36 StAZH, S 226 b 1, Röntgeninstitut des Kantonsspitals 1897–1922, Brief von Sauerbruch an Sekretär des Gesundheitswesens, 5 March 1916.

37 Hans Rudolf Schinz and F. Zollinger, "Materialsammlung von Unfällen und Schäden in Schweizerischen Röntgenbetrieben", p. 59.

38 Hans Rudolf Schinz and F. Zollinger, "Materialsammlung von Unfällen und Schäden in Schweizerischen Röntgenbetrieben", S. 61.

39 Max Hopf, "25 Jahre Schweizerische Röntgen-Gesellschaft", Separatdruck *Schweizerische Medizinische Wochenschrift*, 68.19 (1938), p. 13.

40 These associations were the Swiss Surgical Society (*Schweizerische Gesellschaft für Chirurgie*), the Swiss Dermatological Society (*Schweizerische Gesellschaft für Dermatologie*), the Swiss Society for Accident Medicine (*Gesellschaft Schweizerischer Unfallärzte*), and the Gynecological Society (*Gynäkologische Gesellschaft*).

41 See Hans Rudolf Schinz and F. Zollinger, "Materialsammlung von Unfällen und Schäden in Schweizerischen Röntgenbetrieben", p. 4.

42 Hans Rudolf Schinz and F. Zollinger, "Materialsammlung von Unfällen und Schäden in Schweizerischen Röntgenbetrieben", p. 3.

43 Hans Rudolf Schinz and F. Zollinger, "Materialsammlung von Unfällen und Schäden in Schweizerischen Röntgenbetrieben", p. 19.

44 Hans Rudolf Schinz and F. Zollinger, "Materialsammlung von Unfällen und Schäden in Schweizerischen Röntgenbetrieben", p. 39, 41.

45 Hans Rudolf Schinz and F. Zollinger, "Materialsammlung von Unfällen und Schäden in Schweizerischen Röntgenbetrieben", p. 7.

46 W. Molineus, H. Holthusen and H. Meyer (eds), *Ehrenbuch der Radiologen aller Nationen*, Berlin 1992, pp. ix–x.

47 Daniel Paul Serwer, *The Rise of Radiation Protection {Mikroform}*, pp. 232–6.

48 Hans Rudolf Schinz and F. Zollinger, "Materialsammlung von Unfällen und Schäden in Schweizerischen Röntgenbetrieben", p. 42.

49 "Die gesetzliche Regelung der Röntgentätigkeit in der Schweiz", *Schweizerische Ärztezeitung*, 15.29 (1934), p. 402.

50 MedHistBE (Medizinhistorisches Institut Bern) Archiv der Schweizerischen Gesellschaft für Medizinische Radiologie (SGMR), formerly the Schweizerische Röntgen-Gesellschaft. Richtlinien für die Erstellung und Führung von medizinischen Röntgenanlagen. See also Adolf Liechti, "Die Neuausgabe der 'Richtlinien für die Erstellung und Führung von medizinischen Röntgenanlagen' durch die Schweizerische Röntgengesellschaft", *Schweizerische Ärztezeitung*, 15.29 (1934), pp. 398–401.

51 Hans Rudolf Schinz and F. Zollinger, "Materialsammlung von Unfällen und Schäden in Schweizerischen Röntgenbetrieben", p. 65. Hans Rudolf Schinz, "Röntgenschädigungen", Sonderabdruck aus: *Schweizerische Medizinische Wochenschrift*, 58.8 (1928), p. 2.

52 MedHistBE Archiv der Schweizerischen Gesellschaft für Medizinische Radiologie (SGMR), formerly the Schweizerische Röntgen-Gesellschaft. Richtlinien für die Erstellung und Führung von medizinischen Röntgenanlagen, p. 1.

53 On the history of the pedoscope in the USA and UK, see Jacalyn Duffin and Charles R. Hayter, "Baring the Sole. The Rise and Fall of the Shoe-Fitting Fluoroscope", *Isis*, 91 (2000), pp. 260–82.

54 See, for example, "Wie steht es mit den Aussichten für die Mass-Schuhmacherei?", *Schweizerische Schuhmacher-Zeitung*, 53.13 (1927), pp. 205–6.

55 See the Bally company archive (Schönewerd), campaign for Bally-Vasano-Schuhe including a publicity film. "Die 'Doktor-Stiefel' ", *Schweizerische Schuhmacher-Zeitung*, 51

(1925), p. 376. "Die sog. 'Doktor-Stiefel' ", *Schweizerische Schuhmacher-Zeitung*, 53.23 (1927). "Die moderne Folter", *Schweizerische Schuhmacher-Zeitung*, 57 (1931), pp. 5–6.

56 Bally company archive, Brochure "Hurra ich gehe" (1931), p. 3.

57 Bally company archive, Prospekt Winter 1931/1932.

58 Hans Rudolf Schinz and F. Zollinger, "Materialsammlung von Unfällen und Schäden in Schweizerischen Röntgenbetrieben", pp. 20–1.

59 BAG (Bundesamt für Gesundheit Liebefeld) Strahlenschutz 18.10.–23/63 Pedoskop. Tätigkeitsberichte SEV 1970 and 1971.

60 W. Minder, "Vorläufige Ergebnisse der Strahlenschutzmessungen", *Helvetica Medica Acta*, 1940, pp. 97–9.

61 On the social perception of risk, see Adalbert Evers and Helga Nowotny, *Über den Umgang mit Unsicherheit. Die Entdeckung der Gestaltbarkeit von Gesellschaft*, Frankfurt a. M.: 1987.

62 Susan M. Lindee, *Suffering Made Real. American Science and the Survivors at Hiroshima*, Chicago: 1994. On the history of research on radioactivity, see Lawrence Badash, *Radioactivity in America. Growth and Decay of a Science*, Baltimore/London: 1979. For an overview of the history of radiation damage, see Samuel J. Walker, *Permissible Dose. A History of Radiation Protection in Twentieth Century*, Berkeley: 2000.

63 The following claim is based on Dominique Benjamin Metzler, "Die Option einer Nuklearbewaffnung für die Schweizer Armee 1945–1969", *Zeitschrift des Schweizerischen Bundesarchives. Studien und Quellen*, 23 (1997), pp. 121–69. Peter Hug, "Atomtechnologieentwicklung in der Schweiz zwischen militärischen Interessen und privatwirtschaftlicher Skepsis", in Bettina Heintz and Bernhard Nievergelt (eds), *Wissenschafts- und Technikforschung in der Schweiz. Sondierungen einer neuen Disziplin*, Zürich: 1998, pp. 225–42. Patrick Kupper, *Atomenergie und gespaltene Gesellschaft. Die Geschichte des gescheiterten Projektes Kernkraftwerk Kaiseraugst*, (Interferenzen; 4), Zürich: 2003. Tobias Wildi, *Der Traum vom eigenen Reaktor. Die schweizerische Atomtechnologieentwicklung 1945–1969*, (Interferenzen; 5), Zürich: 2003.

64 Eidgenössisches Gesundheitsamt Bern (ed.), *Schutz gegen Röntgenstrahlen. Auszug aus den Richtlinien für den Schutz gegen ionisierende Strahlen in der Medizin, in Laboratorien, Gewerbe- und Fabrikationsbetrieben*, Bern: 1955. On the social history of the radium industry and radiation, see Claudia Clark, *Radium Girls. Women and Industrial Health Reform. 1910–1935*, Chapel Hill, London: 1997.

65 BAR (Bundesarchiv Bern) 3801 1975/8 Tschudi Band 1975: Eidgenössisches Departement des Innern. Verordnung über den Schutz vor ionisierenden Strahlen. Draft November 1962.

66 The following claims are based on an interview with Gerhart Wagner (Stettlen 22. September 2000). See also Gerhart Wagner, *Wissen ist unser Schicksal. Wir Menschen und die Atomkernenergie*, Ostermundigen-Bern: 1979.

67 These speeches, delivered along with speeches by Colonel A. Ernst and Pastor W. Lüthi from Berne in the Spring of 1958, are published together in A. Ernst, G. Wagner and W. Lüthi, *Schweizerische Atombewaffnung?* Referate gehalten in Basel: 4–6 November 1958, Zollikon: 1958.

68 Schweizerischer Aufklärungs-Dienst (ed.), *Probleme der Schweizer Atombewaffnung I. Mit Texten von Paul Huber, Hans R. Schinz und Eugen Studer*, (Schriften des SAD), Bern: 1959. Schweizerischer Aufklärungs-Dienst (ed.), *Probleme der Schweizer Atombewaffnung II. Auseinandersetzungen*, (Schriften des SAD), Bern: 1961.

69 "Strahlenschutz bei Schuhdurchleuchtungsapparaten", *Neue Zürcher Zeitung*, 22 June 1961.

70 Hans Rudolf Schinz, "Der Mensch im Atomzeitalter", Sonderdruck *Schweizerische Medizinische Wochenschrift*, 92.15 (1962), p. 32.

71 BAG Strahlenschutz 18.1.1.–4k: Vernehmlassung zum definitiven Entwurf der Verordnung über den Schutz vor ionisierender Strahlen (VO).

72 Helga Nowotny, Peter Scott and Michael Gibbons, *Re-Thinking Science. Knowledge and the Public in an Age of Uncertainity*, Cambridge: 2001.

73 BAG Strahlenschutz 18.1.1.–4k: Vernehmlassung zum definitiven Entwurf der Verordnung über den Schutz vor ionisierender Strahlen (VO). Brief des EDI an den Präsidenten der Schweizerischen Gesellschaft für Radiologie und Nuklearmedizin und den Präsidenten der Verbindung für Schweizer Ärzte.

74 StABS SD-REG 5 (1) 1–70–0 Akten des Gesundheitsamtes Basel-Stadt betr. Chiropraktiker. Broschüre: Warum heilt Chiropraktik?

75 Ambrosius von Albertini *et al.*, *Gutachten über die Chiropraktik*, Zürich: 1937.

76 J. Zemp, "Medizin und Chiropraxis", *Schweizerische Ärztezeitung*, 27 (1960), pp. 456–64.

77 BAG Strahlenschutz 18.1.1.–4k: Vernehmlassung zum definitiven Entwurf der Verordnung über den Schutz vor ionisierender Strahlen (VO). Aktennotiz von G. Wagner über die Besprechung vom 26. Oktober mit Dr. med. Renfer und den Herren Lorez, Basel und Sandoz, Genf (Chiropraktikern). 30 October 1962.

78 BAR 3801 1975/8 Tschudi Band 1975: Eidgenössisches Departement des Innern. Verordnung über den Schutz vor ionisierenden Strahlen. Entwurf November 1962.

79 See H. Kopp, "Radiation Damage Caused By Shoe-Fitting Fluoroscope", *British Medical Journal*, December 7 1957, pp. 1344–5.

80 BAG, Strahlenschutz 18.10.–23/13: Schuhdurchleuchtungsapparate. Brief Justiz- und Sanitätsdepartement SG an BAG, 3 August 1959.

81 BAG, Strahlenschutz 18.10.–23/1: Schuhdurchleuchtungsapparate. Brief vom Kantonsarzt Ch. Bavaud an die Schuhgeschäfte, 7 October 1958.

82 BAG, Strahlenschutz 18.10.–23/16: Schuhdurchleuchtungsapparate. Brief von Prof. Dr. J. Müller (Frauenklinik Zürich) an Regierungsrat J. Heusser. 9 October 1959.

83 See, for example, Hans Rudolf Schinz, "Erbmasse und ionisierende Strahlung", Special issue: *Verhandlungen der Schweizerischen Naturforschenden Gesellschaft*, Bern: 1958.

84 BAG, Strahlenschutz 18.10.–23/31: Schuhdurchleuchtungsapparate. Votum von Dr. Sauter, Direktor des Gesundheitsamtes anlässlich der Besprechung mit Vertretern des Schweizerischen Schuhhändlerverbandes, 8 March 1960.

85 BAG, Strahlenschutz 18.10.–23/47: Schuhdurchleuchtungsapparate. Brief der Hug & Co AG an das Eidgenössische Gesundheitsamt, 19 May 1960.

86 BAG, Strahlenschutz 18.10.–23/22: Schuhdurchleuchtungsapparate. Brief von G. Joyet an die Gesundheitsdirektion des Kantons Zürich, 16 October 1959.

87 BAG, Strahlenschutz 18.10.–23/165: Schuhdurchleuchtungsapparate. Vorschriften über den Strahlenschutz bei Schuhdurchleuchtungsapparaten. Entwurf Mai 1963. Eidgenössisches Departement des Innern, "Ab 1. November 1963: Eidgenössische Vorschriften für die Schuhdurchleuchtungsapparate", *Der Schuhhandel*, 45/21 (1963), pp. 389–91.

88 Eidgenössisches Departement des Innern, "Ab 1. November 1963: Eidgenössische Vorschriften für die Schuhdurchleuchtungsapparate", *Der Schuhhandel*, 45.21 (1963), p. 390.

89 Firmenarchiv Bally, Publicity "Orthoscope Modell Ultra" (1963).

90 BAG, Strahlenschutz 18.10.–23/63 Pedoskop. Tätigkeitsberichte SEV 1970 and 1971.

91 BAG, Strahlenschutz 18.10.–23: Pedoskop. Brief von Frieda Studer an das Eidgenössische Gesundheitsamt, 25 January 1969.

92 BAR 3801 1975/8 Tschudi Band 1975: Eidgenössisches Departement des Innern. Verordnung über den Schutz vor ionisierenden Strahlen. Entwurf November 1962.

93 Hans Rudolf Schinz, "Erbmasse und ionisierende Strahlung", p. 35.

7   The population as patient

Alice Stewart and the controversy over low-level radiation in the 1950s

Sarah Dry

Introduction

In early 1956, Alice Stewart, a 50-year-old doctor and assistant director of the Institute of Social Medicine at Oxford, visited the first of 203 local public health departments she would call on that year. Travelling by train and funded by a £1000 grant from the Lady Tata Memorial Fund for Leukaemia Research, she was seeking cooperation in carrying out a survey designed to investigate the causes of leukaemia. The Oxford Survey of Childhood Cancers, as the project would come to be known, had been prompted by a 1955 paper by her colleague, David Hewitt, at the Oxford Centre for Social Medicine that indicated a startling rise in leukaemia rates in developed countries. Hewitt had shown that the chances of a newborn male dying of leukaemia had nearly tripled between 1930 and 1955. Deaths from leukaemia, though a small proportion of total deaths, were noteworthy because, as Hewitt put it, "the years of potential life lost by death from leukaemia were disproportionately great".[1] In other words, many children were dying from leukaemia, especially children between two and four years old, an age when children were traditionally less likely to perish from malignant disease. The rate of increase of leukaemia deaths was also striking, outpacing all other causes of death save lung cancer and coronary thrombosis. This finding was statistically very unusual. As Hewitt put it, "This abrupt, upward change in mortality has no parallel in any other cause of death for which statistics are available ... This phenomenon appears ... to have become more important during recent years."[2]

Hewitt concluded that the rise in leukaemia was most likely due to "some new factor (or factors) in the environment, which has been operating for twenty-five years at least, and possibly since the 1860s".[3] Dietary habits, new pharmaceuticals and X-rays were all mentioned as possible causes, with this last factor receiving special discussion:

> The use of X rays goes back to the beginning of the century. X rays are known to act as a leukaemogen or co-leukaemogen on laboratory animals, and are thought to be responsible for the one established

example of occupational risk of leukaemia. Gamma radiation has also been incriminated as a cause of leukaemia in survivors from the atomic explosions in Japan.[4]

The survey offered Stewart an opportunity to investigate a possible new cause of leukaemia, and she took Hewitt's hint into account. Working with Hewitt and two other colleagues, Josephine Webb and Dawn Giles, she designed an alluringly straightforward survey. Death certificates were searched to identify all children who had died in England between 1953 and 1955 from leukaemia or other malignant disease. Public health departments were contacted and their cooperation was sought in locating the mothers of these children: they were then interviewed to establish their medical history, their child's medical history, and a host of other details. These were the cases with which Stewart's survey was primarily interested. Would there be certain shared experiences among them? A control group was established by pairing a living child, of the same age, sex and home town, with each dead child. The mothers of the paired dead and live children were interviewed by the same person, as a control against any possible recording differences between interviewers. All mothers were asked the same questions about their past health, eating habits, prenatal care, and previous or subsequent pregnancies.

By the late summer of 1956, Stewart's train journeys and the modest grant had yielded a startling result. Based on a preliminary sample of 500 pairs of living and dead children, the results, according to Stewart, were quite clear:

> *Yes* was turning up three times for every dead child to once for every live child, for the question "have you had an obstetric x-ray?" *Yes was running three to one.* It was an astonishing difference. It was a shocker. They were alike in all respects except on that score. And the dose was very small, very brief, a single diagnostic x-ray, a tiny fraction of the radiation exposure considered safe, and it wasn't repeated. It was enough to almost double the risk of an early cancer death.[5]

After the early data had been refined, it appeared that twice (not three) times as many mothers of dead children reported being X-rayed during pregnancy as did mothers of living children, still a remarkable finding. Stewart published her initial findings in a preliminary report in the *Lancet* in September 1956.

Almost immediately the results turned heads. In 1927, H. J. Muller's work on *Drosophila melanogaster* (for which he received the Nobel Prize) had indicated that low doses of X-ray radiation could damage genetic material in flies, but ordinary X-rays had long been considered safe.[6] Recent studies on atomic bomb survivors and fallout from weapons testing had heightened awareness of the deleterious genetic effects caused by even low levels of ionizing radiation – the type of radiation produced by X-rays, atomic bombs and cosmic rays. Stewart's findings suggested that, in addition to this threat to future generations, something as simple and seemingly harmless as a diagnostic X-ray could harm the unborn individual as well. X-rays, previously believed to deliver doses of radiation under a safe threshold, would have to be re-evaluated.

Stewart herself had failed to capture her original statistical quarry: a cause which would account for the *total* rise in leukaemia over the past twenty-five years. What she had uncovered accounted for just 6 to 7 per cent of the increased mortality that Hewitt had identified: of the 547 children in her initial survey who had died of malignant disease, just forty could be counted as "extra" X-ray-related deaths. Five hundred, according to Stewart, had contracted cancer by other means. But as the response to her findings would show, numbers alone did not drive the ensuing debate. Tragic at any moment, the dead children identified by Stewart's findings as potential victims of X-rays took on added importance because of the role they played in an on-going debate over the uses and effects of radiation in both wartime and peacetime.[7]

Disciplinary factors played a central role in the debate over Alice Stewart's findings. Practitioners of clinical medicine, and researchers in social medicine, statistical epidemiology, and government-based health physics responded to the results based on the aims of their research and the questions their training equipped them to answer. Tremendous energy and resources, both intellectual and financial, were expended trying to confirm or deny Stewart's results. But even if some agreement could be reached on what counted as good results, those results were still inadequate for resolving the debate. In fact, those shared results often became central features of bitterly contested disputes over what action was required. Though a definite answer was sought to the question of safe thresholds, an answer based on well-substantiated evidence, I will show that such an answer was in the end insufficient for resolving the question of what constitutes an acceptable risk. The history of Stewart's results and the reaction they produced instead provides an example of the limitations of scientific disciplines in settling matters of fact and guiding decision-making in areas such as medicine and public policy.

Alice Stewart contributed over 40 years of work to the field of radiation epidemiology after publishing her X-ray results in 1956, yet she remains strangely absent from the institutional history of social medicine and the wider history of twentieth-century medicine.[8] Though this chapter centres on Stewart's results and the response to them, I have focused on the disciplinary rather than the biographical issues revealed by this episode. It is to be hoped that further research on Stewart will be undertaken, facilitated by the recent acquisition of Stewart's personal papers by the Wellcome Library for the History and Understanding of Medicine. Readers should consult Gayle Greene's biography, *The Woman Who Knew Too Much*, to learn more about Stewart's long and varied life.

From tolerance to permissibility: setting standards for radiation protection

Standard-setting is at the core of this story. Like other metrological projects, radiation standards are expressions of scientific authority and require tremendous energy to assert and maintain. The making of the atomic bomb, coupled with rising awareness of the genetic risk of low-level radiation, and the somatic risk of higher doses, led to the consolidation of a scientific discipline dedicated to radiation protection, safety and measurement. Health physics, as the new discipline was known, was born on the Manhattan Project, when atomic physicists struggled to create protocols for protecting more people against more powerful radioactive materials than ever before. Many of the first health physicists were members of the two bodies responsible for setting radiation standards, the US-based National Committee on Radiation Protection (NCRP) and the International Committee on Radiation Protection (ICRP), where they exerted considerable influence.[9]

Early standards had been defined as tolerance doses, implying that anything below the given dose would be tolerated and safe. In the first three decades of the twentieth century, the erythema dose, or the amount of radiation required to visibly redden the skin, was considered a basic threshold dose. A given fraction of this amount was considered safe, though sensitivity between individuals was known to vary by up to 1,000 per cent. In 1934, a tolerance dose of 0.2 roentgens per day was recommended. The ICRP advised a lowered limit of 0.1 roentgens per day in 1936, and standards continued to be lowered through the 1950s.[10]

After World War Two, studies on survivors of the atomic bombs at Hiroshima and Nagasaki generated more data for health physics, prompting further changes in standards.[11] Perhaps the most important shift took place in 1949, when the concept of maximum permissible dose per year was introduced, signalling a retreat from an implicit safe threshold and an awareness of the potential for risk presented by any level of radiation. Rather than certifying absolute safety, the "maximum permissible dose" concept implied that even low-level radiation doses posed some risks to humans, but that, in the name of industry, medicine or defence, they could be regulated and sanctioned. For the first time, the balance between risks and benefits became a key concept in radiation protection. In the same year, the NCRP developed new recommendations for workers based on a maximum permissible annual dose of 15 rem.[12]

By 1954, it was clear that man-made radiation posed a hazard to the general public as well as to workers in radiation-related industries. Until then, radiation standards had been designed to protect those who worked with radiation, most commonly in the nuclear, medical or mining professions. The ICRP explicitly stated a new objective to set standards for "larger groups of persons, or whole populations, which might be exposed to radiation by radioactive materials, either natural or artificial, in very small quantities in water or food, as well as irradiation from radioactive materials in the atmosphere and contamination of the earth's surface".[13] Given what the ICRP called "scanty" data on the effects of radiation on large populations, it recommended limiting the reproductive organ dose to what it saw as a conservative limit: "an amount of the order of magnitude of the natural background". This amount was in addition to that received from the natural background radiation. The ICRP also tied the recommended dose for the public to the existing worker limits, suggesting that the public should be exposed, at a maximum, to one-tenth of the occupational limit. Based on the then-current standard, this amounted to 1.5 rem. In 1956, this maximum permissible dose was further lowered to 0.5 rem per year, where it remains today.[14]

The standard-setting activities of the ICRP and NCRP implied authority on a topic which had been, as falling threshold levels revealed, frequently misjudged. Though the language of standard guidelines cautioned against viewing "maximum permissible doses" as "safe" thresholds, the setting of any standard gave a simultaneous impression of danger (the organization feels the need to limit exposure) and safety (the organization assures the citizen that *this* level is harmless). This internal contradiction, especially salient in the low-level radiation debate, would affect the reception of Stewart's findings among health physicists. The suggestion that *any* dose, no matter how small, could be harmful (even if it was acknowledged in the qualified language of the guidelines' fine print) had the potential to undermine the public's trust in organizations such as the ICRP and NCRP, which lent their authority to recommendations on standards. The fact that maximum permissible dose limits remain the same today as they were in 1956 suggests that, Stewart's results and subsequent research notwithstanding, no further rationale for lowering standards could be generated.[15]

The MRC and NAS reports to the public on the hazards of radiation

While international standards organizations like the ICRP made recommendations, widespread concern over radioactive fallout prompted two important reports on the effects of radiation on humans. Published simultaneously in June 1956, reports of the American National Academy of Sciences (NAS) and the British Medical Research Council (MRC) both contained information on the results of studies on survivors of the atomic bomb, patients exposed to high doses of X-rays as part of a therapy, and death rates among radiologists. Both used the level of normal background radiation, caused by cosmic rays and radioactive elements in food and housing materials, as a standard against which to judge 'extra' man-made radiation.[16]

Long-term genetic damage due to radiation-induced mutation received most attention. The NAS genetics committee provided estimates of the total radiation exposure a person living in the United States could be expected to receive over thirty years, the average age at parenthood. They estimated that background radiation, caused by cosmic rays and radioactive elements in homes and food, accounted for 4.3 r[oentgens] over 30 years. Fallout from weapons testing, based on fallout data from the past five years, was estimated at between 0.02 r to 0.5 r over 30 years. Medical X-rays, used for treatment and diagnosis, accounted for an estimated 3 r over 30 years. The NAS report concluded that a dose of 10 r, or double the background radiation level, would be an acceptable "lifetime reproductive (zero to 30 years) limit". This arbitrary dose was considered to be acceptable and thus, in a certain sense, safe, because it was allied to a natural dose, the level of normal background radiation. They recommended that "the general public of the United States be protected, by whatever controls may prove necessary" from receiving more than this dose.[17]

At high doses of radiation, the reports indicated, somatic effects were relatively well catalogued. The highest doses caused acute radiation sickness and death. Early radiologists, exposed to less acute doses but still extremely high levels, had suffered severe inflammation and infection in frequently exposed body parts, such as their arms (often requiring amputation), as well as heightened incidence of leukaemia and acute aplastic anaemia. Patients treated with high doses of X-rays for a variety of conditions had all been documented with higher than normal rates of leukaemia. Despite the evidence for damage to the individual at high doses, the MRC report assured its readers that "relatively heavy doses of radiation are required to impair the health of the individual and such doses are rarely associated with the ordinary circumstances of civilian life".[18]

The reports cautioned against careless use of diagnostic X-rays because of the potential for long-term genetic damage from even very small doses. Though the effects at low doses were correspondingly small, the large numbers of people in developed countries such as Britain and the US receiving diagnostic X-rays each year meant that the total number of mutations was potentially large. In fact, while the reports had been commissioned in response to growing anxiety over fallout, both concluded that, while the radioactivity released from fallout was significant and should be watched, it was still a small fraction, perhaps 1 per cent, of normal background radiation. Low-dose diagnostic X-rays (as opposed to the higher doses used for therapies), on the other hand, amounted to at least 22 per cent of background radiation, according to the MRC report, and were, as the report reminded, "in addition to it" and "possibly much more than this".[19] In the United States, the NAS estimated that medical X-rays accounted for nearly 3 and 4 r per person out of the recommended 30 year reproductive lifetime limit of 10 r. "It is really very surprising and disturbing to realize that this figure is so large, and clearly it is prudent to examine this situation carefully. It is folly to incur any medical X-ray exposure to the gonads which can be avoided without impairing medical service or progress."[20]

The MRC singled out two obstetric X-ray examinations that were responsible for the lion's share of contribution to total dosage in the United

States: pelvimetry and abdominal examinations. Pelvimetry, the measurement of a pregnant woman's pelvis often used to determine any possible delivery difficulties, generated especially high doses to the fetus. One pelvimetry (which required between three and five X-ray exposures) subjected the reproductive organs of the fetus to over 2.5 r of radiation, more than half the average annual background radiation in Britain. Mothers receiving pelvimetry were exposed to a reproductive dose of about 1.3 r, more than twice that received from an abdominal X-ray.[21] The stage was set for a reappraisal of diagnostic radiology in general, and obstetric radiology in particular.

Obstetric radiology: "great accuracy is required"

The practice of pelvimetry was fairly routine, dating back to the first uses of X-rays in the early years of the twentieth century. By the 1920s and 1930s, diagnostic X-rays in general, and pelvimetries in particular, had become a standard element in the modern obstetrician's diagnostic armamentarium. The measuring of pelves can be seen as part of a larger campaign, dating from the early twentieth century and lasting until mid-century, to make the obstetrician and the obstetric consultant hospital crucial elements of all pregnancies and childbirths. As obstetrics struggled to distinguish itself from midwifery, pelvimetry offered the allure of modern technology without the troubling dangers such as increased mortality that seemed to accompany other "modern" interventions such as caesarian sections.[22] In other words, pelvimetries did not seem to harm the mother and child. Furthermore, they generated data that obstetricians could use to establish a quantitative research tradition in line with modern medicine. Whether they accomplished their advertised result – the diagnosis of potentially difficult or dangerous labours – is less clear.

Obstetric X-ray examinations, including pelvimetries, were frequently performed in hospitals in England in the early 1950s. Data incorporated in the 1956 MRC report and later published in the *Lancet*, indicated that roughly 10 per cent of all women who delivered full-term babies in the hospital had pelvimetries and that one quarter of all women had abdominal X-ray examinations. In 1954, an estimated 26,000 X-ray pelvimetries and 86,000 obstetric abdominal examinations were performed in England and Wales.[23]

Radiological staff at Queen Charlotte's Maternity Hospital had seemed almost apologetic in reporting that just under 2,000 X-ray exams had been carried out in 1953: "although this number is not very great," they explained in the annual clinical report for that year, "much of the work (pelvimetry and placentography, etc.) is highly specialized and is time consuming because great accuracy is required."[24] Of the 3,045 patients delivered that year, roughly one-third received at least one obstetrical X-ray. Over the next three years, the hospital reported a gradual increase in the use of X-rays.

The MRC and NAS reports occasioned immediate response from physicians. In July 1956, J. Blair Hartley, a doctor at St Mary's Hospital in London, had expressed concern in a letter to the editor of the *Lancet* following the recent publication of the MRC report and the NAS report:

> It is clear from your summaries [of the reports] ... that immediate attention must be given to reduction of X-radiation dosage to patients, under the age of 30 years, from X-ray diagnostic examinations. There is one important step which we can take immediately; and this letter is to implore all British radiologists to take it voluntarily today, now, at once. It is, simply, to forbid absolutely in all X-ray departments under their control the taking of Thoms' brim view of the pelvis *during pregnancy*.[25]

The writer's primary concern, as evidenced by his mention of the age of relevant patients, was with genetic rather than somatic effects. The growing awareness of the risks to patients, including unborn children, of diagnostic X-rays would soon take on a new urgency with the publication of Stewart's findings.

Findings in context: the response to Stewart's results

Response to the publication of Stewart's initial results in the *Lancet* of 1 September 1956 was prompt.[26] The publication was, for one thing, well-timed, appearing just three months after the influential and high-profile MRC and NAS reports. *Lancet* editors drew attention to the report in a leading article as "the first published epidemiological evidence of the hazards of diagnostic radiography to the patient (in this case the unborn)".[27] The central finding of the one-page report was the "one important difference between the children who died and their controls: the number of mothers who had an X ray of their abdomen during the relevant pregnancy was 85 for the cases and only 45 for the controls". According to Stewart and her colleagues, this difference could "hardly be fortuitous". They closed their brief report with the suggestion that "besides causing genetic damage, this apparently harmless examination may occasionally cause leukaemia or cancer in the unborn child".[28] Stewart and her collaborators did not advocate a ban on prenatal X-rays, which they considered a "valuable and essential means of saving life". But despite this clinical judgement, Stewart reiterated the statistical and aetiological significance of her findings on the matter of delayed effects of low-level radiation: "we cannot accept [the] view that the dose of X rays received during a single prenatal examination is too small to be regarded as a plausible cause of later malignant changes".[29] Though she agreed that "the risk to life associated with irradiation *in utero* must be small," Stewart wrote later, "nevertheless our report has a practical implication if the risk of *not* performing an antenatal X ray is also small".[30] In the weeks and months following its publication, the report was the subject of lively correspondence in the *Lancet*. Not everyone was convinced by the "new and extremely powerful" method used by Stewart.

Medical response: "the risk to the fetus"

Some drew attention to the need to balance the risk of a dangerous labour against the very small risk to the unborn child. Rohan Williams, the consultant radiologist at Queen Charlotte's Maternity Hospital, and a colleague wrote forcefully in a letter to the editor of the *Lancet*: "The broad and sweeping condemnation of antenatal radiology [in Stewart's paper] is without justification: the very slight apparent risks of this procedure (as yet unproven) must be weighed against the considerable advantages afforded by the information gained from radiological examination."[31] For others, the risk to the unborn child, however small, was unacceptable. A *Lancet* reader reported that his own wife had been X-rayed while pregnant. "It seems probably that the X-ray examination of my wife has definitely increased the risk of leukaemia in the child. The risk in a particular case, even after irradiation, may not be great; but if this story continues to be repeated, who dare say that the incidence of leukaemia will not be materially increased?"[32]

Other physicians objected to the design of Stewart's study. How could the mothers be trusted to remember events up to ten years earlier? Would the mothers of children who had later died remember certain events, such as prenatal X-rays, more vividly than the mothers of healthy children? One writer cautioned that the study did not take into account "that a pregnancy X-ray examination is not a routine examination" but is a specialized procedure "confined to a highly selective group of mothers". Rather than X-rays causing leukaemia, he asserted, "it seems much more likely that there is some inherent abnormality or morbidity in the mother or fetus which predisposes to the latter development of leukaemia".[33] Underlying disease, he argued, could account for the symptoms leading to the use of X-rays in the first place and its later onset might be completely unrelated to the small dose of radiation received *in utero*.

The response of radiologists and obstetricians at Queen Charlotte's Maternity Hospital indicate that many medical practitioners were quickly convinced to drop the technique based on these preliminary results, suggesting that, for them, the perceived risk of *not* performing an X-ray was indeed small. In 1957, according to the annual clinical report for that year, "there was a striking change in the radiological work at Queen Charlotte's Maternity Hospital". Mentioning Stewart's preliminary study, the radiology department reported that "the effect of this publication has been sharply to limit the number of patients referred for X-ray examination in the antenatal period, and thus the amount of radiological work dropped sharply in 1957".[34]

The dampening effect on the use of prenatal X-rays was lasting. In 1958 and 1959, radiological staff reported considerably lowered use of prenatal

X-rays. By 1960, the separate radiological report had disappeared from annual clinical reports and levels of obstetric X-rays at the hospital were no longer reported.[35]

While many doctors expressed doubt over the causal relationship between prenatal X-rays and childhood cancers, the practical response for many was to act as if there was a link. Disagreement over the validity of Stewart's methods and results existed in conjunction with a widespread desire, based on the findings, to limit prenatal X-rays. Had diagnostic X-ray usage been the subject of an earlier reform, there might not have been room for such *ad hoc* judgements. But given the relatively widespread and casual use of obstetric X-rays, and the recent information on the genetic effects of very small doses of radiation, the decision to limit X-ray use by doctors (who may or may not have been responding to their patients' anxieties) appears to have been fairly straightforward to make and implement.

The epidemiological turn: drawing the dose–response curve

While doctors may have responded to patient anxiety and ambiguous results by applying a precautionary principle, the debate over the relationship between X-rays and childhood cancer continued in epidemiological terms with all the force of a debate over realism. Did X-rays really cause cancer? Or were they merely associated with it? It was conceivable that the need to have an X-ray implied poor health in the mother, which could, in turn, account for the development of leukaemia in the unborn child. In the medical context, the personal judgement of the physician proved adequate for resolving the debate in practical terms. In contrast, the epidemiological debate turned on differing philosophies of survey design and the interpretation of results which hovered at the edge of statistical visibility. Methodological preferences were directed towards solving quantitative problems. Resolution of this debate proved elusive.

One man in particular would play a central role in the epidemiological debate. Richard Doll, then deputy director of the MRC's Statistical Research Unit at the London School of Hygiene and Tropical Medicine, had already carried out an important study on the incidence of leukaemia in patients treated with high doses of X-rays for a painful back condition called ankylosing spondylitis. Doll's study, completed with his boss, William Court Brown, had attempted to determine the so-called "dose–response curve" for radiation, a graphical representation of the relationship between a given dose of radiation and subsequent disease.[36] But while Doll and Court Brown sought the holy grail of one cause and one effect, it was elusive. Based on 13,000 patient records from 81 radiotherapy centres, the study provided evidence of links between high doses of radiation and cancer, but was ultimately inconclusive for low dose levels of X-rays, the very levels Stewart's survey had investigated.[37]

By eliminating the confusion of what were seen as irrelevant factors that create a misleadingly complex epidemiological picture, the dose–response curve was attractive to those such as Doll and Court Brown who thought of epidemiological surveys as experiments. The curve, plotting one dose against one response, suggested clarity and a causal link. Stewart, who made use of subjective patient interviews and emphasized complex environmental factors that resisted precise quantification, was agnostic about such curves. For her, the aim had always been for a greater understanding of the complex aetiology of cancer. The dose–response curve, "often regarded by physicists and biologists as the only epidemiological proof that low-level radiation causes human cancers … is regarded by me and my statistical colleagues as no more than an important link in a relatively long chain of evidence".[38] The paradox for Stewart was to design a study that would balance the multiple background factors in order to reveal their "true" relationship. She saw entire populations as both individual cases and conglomerations of individuals with variable risk profiles, and then attempted to use the tools of individual medicine (i.e. the case history method) to analyse large groups. For the advocates of an experimental approach, this method was messy, unreliable, and could not support valid conclusions of cause and effect, the ultimate point of the project.

Meanwhile, Stewart published a full report in 1958, which bore out her preliminary findings. Out of 1,416 pairs of living and dead children, 107 mothers of dead children had received prenatal X-rays, while just 58 mothers of living children had received them.[39] Doll and Court Brown read these results with interest. They guessed that using their large-scale techniques designed to uncover precise dose–response relationships, they would need to study in the order of twenty million people over ten years. Only with such vast numbers would it be possible to detect an effect at very low doses. Though there were undeniable practical challenges to be overcome in such a study, Doll and Court Brown believed it should be undertaken. "In this era when the medical and industrial uses of atomic energy are expanding so rapidly," they wrote in the *Lancet*, "it is of basic importance to determine whether threshold doses for the induction of these delayed somatic effects exist."[40]

They initiated a study on the very same topic: the incidence of leukaemia after exposure to diagnostic radiation *in utero*. But where Stewart's study had been retrospective, starting with a group of already identified cases, Doll and Court Brown's study was prospective. Rather than starting with a small group of already fatal cases of childhood cancer, Doll and Court Brown started with a large group of women who had been X-rayed while pregnant (though well under the 20 million they had earlier mentioned). Selecting eight hospitals, the pair compiled lists of all the women who had been X-rayed between 1945 and 1956 while pregnant at these hospitals. From radiological records (which eliminated the problem of faulty memory), they gathered information about the date and type of X-ray exam. They then followed the nearly 40,000 children born to these women for up to fourteen years, searching death entries of children who had died of leukaemia between 1945 and 1958 for matching names. They found a total of nine children out of the original 40,000 who had died of leukaemia. The expected number, based on leukaemia death rates for the entire population at the various ages records, was 10.5. In other words, Doll and Court Brown failed to show any increase in leukaemia mortality among children X-rayed prenatally and had, in fact, found slightly fewer than might have been expected. They concluded that while "the existing evidence of the effect of irradiation *in utero* is conflicting", their own results led them to believe that "an increase of leukaemia among children due to radiographic examination of their mother's abdomen during the relevant pregnancy is not established".[41]

By designing a large prospective survey, Doll and Court Brown sought to lay to rest one side of the debate. Their results, if inconclusive, suggested that even if the effect was real, it was too small to measure and thus, in some sense, too small to be of concern. Even starting with 40,000 children, the incidence of leukaemia, radiation-induced or otherwise, was still so low that Doll and Court Brown's results could be attributed to statistical variation rather than the absence of an effect. Their report did not halt research into the problem. The most impressive support for Stewart's finding was the 1962 study by Brian MacMahon, which traced 734,243 babies born in thirty-seven hospitals between 1947 and 1954. Based on a sample of 1 per cent of these babies, MacMahon concluded that prenatal X-rays increased the chances of malignant childhood disease by 42 per cent, less than half what Stewart had found, but still a significant result. Stewart herself continued to publish on the data collected in the Oxford Childhood Cancer Survey, generating dozens of papers. Today, Tom Sorahan, an occupational epidemiologist at the University of Birmingham, continues to mine the data.

Attitudes towards the findings seem to hinge on a version of the scientific realism debate. Were the effects of the X-rays on the unborn children producing real cancers that were, statistically, barely perceptible? Or were the studies producing statistical artifacts? By focusing on dose–response curves, Doll and other epidemiologists sought to frame the debates in terms that only their methods would be suited to answer. Though Stewart and Doll and Court Brown shared more methodological tools with each other than either did with clinical doctors, they disagreed on the best way to measure risks. For Stewart, interviews with the mothers of dead children were powerful devices for uncovering otherwise hidden effects. For Doll and Court Brown, the machinery of a well-funded and cooperative state health-care system could support large prospective studies that sought to eliminate individual variability.

Specifying the dose–response curve at low doses proved to be an abiding concern. In a 1961 report of their own study on the relationship between leukaemia and prenatal X-rays, Josephine Wells and Charles Steer reviewed the state of the research. Two reports indicated a link between X-rays and childhood cancer; four others did not. "It seems to us," they wrote, "therefore, that a causal relation between X-ray examination of the pregnant woman and the development of malignant disease in her offspring has not been demonstrated. On the other hand, one may say just as certainly that a lack of relation has not been demonstrated. Our figures do not allow us to answer this question at present."[42] Conflicting results continued to be published, with Stewart and her colleagues contributing a 1970 paper based on 7,600 case/control pairs that asserted a linear relationship between dose and response down to one X-ray,[43] and a report by scientists at the Atomic Bomb Casualty Commission that found no extra cancer deaths among children exposed prenatally at Hiroshima and Nagasaki.[44]

Despite these differing results, the weight of opinion gradually shifted towards the Stewart results. By 1973, Doll told an audience at the Leukaemia Research Fund that objections to the linear non-threshold dose–response relationship, as it was technically called, were no longer significant. "That children who were irradiated in the third trimester of intra-uterine life develop more leukaemia, and indeed more cancers of all the types that characteristically occur in childhood – has now been demonstrated so often and so consistently that it cannot be challenged."[45]

In the past two decades, the prenatal X-ray issue has gradually dropped from public view, not because the link between low-level radiation and cancer was clearly defined, but because radiologists found other, less controversial ways to image the developing foetus. This elimination of prenatal X-rays from obstetric radiology means that there is no more data to examine. The window on this practice closed with the publication of Stewart's paper, as doctors dramatically reduced their use of prenatal X-rays. Studies of the effects of low-level radiation on animals, which require thousands of research subjects in order to approach meaningful results for very low dose levels, have also failed to provide statistical closure. But even if there was more data, the response to the initial findings indicates that more information would not guarantee agreement on what a safe level of radiation would look like.

Conclusion: science and a risk society

Stewart's results emerged at a precarious moment in the history of radiation when post-war fears clashed with technological optimism. They were controversial, both because they were possibly unfounded and because if they were accurate they had serious ramifications for nuclear testing, occupational safety standards, and medical practice. Disciplinary membership and socio-political profiles help understand the competing approaches to the results and the issues of the day. The medical X-ray issue raised by Stewart's paper was resolved by the medical community fairly fluidly because X-rays were administered in the context of an individual cost–benefit analysis. The issue of fallout was resolved, at least in part, by the Partial Test Ban Treaty of 1963. With the elimination of the main source of political tension, as well as the main source of man-made radiation (save for medical uses), public attention shifted to the safety of nuclear reactors. The epidemiological challenge of identifying any "extra" deaths caused by X-rays gradually dropped from view, not because it was resolved, but because it could not be. No one paper or fact swung opinion in favour of Stewart's camp, but the gradual accretion of supporting results in an atmosphere of continued anxiety about radiation served to ratify her results *de facto*.

The debate over very low levels of radiation and cancer suggests the durability of different philosophies of risk, and their insusceptibility to increased information. But while it reveals the importance of disciplinary factors in debates over what gets to count as evidence, this episode also reveals the limits of using disciplines, particularly scientific disciplines, as units of analysis. While the medical, epidemiological and health physics disciplines helped to shape the debate over Stewart's findings by providing training, motivation and the venues for discussion, action was often based on extra-disciplinary factors.

One surprising result of the disagreement over low-level radiation has been to divorce standard-setting from "scientific" methods in favour of a more moral reasoning. Radiation controls in industry are now associated with the highest costs per year of life saved by "life-saving interventions".[46] The belief that it "can never be too expensive to reduce [radiation] risks" has, somewhat ironically, diminished the importance of radiation protection standards as the desire to keep radiation exposure "as low as reasonably achievable" has led, in some instances, to standards for specific practices that are lower than the dose from natural background radiation. The end result, according to some health physicists, is that radiation protection has become "increasingly distanced from any radiobiological or epidemiological basis".[47] In the end, epidemiological data have become not merely insufficient but irrelevant to radiation safety.

Alice Stewart had been prompted to undertake her survey by a startling and unexplained rise in leukaemia that was occurring in developed countries. The association between technological development and new risks in the modern world lies at the heart of this story, but it does not suggest that scientific solutions are the only acceptable solutions to technological problems, or the only solutions sought.

Notes

1 D. Hewitt, "Some features of leukaemia mortality", *Br J Prev Soc Med*, 9, 1955, p. 81.
2 Hewitt, "Some features", p. 83.
3 Hewitt, "Some features", p. 87.
4 Hewitt, "Some features", pp. 87–8.
5 Gayle Greene, *The Woman Who Knew Too Much: Alice Stewart and the Secrets of Radiation*, Ann Arbor: University of Michigan, 1999, p. 83.

6 H. J. Muller, "Artificial transmutation of the gene", *Science*, 66, 1928, pp. 84–7.
7 There is an extensive literature on the history of atomic radiation in the United States. For authoritative histories on radiation safety and the United States military see: B. Hacker, *The Dragon's Tail: Radiation Safety in the Manhattan Project, 1942–46*, Berkeley: University of California, 1987; and B. Hacker, *Elements of Controversy: The Atomic Energy Commission and Radiation Safety in Nuclear Weapons Testing 1947–1974*, Berkeley: University of California Press, 1994. See also J. Samuel Walker, "The Controversy Over Radiation Safety", *JAMA*, August 4, 1989, 262(5), pp. 664–8; J. Samuel Walker, *Permissible Dose: A History of Radiation Protection in the Twentieth Century*, Berkeley: University of California Press, 2000; J. Samuel Walker, "The Atomic Energy Commission and the Politics of Radiation Protection, 1967–1971" *Isis*, 1994, 85, pp. 57–78; and J. Samuel Walker with G. Mazuzan, *Controlling the Atom: The Beginnings of Nuclear Regulations, 1946–1962*, Berkeley: University of California Press, 1984. For an overview of the history of radiation in the twentieth century, see C. Caulfield, *Multiple Exposures: Chronicles of the Radiation Age*, London: Secker and Warburg, 1989.
8 For the origins of social medicine in the 1940s, see N. T. A. Oswald, "A Social Health Service Without Social Doctors", *The Society for the Social History of Medicine*, 4(2), 1991, pp. 295–315; and D. Porter, "Changing Disciplines: John Ryle and the Making of Social Medicine in Britain in the 1940s", *History of Science*, Vol. 30, 1992, pp. 137–68. See also D. Porter (ed.), *Social Medicine and Medical Sociology in the Twentieth Century*, Amsterdam: Rodopi, 1997.
9 For the history of protection standards, the classic reference is L. Taylor, *Radiation Protection Standards*, Cleveland: CRC Press, 1971. See also A. Brodsky, R. Kathren and C. Willis, "History of the Medical Uses of Radiation: Regulatory and Vol.untary Standards of Protection", *Health Physics*, November 1995, Vol. 69, No 5, pp. 783–823; Stewart Bushong, "History of Standards, Certification, and Licensure in Medical Health Physics", *Health Physics*, November 1995, Vol. 69, No 5, pp. 824–36; and D. C. Kocher, "Perspective on the Historical Development of Radiation Standards", *Health Physics*, Vol. 61, No 4, October 1991, pp. 519–27. For the institutional and political affiliations of members of the NCRP, see Gilbert Whittemore, "The National Committee on Radiation Protection, 1928–1960: From professional guidelines to government regulation", PhD dissertation, Harvard University, 1986. For the same for the ICRP, see Patrick Green, "The Controversy Over Low Dose Exposure to Ionising Radiations", Graduate Thesis, University of Aston, Birmingham, 1984.
10 Bushong, "History of Standards", p. 828. Radiation doses and exposures are measured in a variety of units. The *roentgen* measures the ionization of the air caused by gamma radiation, such as X-rays, without reference to biological effects. The *rad*, or radiation absorbed dose, measures the amount of radiation received by a person. The *rem* takes into account the different biological effects of different kinds of ionizing radiation. Alpha radiation, for example, is approximately ten times more biologically damaging than gamma radiation, so that 1 *rad* of alpha radiation is equivalent to 10 *rems*, while 1 *rad* of gamma radiation is only 1 *rem*. For doses of X-radiation (mostly gamma radiation), the *roentgen*, the *rad* and the *rem* can be considered roughly equivalent, i.e. 1 *roentgen*= 1*rad*=1*rem*.
11 Nearly 1,000 papers were published between 1947 and 1974 on the effects of radiation on the survivors, according to M. Susan Lindee's *Suffering Made Real: American Science and the Survivors at Hiroshima*, Chicago: University of Chicago, 1994, p. 256. For a review of the findings, see W. Schull, *Effects of Atomic Radiation: A Half-century of Studies from Hiroshima and Nagasaki*, New York: Wiley-Liss, 1995.
12 Kocher, "Perspective", p. 520.
13 ICRP Press release 1956, quoted in S. B. Osborn and E. E. Smith, "The Genetically Significant Radiation Dose from the Diagnostic Use of X Rays in England and Wales: A Preliminary Survey", *Lancet*, 16 June 1956, pp. 949–53.

14 Kocher, "Perspective", pp. 520–2. For current standards, see Faiz Khan, "The Physics of Radiation Therapy", 2nd edn, Baltimore: Lippincott Williams and Wilkins, 1994, p. 480.

15 See Kocher, "Perspective", p. 527 for a discussion of the increasing importance of the ALARA (as low as reasonably achievable) principle.

16 National Academy of Sciences, *The Biological Effects of Atomic Radiation Summary Reports*, Washington: National Academy of Sciences/National Research Council, 1956; Medical Research Council, *The Hazards to Man of Nuclear and Allied Radiations*, London: HMSO, June 1956.

17 National Academy of Sciences, "Biological Effects", p. 29.

18 Medical Research Council, "Hazards", p. 48.

19 Osborn and Smith, "Genetically Significant", p. 949, and Medical Research Council, *Hazards to Man*, Appendix K.

20 National Academy of Sciences, *Biological Effects*, p. 30.

21 Osborn and Smith, "Genetically Significant", p. 949.

22 There is an ample literature on twentieth-century developments in pregnancy and childbirth in Britain. See, for example, J. Garcia, R. Kilpatrick and M. Richards (eds), *The Politics of Maternity Care: Services for Childbearing Women in Twentieth-Century Britain*, New York: Clarendon Press, 1990; J. Lewis, *The Politics of Motherhood: Child and Maternal welfare in England, 1900–1939*, Montreal: McGill-Queen's University Press, 1980; and M. Tew, *Safer Childbirth? A Critical History of Maternity Care*, London: Chapman and Hall, 1990.

23 Osborn and Smith, "Genetically Significant", p. 949.

24 London Metropolitan Archives (hereafter LMA) Clinical Report of Queen Charlotte's Maternity Hospital for 1953, H27/QC/A/027/125, p. 7.

25 J. Blair Hartley, Correspondence, *Lancet*, 7 July 1956, p. 46.

26 A. Stewart *et al.*, "Malignant Disease in Childhood and Diagnostic Irradiation *In Utero*", Preliminary Communication, *Lancet*, 1 September 1956, p. 447.

27 Leader, *Lancet*, 1 September 1956, p. 449.

28 Stewart *et al.*, "Malignant Disease", p. 447.

29 A. Stewart *et al.*, Correspondence, *Lancet*, 29 December 1956, p. 1355.

30 A. Stewart *et al.*, Correspondence, *Lancet*, 9 March 1957, p. 528.

31 R. Williams and H. Arthure, Correspondence, *Lancet*, 8 December 1956, p. 1211.

32 Anonymous correspondence, *Lancet*, 8 September 1956, p. 513.

33 J. Rabinowitch, Correspondence, *Lancet*, 15 December 1956, pp. 1261–2.

34 LMA, Clinical Report of Queen Charlotte's Maternity Hospital for 1957, H27/QC/A 027/129, p. 7.

35 LMA, Clinical Report of Queen Charlotte's Hospital for Women 1980, H27/QC/A/ 027/140, p. 18.

36 W. M. Court Brown and R. Doll, "Leukaemia and Aplastic Anaemia in Patients Irradiated for Ankylosing Spondylitis", MRC Special Report Series, No 295, London: HMSO, 1957, p. iii.

37 Court Brown and Doll, "Ankylosing", pp. iii–iv.

38 A. Stewart, "An Epidemiologist Takes a Look at Radiation Risks", US Department of Health, Education and Welfare, Public Health Service, FDA, Bureau of Radiological Health, Rockville, MD, 1973, p. 71.

39 A. Stewart, J. Webb and D. Hewitt, "A Survey of Childhood Health Malignancies", *British Medical Journal*, 28 June 1958, pp. 1495–508.

40 W. M. Court Brown and R. Doll, Correspondence, *Lancet*, 12 January 1957, pp. 97–8.

41 W. M. Court Brown, R. Doll and A. Bradford Hill, "Incidence of Leukaemia After Exposure to Diagnostic Radiation *In Utero*", *British Medical Journal*, 26 November 1960, pp. 1539–45.

42 J. Wells and C. Steer, "Relationship of Leukemia in Children to Abdominal Irradiation of Mothers During Pregnancy", *Am J. Obst. Gynec*, May 1961, p. 1061.

43 As technology improved, single X-ray doses for the twenty-two-year period studied fell from 0.46 rad in 1943 to 0.2 rad in 1965. See A. Stewart and G. Kneale, "Radiation Dose Effects In Relation to Obstetrics X-rays and Childhood Cancers", *Lancet*, 6 June 1970, p. 1186.

44 S. Jablon and H. Kato, "Childhood Cancer in Relation to Prenatal Exposure to Atomic Bomb Radiation", *Lancet*, 14 November 1970, pp. 1000–3.

45 Wellcome Library for the History and Understanding of Medicine Archives, Richard Doll "The Epidemiology of Leukaemia", Leukaemia Research Fund Lecture, December 1971, PP/DOL/D/1/18.

46 Cited in Paul Slovic, "The Perception of Risk" in Paul Slovic (ed.), *The Perception of Risk*, London: Earthscan Publishing, 2000; p. 266.

47 Kocher, "Perspective", p. 526.

8   To treat or not to treat

Drug research and the changing nature of essential hypertension

Carsten Timmermann

Hypertension underwent a remarkable transformation in the mid-twentieth century, a transformation that was linked both to demographic changes and to a number of new therapies developed in the decades following World War Two. This chapter is an attempt to trace the trajectory of moderate essential hypertension, from a mysterious risk which may or may not be responsible for early deaths and could only be tackled through lifestyle changes, towards today's multi-factorial disease and risk factor, which is managed and controlled with a variety of drugs, despite unclear and disputed boundaries between normal and pathological blood pressures.[1]

Hypertension as we know it today is largely a product of post-war medical innovations. Prior to World War Two, evidence was mounting, indicating that, as people lived longer lives, degenerative diseases would replace infections in the West as the leading cause of premature deaths. Between 1945 and 1960, governments dedicated increasingly large funds to research efforts into the causes of coronary heart disease. As evidence emerged for a statistical association between high blood pressure and shorter life expectancies, it was tempting to infer a causal link to the epidemic rise of heart disease. While exact mechanisms of causation remained unknown, hypertension was increasingly treated, de facto, as a cause of stroke and coronary heart disease. During the 1950s and 1960s clinicians debated whether hypertension itself was merely the symptom of an underlying disease whose true causes first had to be established to treat it. Since the 1970s, it has been more and more widely assumed that high blood pressure, even in relatively mild cases, needed to be treated to reduce the associated risks.[2] Continuing debates over the safety and efficacy of antihypertensive drugs did not change this general assumption.

This chapter deals with three different but intermeshed notions of risk related to high blood pressure: the probability that individuals were going to suffer serious illness later in life if diagnosed with higher-than-normal blood pressure; the possibility that the consequences of drug therapy were worse than the long-term consequences of hypertension; and the balance of insecurity and opportunities associated with developing drugs for a phenomenon for which the desirability of treatment was contested. All three link statistically quantifiable probabilities – epidemiological, clinical, and commercial – with perceptions of safety and danger. Informed by psychological, social, political, and economic considerations, these probabilities and perceptions were feeding into a complex assessment process that fundamentally redefined the meaning of hypertension and reflected changing understandings of causality.[3]

The chapter is divided into five sections. First I will reflect briefly on concepts of essential hypertension as a disease and a risk in the interwar years. Then I will discuss the changes in the nature of research undertaken into essential hypertension and heart disease in the wake of World War Two, as well as the consequences this had for the choices available to patients and drug companies. Drug development in the 1950s and contemporary discussions over how appropriate it was to treat high blood pressure with pharmaceuticals are the subject of the following, third part of the chapter. In the last two sections I will use the example of beta blockers to discuss changes in the drug culture of the Western world in the 1960s and 1970s and their consequences for the treatment of high blood pressure and the assessment of health risks.

Modern life, early deaths, and the problem of causation

The 1930s saw the beginning in the industrialized world of what has been termed an "epidemiological transition".[4] It became increasingly obvious to epidemiologists that "degenerative" diseases were overtaking infectious diseases in the mortality statistics. Medical science since the late nineteenth century was dominated increasingly by laboratory-based approaches from physiology and bacteriology and concerned with the direct causes of disease.[5] Chronic, "degenerative" disorders, such as hypertension, which developed over long periods of time, posed new problems which were difficult to solve with these laboratory tools. Some medical authors suggested that high blood pressure was simply an adaptation mechanism, a response to arteriosclerosis and therefore to the process of ageing. Others were puzzled by the fact that the statistics of insurance physicians pointed to higher mortality rates for hypertensives, while many of their patients with severely increased blood pressures lived to old age.[6]

As Postel Vinay and Rothstein have pointed out, physicians employed by life insurance companies pioneered the routine measurement of blood pressure, and they were the first to collect and evaluate blood pressure data and explore the association with mortality rates in a systematic fashion.[7] For life insurance companies, the fate of individual patients did not matter, but rather the establishment of parameters that allowed an accurate estimation of the statistical probability for an individual applicant to die earlier than the average insurance client. While in the US, it seems, life insurance medical directors introduced the notion of risk factors to medicine, the story is slightly different in the UK. Here the biometrics tradition pioneered by the eugenicist and statistician, Karl Pearson, and further pursued by human geneticists and epidemiologists associated with the Medical Research Council (MRC), played a central part in introducing statistical models to clinical medicine.[8]

While the statistical evidence was mounting, it remained unclear why exactly people with high blood pressure died earlier. Did hypertension give rise to other diseases or was hypertension the disease itself? For the malignant phase of hypertension, the answer was easier than for mild and moderate hypertension. Malignant hypertension had obvious clinical symptoms, and in most cases life-threatening consequences. Mild or moderate hypertension, in contrast, did not produce any immediate pathological lesions or symptoms, but was nevertheless statistically associated with lowered life expectancy.

To make sense of illness, since the early nineteenth century, medical science has increasingly embraced more restricted and localized notions of causality. Holistic approaches have become increasingly marginal and are today often associated with alternative medicine (they have never really disappeared, though, and remain popular with those who see modern medicine in crisis).[9] Reductionism resonated with the new, managerial and administrative functions of medicine in industrializing states, and it was better suited to forms of practice where patients were no longer patrons. Measuring a patient's blood pressure, a practice that allowed quick and easy access to a quantifiable physiological parameter, matched the administrative role of modern medicine well. As far as therapy was concerned within this new form of medicine, surgery was the appropriate way of dealing with localized complaints, and new magic-bullet drugs got rid of identifiable pathogens.

For hypertension as well as many other non-communicable diseases, however, the precipitating causes were difficult to identify. In order to establish causal links between factors that were statistically correlated, strong corroborating evidence was needed. For smoking and lung cancer such a causal link is now widely accepted.[10] The story that Allan Brandt has told about the development of attitudes towards smoking in the US since the 1930s shows similarities with the changing attitudes towards hypertension.[11] Brandt has argued that post-war epidemiological studies linking lung cancer and smoking implicitly critiqued conventional notions of causality and touched off "an important debate within the scientific community about the nature of causality, proof and risk".[12] Mild and moderate hypertension was increasingly treated like a cause of further cardiovascular complications, while mechanisms of causation remained unknown, and it became acceptable to lower blood pressure with drugs that in turn produced new risks.

We may think that we are talking about two different types of risk: (1) the statistical probability of becoming ill later in life after being diagnosed with high blood pressure today; and (2) the benefits and dangers associated with taking a drug. However, both are calculated by related methods.[13] In fact, effective drugs provided researchers with corroborating evidence for causal links between high blood pressure and cardiovascular disease. Large-scale treatment trials, first for modest and later for mild hypertension, in the 1960s and 1970s were in effect very expensive experiments designed potentially to prove such causal links. The results, however, were not always conclusive. The Veterans Administration Trial, for example, demonstrated that the treatment of moderate hypertension produced evident benefits for the patients.[14] Studies undertaken in the UK and Australia for the treatment of mild hypertension, in contrast, failed to do so.[15] But before we turn to treatment, let us revisit the epidemiological studies that made statistical claims about the links between hypertension and early deaths credible.

Making statistics credible

The largest and best known amongst the studies that converted an actuarial into a scientific hypothesis was the Framingham Heart Study, initiated in 1947 by the United States Public Health Service and since 1949 part of the intramural programme of the National Heart Institute. The objective of the study was to survey the population of a typical American city for arteriosclerotic heart disease (ASHD, later ischemic heart disease or coronary heart disease, CSD) and its possible causes over a twenty-year period. The organizers of the study considered Framingham, a Massachusetts town with a population of 28,000, to be representative of the American urban way of life. The town had been the site of a tuberculosis community study in the inter-war years and was located conveniently close to the Boston medical schools. The first Framingham reports were published in 1957. The authors presented statistical evidence for claims that high blood pressure (besides overweight and hypercholesteremia) "is clearly associated with the incidence of ASHD".[16]

In the UK, research into the risks of hypertension was pursued in somewhat different ways. Like Framingham, such studies were funded by the government. During three months in the winter of 1953, William Miall and his colleagues at the MRC Pneumoconiosis Research Unit at Llandough Hospital (near Cardiff) performed blood pressure measurements on a random sample of the general population of the Rhondda Fach, one of the mining valleys in South Wales. Exactly five years later, in a follow-up study, they revisited the survivors of the first survey.[17] Miall studied the correlation between occupation and blood pressure and found that middle-aged men who worked in physically demanding jobs were most likely to have increased blood pressure. They also found a correlation between high blood pressure and heart disease. In 1959, S. L. Morrison and J. N. Morris of the MRC Social Medicine Research Unit at London Hospital published the results of a study in which they measured the blood pressures of a sample of

London bus drivers and conductors.[18] Studies like Framingham or the research undertaken by the two MRC units indicated that hypertension was common all over the industrialized world throughout the population. They supplemented the statistics of the insurance physicians with what was considered credible, neutral science.

The studies undertaken by the two MRC units were part of a lively controversy over "the nature of essential hypertension" between the British clinicians Robert Platt and George Pickering, who debated whether essential hypertension was a distinct disease entity or just the upper end of a normal distribution of blood pressures.[19] Interest grew within governments as well as amongst representatives of the pharmaceutical industry in the causes and consequences of hypertension. Moderate hypertension began to look like a health issue that could have political repercussions and a potentially lucrative market for the pharmaceutical industry.

Drugs against the pressure

Until the late 1950s, the only real choice of treatment available to patients with moderate hypertension was a change of lifestyle. New drug therapies were being developed, but their side effects made them unsuitable unless a patient's hypertension had become life threatening. "When it comes to detailed therapy, the position is not so easy", George Pickering reasoned in his influential 1961 book on essential hypertension:

> The specified cause of essential hypertension has not been demonstrated and so the doctor has to fall back on what are called general principles, and on symptomatic treatment. Thus the patient whose pressure approaches the critical level is commonly told not to smoke, or drink, he is told to avoid red meat, not to eat salt, to restrict his exercise and to avoid acts resulting in the propagation of his race. Symptomatic treatment at one time was surgical – section of the anterior roots, sympathectomy and adrenalectomy. Now it takes the form of drugs, whose ability to cause disturbing symptoms in the recipient has been amongst their most remarkable properties.[20]

Each of these drugs seemed to produce a disease of its own. Hexamethonium, for example, a so-called ganglion blocker and in the late 1940s one of the first antihypertensive drugs in clinical use, frequently affected patients' visual accommodation, made them feel cold, caused constipation, slowed down kidney and bladder function, and made male patients impotent.[21] The unwanted side effects of other drugs such as Hydralazine or Reserpine could also be quite drastic, depending on the dosage.[22] Still, it became clear in the early 1950s that these drugs produced long-term benefits for patients with life-threatening, malignant hypertension, even if they had to be administered over long periods of time. However, using these drugs in the treatment of symptom-free, mild or moderate hypertension was clearly problematic.

Still, increasingly more experts called for the preventive treatment of high blood pressure.[23] What was needed, according to the clinicians and pharmacologists participating in a discussion on prophylactic treatments during the First US National Symposium on Hypertension in 1958, was a drug whose limited side effects justified its use for treating moderate hypertension:

DR. SCHMIDT: Should antihypertensive drug therapy be limited to the more severe cases of hypertension which already show organic damage?

DR. FINNERTY: I am sure that the average patient who comes to the doctor's office shows very little vascular disease. ... What does the doctor do with this patient?

DR. BEYER: I have been interested in this question from the standpoint of a pharmacologic approach to preventive medicine. ... If therapy is started early, you can arrest the progression of the disease at an early stage rather than trying to reverse a disease process which has already progressed to the point that you know you can't do anything about it.

DR. HEIDER: If we were to subscribe to the idea that hypertension ultimately ends up in producing damage to one organ or another, we are forced into having to treat it. This disease starts somewhere and it progresses – it's not here today and gone tomorrow. I believe that the sooner you treat it the better.

DR. BEYER: This is in large measure contingent on a safe mode of therapy.

DR. SCHROEDER: I think that is right, Dr. Beyer, but we haven't got a completely safe form of therapy yet. So, I think we have to progress in stages. Obviously, when we evaluate the status of a patient we take our chances with the severe or fatal side effects of any regimen. ... And when the chances of the drug doing harm are less than the disease, then we take the chance and treat the disease.[24]

Beyer had reasons to expect that drugs would be available soon that justified the treatment of moderate hypertension. He was the researcher responsible at Sharp & Dohme (later Merck Sharp & Dohme, MSD) for the development of the diuretic chlorothiazide (trade name: Diuril).[25] The introduction of the thiazide diuretics, according to the British clinician Colin Dollery, represented "the real revolution" in the treatment of high blood pressure.[26] To the present day they are included amongst the safest, most effective and inexpensive treatments of hypertension, despite the fact that their precise mechanism of antihypertensive action remains unclear.[27]

A major promoter of the treatment of high blood pressure was Edward Freis, who in 1958 published the results of a first clinical study on the effects of thiazides on hypertensive and normotensive patients.[28] Freis argued that blood pressure should be "controlled at normotensive or nearly normotensive levels" even if the exact causes were not known and a cure was not going to be available in the foreseeable future, to prevent the blood pressure from causing organic damage.[29] The influence of Freis was considerable. He headed what many saw as the definitive study establishing the benefits of treating hypertension, the already-mentioned large-scale cooperative trial at the US Veterans Administration Hospitals whose results were published in 1967.[30] According to another therapeutic enthusiast, Irvine Page, this study "showed that severe essential hypertension could be practically controlled by combinations of thiazides, reserpine, and hydralazine, and therefore that drug treatment was beneficial".[31]

Groups in Europe had developed new heart drugs since the 1940s. One of these was a team at the Pharmaceuticals Division of Imperial Chemical Industries, pursuing work that led to the iconic beta blockers. In July 1958, the physiologist James Black joined this group at ICI's new site in Alderley Edge, Cheshire, to develop a drug for angina pectoris.[32] The ideas leading to the beta blockers were based firmly on pharmacological rationalities and mechanistically oriented, physiological concepts of disease causation, but, ironically, these failed completely to explain the drugs' effects on blood pressure. This turns beta blockers into an interesting case for studying notions of risk and safety in drug development within a context that was undergoing changes regarding both the understanding of high blood pressure and public attitudes to drugs.

Beta blockers

In 1957, the ICI researchers were completing work on a new ganglion blocker. It was clear at this point, though, that ganglion blockers, due to their side effects, did not have much of a future in hypertension treatment. Black, who held an appointment at the University of Glasgow Veterinary School, gave the research in Alderley Park a new direction. Black's work on coronary circulation was influenced by W. B. Cannon's theories on homeostasis and the function of the sympathetic nervous system.[33] Could it be "that the activity of the sympathetic nervous system would not necessarily or always (in cardiac disease for example) have survival value"?[34] What would happen if a drug blocked the effect of adrenaline on the heart? Would the organ's oxygen demand decrease, alleviating the symptoms of angina? Black drew on the controversial receptor theories of Raymond Ahlquist, who in 1948 had suggested that there were two distinct types of adrenotropic receptors, which he designated *alpha* and *beta*.[35] With his colleagues at Alderley Park, Black experimented with the substance dichloroisoprenaline (DCI). Researchers at Lilly Research Laboratories in Indianapolis had synthesized DCI in 1956 and found that it inhibited tissue reactions to adrenaline. After initial problems with the test set-up, in 1959 the ICI group decided to choose DCI as a lead compound and to screen DCI derivatives for better efficiency and selectivity. Research on ganglion blockers was dropped and all energies concentrated on the beta-adrenoreceptor blockers.

Risk and safety had different meanings for pharmacological reasearchers than for clinicians, legislators and the public. The researchers at ICI were looking for a pure mechanism, a drug whose action was rational and clean, as one of them conceded in an interview:

> Well, I think people always have an attraction to pure, simple action, I mean, just as in mathematics, the elegance of a simple formulation is an attraction to mathematicians. And I think to a pharmacologist a drug which does one single thing is always more wonderful than a drug which ... I mean, they talk of clean and dirty drugs. ... So a drug which is very specific for a single receptor and has no stimulating activity is like a very fine bullet. It appeals to people from an aesthetic point of view that a drug has very pure action. That is pure aesthetics and emotion.[36]

Such sentiments were fairly common amongst pharmacologists, as the example of William Paton shows, who a decade earlier marvelled in similar ways over the clean action of hexamethonium.[37]

The first promising DCI derivative was pronethalol. ICI submitted the patent application in May 1960, clinical trials started late in 1961 and the results were published in the *Lancet* in 1962. Simultaneously, the ICI team screened further compounds, about 800 by the time pronethalol was marketed in November 1963. By accident, during a double-blind trial of pronethalol with angina pectoris patients, the pharmacologist Brian Prichard observed that the drug lowered the blood pressure of hypertensive patients (although theoretically it should not have done so). Was pronethalol the cardiovascular wonderdrug many people had been waiting for?

It was not. ICI interrupted the clinical evaluation of the compound when pronethalol was found to produce tumours in mice. The company delayed the marketing of the drug until November 1963 and then only received a licence for "the treatment of conditions which themselves threaten life immediately or cause such morbidity that only a short survival may be expected".[38] Prichard's report in 1964 recommended that "when a non-carcinogenic beta-receptor blocker is produced it would be worth trying in the treatment of hypertension".[39] Links with cancer were not the only problems associated with pronethalol. Experiments with cats and dogs showed effects on the central nervous system, and after the Thalidomide disaster this was a particularly sensitive issue.[40] Clinical tests also revealed side effects of central nervous origin in humans: paraesthesia, "walking on air", visual disturbances, dreams, fatigue, nausea, vomiting and dizziness. Pronethalol was definitely not an attractive remedy for a disease which was mainly defined as a risk and which had no direct impact on the immediate wellbeing of patients.

The compound which would bring some kind of a breakthrough for beta blockers was propranolol. Shanks, who had joined ICI from Belfast, first administered it to a cat in November 1962. Propranolol proved to be about ten times as powerful as pronethalol when bringing about the desired effects, while the dose required to produce the toxic side effects was comparable. This meant that the so-called therapeutic ratio (therapeutic dose/toxic dose) was significantly better than that of pronethalol. Clinical trials with the new drug started in 1964 and in July 1965 ICI marketed propranolol under the brand name Inderal. However, beta blockers were not an instant success for ICI, which partly had to do with a changed public attitude towards drugs.

Adverse reactions

Public attitudes towards the risks and benefits of science in the early postwar years were ambiguous. Science was seen as a powerful force which could produce miracles as well as destruction. "Many thought that research had allowed development of the weapons that had been so effective in defeating Nazi Germany," reminisces Harriet Dustan, the long-time president of the American Heart Association, and "manufacturers and businessmen had the heady feeling that they could address and solve problems previously considered insoluble."[41] While the claims of medical scientists remained ambitious, people were becoming suspicious about the claims of drug companies. This change was partly triggered by the Thalidomide disaster. In November 1961, the sedative Thalidomide, developed by the German pharmaceutical company Chemie Grünenthal and produced under licence worldwide, was withdrawn from sale. The drug had been marketed as a particularly safe choice, because unlike barbiturates even large doses were not lethal. However, Thalidomide was found to cause neural disorders in elderly patients. Grünenthal withdrew the drug when it became clear that it was also responsible for a large number of birth defects in children.[42] In the wake of the disaster, governments re-examined the legal mechanisms of drug regulation and long, highly publicized lawsuits followed.[43] Thalidomide turned into a powerful cultural symbol for the risks associated with legal drugs.[44]

In the light of the Thalidomide scandal, let us return to the beta blockers. Amongst the reasons why it took so long for beta blockers to be generally accepted by clinicians and regulatory agencies may have been that a worried public was losing trust in the claims of drug manufacturers at the same time when pronethalol ran into trouble. The anti-hypertensive effect of the beta blockers, furthermore, had not been described in animals and the mechanism by which it lowered blood pressure was unknown.[45] But nobody could explain satisfactorily how diuretics lowered the blood pressure of patients, either. Why then did the world accept these more or less instantly, and beta blockers only after two decades?

While the timing of the introduction of the diuretics before the Thalidomide disaster may have had an effect on acceptance, we may also want to take into account the cultural significance of the organs which either drug targeted. Beta blockers directly interfered with the function of the heart, while diuretics urged people to urinate more often. Most people would locate the kidneys in the cultural hierarchy of bodily organs below the heart, and most people would consider stimulating kidney function as less worrying than slowing down the heart rate. After all, we are all familiar with the diuretic effects of everyday drugs such as alcohol or caffeine.

How did experts explain the slow uptake of beta blockers in clinical practice? Brian Prichard, one of the authors of the 1964 report that first described the antihypertensive effect of beta blockers, blamed their delayed acceptance on conservative attitudes in the medical profession.[46] Beta blockers inhibited cardiac contraction, and clinicians viewed this "as a basically undesirable effect" which in addition was associated with adverse reactions in acutely ill patients. In his book *Drugs Looking for Diseases*, Rein Vos argues that propranolol turned into an "endangered drug", paradoxically, while more potential therapeutic uses for the drug became established through clinical trials.[47]

Ironically, the ambitious claims of propranolol's creators, who insisted that they had created a fully rational drug whose mechanism was clean, pure and controllable, may also have been counterproductive. Many clinicians had their doubts as to whether beta blockage was responsible for the anti-arrhythmic and anti-anginal effects of the drug, or rather a local anaesthetic activity of propranolol. Vos suggests that the ICI team countered such doubts by drawing parallels between the action of the beta blockers and surgical sympathectomy, pointing to "the analogy between the surgical knife and the purity of chemical blockade exhibited by *propranolol*".[48]

While certainly powerful, propranolol turned out to be rather difficult to manage in clinical situations. It seemed impossible to design general treatment schemes. Neither the intravenous nor the oral administration of propranolol was unproblematic. One interview partner told Vos that he thought the intravenous administration was too dangerous for general practice. When propranolol was administered orally in comparatively low (and safe) doses, on the other hand, the results were unimpressive. In order to get good responses in the treatment of angina, Prichard and Gillam used a variable dose approach individualizing the doses after run-in periods (from 10 milligrammes up to an impressive 4 grammes per day).[49] A demanding undertaking, as Vos remarks: "The clinician needed to take some time to search for the optimal dose, to achieve the best possible therapeutic result in each individual patient and to evaluate the adaptive mechanisms of the patient's body."[50]

Propranolol acquired what Vos calls the "mystique" of a difficult and dangerous drug. In addition, ICI faced competition in 1964 from the Ciba beta blocker, oxprenolol. The ICI researchers were not impressed with it, but

Ciba had well established relationships with physicians in continental Europe and was trusted as a drug manufacturer.[51] In this situation, the ICI team came up with another beta blocking drug, practolol. Practolol was a far less aggressive drug than propranolol. It was much easier to administer, non-toxic, its potency was only a third or a forth of propranolol, and it produced less cardiac depression than equivalent doses of the older drug. Practolol became generally available in the UK in 1970. Its career as a safe and easy beta blocker, however, was over when in 1974 the drug itself turned into a risk factor: it was found to cause a set of serious adverse reactions, collectively termed the "oculomucocutaneous syndrome".[52] In 1976, ICI withdrew practolol from the market.

Conclusion

I am aware that with this chapter I may have posed more questions than I have answered. I have tried to trace the processes through which high blood pressure was transformed from a "risk factor" in the statistics of life insurance actuaries into something which almost amounted to an accepted cause of heart disease, while mechanisms of causation remained in the dark. Aspects of manageability, I have argued, played a central role in this transition, as did treatment trials, despite their inconclusive results for mild and moderate hypertension. I have then attempted to throw light on the debates in the 1950s and 1960s over the question whether moderate, symptom-free hypertension should in fact be treated with the newly available diuretics and beta adrenoreceptor blockers.

It is difficult to come to real conclusions over these issues, as many of the controversial questions in the debates remain unresolved. I have used a broad sweep for this chapter; my main aim was to depict a long-term trend, and in some points my treatment may be superficial. I could have said more about the history of hexamethonium and its effects on the budding market for antihypertensives, but I will leave this for a future publication. I also look forward to a number of forthcoming accounts by other historians on other aspects of this story. The beta blockers, for example, despite all the problems they faced, turned into one of the biggest selling classes of antihypertensive drugs.[53] The question of how a statistical correlation turned into a recognized cause also calls for detailed historical case studies.[54]

Today physicians, patients, pharmacologists and legislators are faced with far more choices regarding the management of blood pressure than those living in the inter-war period. However, this also makes managing the risks involved more complicated. High blood pressure may pose risks, but so do the drugs which lower it. Adequate risk assessment has to take both into account, which is difficult for novelty drugs that have just come onto the market, and much easier for "veterans" such as the thiazide diuretics. The latter, though, are far less lucrative for the manufacturers than freshly patented new remedies. Furthermore, there is ongoing controversy over the question whether lowering blood pressure consistently results in a lowered risk of cardiovascular disease.[55] The decisions are difficult ones.

It is too early to tell how the story of hypertension and of the drugs designed for treating it is likely to end. Still, it is worth studying, as it teaches us much about the ways in which medical research and practices have developed since World War Two. The epidemiological transition in the developed world triggered interest in "diseases of civilization", and studies like the Framingham Heart Study gave scientific credit to the notion of risk factors, which fell on fertile ground in the increasingly individualist and consumerist societies of the West. We are all responsible, we are told, for managing our health risks. And if, in order to avert the danger of dying early, we have the choice to either change our lifestyles or take a few pills, what are we more likely to do? While we may think that lifestyle change might be better, many would choose the convenience of the magic bullet.

Notes

I would like to thank John Pickstone, Michael Worboys and Jonathan Harwood for reading and commenting on earlier versions of this chapter. I am grateful also to the partipants and audiences of the two workshops in Freiburg and Philadelphia, and not least to the editors of this volume for their valuable suggestions. Finally I would like to thank the Wellcome Trust for financing my research with a postdoctoral fellowship.

1 On the increasingly central role of the risk factor in twentieth-century medicine, see W. G. Rothstein, *Public Health and the Risk Factor: A History of an Uneven Medical Revolution*, Rochester: University of Rochester Press, 2003; R. A. Aronowitz, *Making Sense of Illness: Science, Society, and Disease*, Cambridge: Cambridge University Press, 1998. See also D. Armstrong, "The Rise of Surveillance Medicine", *Sociology of Health and Illness* 3, 1995, 393–404.

2 Medical Research Council Working Party, "MRC trial of treatment of mild hypertension: principal results", *British Medical Journal* 291, 1985, 97–104.

3 Much of the literature on risk in recent years has been informed by Ulrich Beck's socio-logical analysis of late modernity (U. Beck, *Risk Society: Towards a New Modernity*, London: Sage, 1992). Influential also were writings by Mary Douglas (for example M. Douglas, *Risk and Blame: Essays in Cultural Theory*, London and New York: Routledge, 1992) and post-structuralist approaches, focusing on questions of surveillance, norm and deviance (for example Deborah Lupton, *The Imperative of Health: Public Health and the Regulated Body*, London: Sage, 1995). See also S. Olin Lauritzen and L. Sachs, "Normality, risk and the future: implicit communication of threat in health surveillance", *Sociology of Health & Illness* 23, 2001, 497–516, an ethnographic study which for the realm of medical advice demonstrates how modern risk assessments, while claiming to secure purity in decision making, are met by patients with very subjective perceptions of danger.

4 See A. R. Omran, "The Epidemiological Transition: a Theory of the Epidemiology of Population Change", *Milbank Memorial Fund Quarterly* 49, 1971, 509–38.

5 C. Gradmann and T. Schlich (eds), *Strategien der Kausalität: Konzepte der Krankheitsverursachung im 19. und 20. Jahrhundert*, Pfaffenweiler: Centaurus, 1999.

6 D. Riesman, "High Blood Pressure and Longevity", *Journal of the American Medical Association* 96, 1931, 1105–11.

7 N. Postel-Vinay (ed.), *A Century of Arterial Hypertension 1896–1996*, Chichester: Wiley, 1996; Rothstein, *Public Health and the Risk Factor*. This observation is supported by early publications on the National Heart Institute's Framingham Study and by conversations

of the author with researchers in the Framingham project office at the National Institutes of Health, who cited the Life Insurance Industry's "Blood Pressure and Build Study" as one of the starting points for their enterprise.

8 Cf. E. Magnello, "The Introduction of Mathematical Statistics into Medical Research: the Roles of Karl Pearson, Major Greenwood and Austin Bradford Hill", in E. Magnello and A. Hardy (eds), *The Road to Medical Statistics*, Amsterdam and New York: Rodopi, 2002, 95–123.

9 Cf. C. Lawrence and G. Weisz (eds), *Greater than the Parts: Holism in Biomedicine 1920–1950*, New York and Oxford: Oxford University Press, 1998; C. Timmermann, "Constitutional Medicine, Neo-Romanticism, and the Politics of Anti-Mechanism in Interwar Germany", *Bulletin of the History of Medicine* 75, 2001, 717–39. See also T. Schlich, "Die Konstruktion der notwendigen Krankheitsursache: Wie die Medizin Krankheit beherrschen will", in C. Borck (ed.), *Anatomien medizinischen Wissens*, Frankfurt: Fischer, 1996, 201–29.

10 S. A. Lock, L. A. Reynolds and E. M. Tansey (eds), *Ashes to Ashes: The History of Smoking and Health*, Amsterdam and Atlanta: Rodopi, 1998.

11 A. M. Brandt, "The Cigarette, Risk, and American Culture", in J. W. Leavitt and R. L. Numbers (eds), *Sickness and Health in America: Readings in the History of Medicine and Public Health*, Madison: University of Wisconsin Press, 1997, 495–505.

12 Brandt, "The Cigarette, Risk, and American Culture", p. 498.

13 Cf. J. Rosser Matthews, *Quantification and the Quest for Medical Certainty*, Princeton: Princeton University Press, 1995; H. M. Marks, *The Progress of Experiment: Science and Therapeutic Reform in the United States, 1900–1990*, Cambridge: Cambridge University Press, 1997.

14 E. D. Freis, "The Veterans Trial and sequelae", *British Journal of Clinical Pharmacology* 13, 1982, 67–72; E. D. Freis, "Reminiscences of the Veterans Administration Trial of the treatment of hypertension", *Hypertension* 16, 1990, 472–5.

15 See Rothstein, *Public Health and the Risk Factor*, pp. 267–70, for a discussion of these studies and some of their methodological problems.

16 T. R. Dawber, F. E. Moore and G. V. Mann, "Coronary Heart Disease in the Framingham Study", *American Journal of Public Health* 47, 1957, 4–24; p. 13. See also W. B. Kannel *et al.*, "Factors of Risk in the Development of Coronary Heart Disease: Six-year Follow-up Experience", *Annals of Internal Medicine* 55, 1961, 33–50; T. R. Dawber, *The Framingham Study: The Epidemiology of Atherosclerotic Disease*, Cambridge, MA: Harvard University Press, 1980.

17 M. B. Miall, "Follow-up Study of Arterial Pressure in the Population of a Welsh Mining Valley", *British Medical Journal* ii, 1959, 1204–10.

18 S. L. Morrsion and J. N. Morris, "Epidemiological Observations on High Blood-pressure Without Evident Cause", *Lancet* ii, 1959, 864–70.

19 J. D. Swales (ed.), *Platt Versus Pickering: An Episode in Recent Medical History*, London: The Keynes Press, 1985; G. W. Pickering, *The Nature of Essential Hypertension*, London: Churchill, 1961.

20 Pickering, *The Nature of Essential Hypertension*, pp. 140–1.

21 C. Timmermann, "Drugs and Chronic Disease: the Trajectory of Hexamethonium, from Research Tool to High Blood Pressure Drug", forthcoming.

22 Cf. Pickering, *The Nature of Essential Hypertension*, p. 141; I. H. Page, *Hypertension Research: A Memoir 1920–1960*, New York: Pergamon Press, 1988, pp. 134–5; M. Moser, "Historical perspective on the management of hypertension", *American Journal of Medicine* 80, 1986, 1–11; M. Weatherall, *In Search of a Cure: A History of Pharmaceutical Discovery*, Oxford: Oxford University Press, 1990, pp. 239–40.

23 Cf. Page, *Hypertension Research*, pp. 126–7.

24 Quoted in R. M. Kaiser, "The Introduction of the Thiazides: a Case Study in Twentieth-Century Therapeutics", in: G. J. Higby and E. C. Stroud (eds), *The Inside Story of Medicines: A Symposium*, Madison: University of Wisconsin Press, 1997, 121–37; p. 130.

25 K. H. Beyer, "Chlorothiazide: How the Thiazides Evolved as Antihypertensive Therapy",
    Hypertension 22, 1993, 388–91; K. H. Beyer, "Chlorothiazide", *British Journal of Clinical
    Pharmacology* 13, 1982, 15–24; K. H. Beyer, "Discovery of the Thiazides: Where Biology
    and Chemistry Meet", *Perspectives in Biology and Medicine* 20, 1977, 410–20.

26 C. Dollery, "Hypertension" *British Heart Journal*, 58, 1987, 179–84; p. 181.

27 Jeremy Greene, "Releasing the Flood Waters: Thiazide Promotion and the Renegotiation
    of Hypertension, 1958–1968", forthcoming. See also A. G. Dupont, "The Place of
    Diuretics in the Treatment of Hypertension: a Historical Review of Classical Experience
    Over 30 years", *Cardiovascular Drugs and Therapy* 7, 1993, 55–62. See also A. V.
    Chobanian *et al.*, "The Seventh Report of the Joint National Committee on Prevention,
    Detection, Evaluation, and Treatment of High Blood Pressure: the JNC 7 Report",
    Journal of the American Medical Association 289, 2003, 2560–72.

28 E. D. Freis, "Chlorthiazide in Hypertensive and Normotensive Patients", *Annals of the
    New York Academy of Science* 71, 1958, p. 450.

29 E. D. Freis, "Rationale and Methods for the Treatment of Early Essential Hypertension",
    Journal of the National Medical Association 50, 1958, 405–12; pp. 411–12.

30 E. D. Freis, "The Veterans Trial and Sequelae".

31 I. H. Page, *Hypertension Research*, p. 127. Page was co-founder in 1945 of the National
    Foundation for High Blood Pressure, and in 1949 of the American Heart Association's
    (AHA) Council for High Blood Pressure Research. See also H. P. Dustan, "A History of
    the Council for High Blood Pressure Research: the First 50 Years", *Hypertension* 30, 1997,
    1307–17.

32 J. A. Woodbridge, *Social Aspects of Pharmaceutical Innovation: Heart Disease*, Birmingham:
    unpublished PhD dissertation, University of Aston, 1981; R. Vos, *Drugs Looking for
    Diseases: Innovative Drug Research and the Development of the Beta Blockers and the Calcium
    Antagonists*, Dordrecht: Kluwer, 1991; J. M. Cruickshank and B. N. C. Prichard, *Beta-
    Blockers in Clinical Practice*, Edinburgh: Churchill Livingstone, 1987, pp. 1–8; R. G.
    Shanks, "The Discovery of Beta Adrenoreceptor Blocking Drugs", in M. J. Parnham,
    J. Bruinvels (eds), *Discoveries in Pharmacology*, Amsterdam: Elsevier, 1984, 38–72.

33 On Cannon, see S. J. Cross and W. R. Albury, "Walter B. Cannon, L. J. Henderson, and
    the Organic Analogy", *Osiris* 3, 1987, 165–92.

34 Black, interview in Woodbridge, *Social Aspects of Pharmaceutical Innovation*, p. 149.

35 Cf. Shanks, "The Discovery of Beta Adrenoreceptor Blocking Drugs", pp. 39–40.

36 Robinson, interview with Rein Vos, quoted in Vos, *Drugs Looking for Diseases*, p. 89.

37 W. D. M. Paton, "The Principles of Ganglionic Block", *Lectures on the Scientific Basis of
    Medicine* 2, 1954, 139–64; W. D. M. Paton, "Hexamethonium," *British Journal of Clinical
    Pharmacology* 13, 1982, 7–14; Timmermann, "Drugs and Chronic Disease".

38 Quoted in Cruickshank and Prichard, *Beta-Blockers in Clinical Practice*, p. 4.

39 Quoted in Cruickshank and Prichard, *Beta-Blockers in Clinical Practice*, p. 4.

40 More on the Thalidomide case in the following section.

41 Dustan, "A history of the Council for High Blood Pressure Research", p. 1308.

42 H. Sjöström and R. Nilsson, *Thalidomide and the Power of the Drug Companies*, Harmondsworth:
    Penguin, 1972; B. Kirk, *Der Contergan-Fall: eine unvermeidliche Arzneimittelkatastrophe?
    Zur Geschichte des Arzneistoffes Thalidomid*, Stuttgart: Wissenschaftliche Verlagsgesellschaft,
    1999.

43 Cf. P. Knightley *et al.*, *Suffer the Children: The Story of Thalidomide*, London: Andre
    Deutsch, 1979; O. L. Wade, *When I Dropped the Knife*, Durham: Pentland Press, 1996.

44 For effects of the Thalidomide disaster on drug regulation practices in the US and
    Germany, see A. Daemmrich and G. Krücken, "Risk Versus Risk: Decision-making
    Dilemmas of Drug Regulation in the United States and Germany," *Science as Culture* 9,
    2000, 505–34. See also S. Timmermans and V. Leiter, "The Redemption of Thalidomide:
    Standardizing the Risk of Birth Defects", *Social Studies of Science* 30, 2000, 41–71.

45 B. N. C. Prichard, "Propranolol and Beta-adrenergic Receptor Blocking Drugs in the
    Treatment of Hypertension", *British Journal of Clinical Pharmacology* 13, 1982, 51–60.

46 B. N. C. Prichard, "Beta-adrenergic Receptor Blockade in Hypertension, Past, Present and Future", *British Journal of Clinical Pharmacology* 5, 1978, 379–99.

47 Vos, *Drugs Looking for Diseases*, pp. 91–3.

48 Vos, *Drugs Looking for Diseases*, p. 92. Again, this comparison had already been drawn by Paton for the ganglion blockers.

49 P. M. S. Gillam and B. N. C. Prichard, "Use of Propranolol in Angina Pectoris", *British Medical Journal* ii, 1965, 337.

50 Vos, *Drugs Looking for Diseases*, p. 93. Vos argues that Gillam's and Prichard's experimental approach was in itself an innovation in clinical research.

51 Vos, *Drugs Looking for Diseases*, p. 102.

52 M.-A. Wallander, "The Way Towards Adverse Event Monitoring in Clinical Trials", *Drug Safety* 8, 1993, 251–62; Cruickshank and Prichard, *Beta-Blockers in Clinical Practice*, pp. 835–9.

53 A number of studies on related issues are currently in progress. Viviane Quirke at Oxford Brookes University is working on the history of the beta blockers, and Jeremy Greene at Harvard is completing a PhD dissertation which deals, amongst other issues, with the impact of the thiazide diuretics.

54 Luc Berlivet at CERMES in Paris is currently pursuing a detailed study into the work of the epidemiologist Richard Doll and his colleagues.

55 F.H. Messerli and E. Grossman, "Beta-blockers and Diuretics: To Use or Not To Use", *American Journal of Hypertension* 12, 1999, 157S–163S.

9 Hormones at risk

Cancer and the medical uses of industrially-produced sex steroids in Germany, 1930–1960

Jean-Paul Gaudillière

Introduction

In 2003 the French daily paper *Le Monde* published a full-page article on "hormone replacement therapy" (HRT) for post-menopausal women. The official motive for this initiative was the publication of a new set of recommendations for doctors by the *Agence française de sécurité sanitaire des produits de santé* (Afssaps), a recently established government agency for the safety of health products.[1] Referring to epidemiological studies released during summer 2002, the government experts working with the agency concluded that, given the risks associated with hormone replacement therapy, sex steroids should not be prescribed to women not suffering from significant post-menopausal symptoms, and in any case for no more than five years. Two types of risks were mentioned by the agency: vascular problems and breast cancer. This official statement was immediately opposed by a group of specialists in reproductive medicine gathered together in the *Association française pour l'étude de la ménopause*. They stressed the fact that epidemiological studies conducted in the United States could not be generalized to France since the US approach did not match French clinical practice, and the cohort in question was not representative of the population of women using HRT in France.

Pointing out the risks of hormonal therapies, and more particularly the putative relationship between estrogens and (breast) cancer, is nothing new. Both the "medicalization" of the menopause and the use of sex steroids for contraceptive purposes had already sparked medical controversies and public debates in the 1960s.[2] The aim of this chapter, however, is not to illustrate the continuity of risk cultures but rather to point out the discontinuities in the conception of therapeutic risk in twentieth-century medicine. These discontinuities revolve around the nature of the risks associated with reproductive medicine, the way they were framed and managed, and how they were articulated with other social practices. The context selected for this purpose is Germany between the 1930s and the 1950s. During this time, Germany was a central locus both for the development of sex steroids and for the control of reproduction. From the mid-1930s onward, the purification and preparation of sex steroids became routine industrial practice, while their clinical use rapidly gained momentum and triggered a decade-long discussion over the possible relationship between the medical consumption of sex steroids and the risk of cancer. Focusing on this German discussion of what may be termed the steroids-and-cancer problem offers several advantages.

First, there is already significant historical work on the medical uses of these steroids.[3] The general picture that emerges from this work is one of medicalization, a trend rooted in the growth of biochemistry, and the molecularization of medicine which preceded the emergence of molecular biology. Local developments were sometimes complex, especially in the United States where the tradition of private scientific patronage left some space open for unusual alliances between biologists and birth-control activists. Nevertheless, despite local differences, the general overall picture that emerges is of the medical profession assuming control over a whole range of reproductive issues. When the sex steroids first appeared on the market, the medical landscape was already occupied by influential women-centred specialities like gynecology and obstetrics, and so the initial uses of the new preparations were heavily gender-biased, centred on the management of women's bodies. While these early uses of sex steroids were confined to reproductive medicine, the linkage with cancer paradoxically opened up new therapeutic opportunities for the same compounds. One unexpected consequence was the fact that the sex hormones shifted back and forth across the boundaries between preventive and curative medicine, as well as between chemical therapies and biological means for enhancing one's quality of life.

Second, the following debate over hormones and cancer reveals a culture substantially different from what the historiography of post-war biomedicine has taken to be characteristic of the era of medical risks, i.e. the use of statistics, definition of populations, mobilization of the vocabulary of chance, etc. If one thinks of it in terms of an organized hierarchy of future events, whose occurrence can be avoided or mitigated by means of appropriate medical action, risk was certainly present in the 1930s. Nevertheless, if one restricts the notion to its formal, quantitative and probabilistic definition, risk does not appear to have existed at the time.

Third, the German configuration offers an original perspective on the relationship between professional and lay expertise in medicine. Sex hormones were initially perceived as natural entities, which could be sold "over the counter" just like vitamins. Free access facilitated particular types of use, especially the treatment of menopausal symptoms. Many gynecologists viewed this practice as highly problematic, and they finally managed to have the legal status of sex hormones changed. State regulation did not, however, succeed in eliminating the tensions that existed between professional and lay uses of steroids, nor did it solve the problems raised by the debate over the risk of cancer.

I will develop my argument in three parts corresponding to three different sections of the chapter. The first one presents the medical status of industrially produced sex steroids in the 1930s. It concentrates on the role played by the Schering pharmaceutical company and its scientific associates in defining the most important sex hormones and their uses. The second part follows the development of the debate about steroids and cancer in the late 1930s and early 1940s, focusing on the "experimentalization" of the evaluation of risk and the procedures by means of which the same techno-scientific network presented in the first part argued that estrogens were not carcinogenic. Finally, the third section deals with the disappearance of the issue of the carcinogenic risk of hormones after the war, and in particular the role played by the post-war boom of cancer chemotherapy in this development.

Sex steroids and reproductive medicine in 1930s Germany

In December 1938, Walter Schoeller, then director of Schering's *Hauptlaboratorium*, presented his colleagues with an internal report on the status of the firm's hormone research.[4] The text focused on the four steroids then produced by Schering (three sex hormones and one product of the adrenal glands, corticosterone). It included a chronological table of the main research achievements in the field. This table alluded to several results obtained in collaboration with the biochemists at the Berlin *Kaiser Wilhelm Institute für Biochemie* under the leadership of Adolf Butenandt. The research outcomes singled out by Schoeller ranged from the crystallization of estradiol to the partial synthesis of progesterone and testosterone. The table mentioned two sorts of products produced by Schering. In chronological order these were: first, extracts of placenta, ovaries or men's urine; and, second – following the crystallization (by Butenandt and his colleagues) of the three sex hormones – pure preparations designated by their brand names, Progynon, Proluton, and Proviron.

The purification paradigm that characterized the decade-long research program conducted within the network that linked the *Kaiser Willhelm Institute für Biochemie* (KWIB) to Schering did not simply involve collecting and handling large amounts of biological material in order to prepare homogeneous (if not pure) glandular extracts. The biochemical utopia that lay behind this work on the sex steroids was the perspective of developing a rational series of chemical reactions that could transform the naturally occurring steroids into cheap, easy to produce, and biologically effective versions. In other words, the aim of the research was not total chemical synthesis of the sex steroids, but the systematic production of analogues, and their partial synthesis. Within this perspective, the most important outcome of Butenandt's work was less the deciphering of chemical structure than the elucidation of biochemical reactions and the description of natural pathways. Thus, artificial synthesis and metabolic studies were intimately connected. Within the KWIB-Schering *Arbeitskreis*, the complex circulation of personnel, material, and information reinforced these investigations that focused on biotechnological processes. As Schoeller reminded his colleagues, this collaboration, starting in the mid-1930s, had resulted in numerous patents, increased production, and a greater availability of estrogens, progesterone and testosterone on the medical market.[5]

The experts at Schering envisioned a remarkably wide range of indications for their hormone preparations. A widely circulated table from 1934 classified the uses of Progynon, the follicular hormone, into three categories: first the genital domain, aimed at the regularization of menstruation or the treatment of various menstrual disorders; second, hormonal regulation focused on problems associated with pituitary secretion or the side-effects of thyroid disorders; and third, more general indications including skin and articulation disorders, insomnia, menopause, and depression. The use of hormones and sex steroids in these indications was not entirely unsubstantiated. The main booklet on hormone therapy distributed by Schering in the mid-1930s listed the same uses with indications of dosages, and references to the medical literature.[6] These indications were also presented in the reports published in *Medizinische Mitteilungen*, the company's own scientific periodical, the majority of whose articles originated within the company's small network of collaborating clinical researchers. For the trials of estrogens and progesterone, two clinics played a critical role. C. Clauberg's clinic at Königsberg University and C. Kaufmann's Frauenklinik der Charité at the Humbold University in Berlin. The former focused on the management of sterility, while the latter specialized in the treatment of amenorrhea.

Kaufmann's career was shaped early on by his collaboration with Schering. His first noteworthy article was a 1933 publication in which he reported the treatment of a "sterile" woman with a combination of Progynon and Proluton intended to mimic the changing hormonal concentrations during the ovarian cycle. This regimen was a success in the sense that menses could be induced.[7] Developed in the course of a dozen cases, Kaufmann's regimen was then adopted as reference for the treatment of amenorrhea.[8] Throughout the 1930s, Kaufmann continued to test the company's products, looking for optimal dosages and broader indications. The most significant innovations were the molecularization of the menopause and the management of its adverse effects. Kaufmann's list of symptoms ranged from circulatory problems to bleeding, headaches, rheumatism, and nervous hypersensitivity, all of them attributed to an insufficient secretion of steroids. By the late 1930s, Kaufmann had become accustomed to the manipulation of artificial hormones and considered the administration of estrogens the simplest and most efficient way of handling the physiological problems experienced by aging women.[9]

The clinical work pursued during the 1930s certainly resulted in a significant expansion of the proposed medical uses of sex hormones. This growth was reflected in a growing number of reports that appeared in gynecological journals advocating such use, as well as in the thickness of Schering's new booklet on Progynon and Proluton published before the war.[10] Schering's production records also bear witness to the expanded use of these hormones, particularly after the beginning of the war. In the autumn of 1945, following the occupation of Berlin by the allied forces, Schering's directors were ordered to review their range of products and their production capacities, and so a memo was circulated and annotated to determine the status of the *Follikelhormone*. It summarized the production data for the war years, asserting that the global production of estrogens had tripled between 1939 (18 kg) and 1943 (58 kg).[11] For testosterone, the figures were of the same order of magnitude: 12 kg in 1939, and 72 kg in 1943.

One may suspect that segments of the profession began to consider broader uses of artificial sex steroids in connection with Nazi reproductive policy, which induced significant changes in medical practice in Germany, including a strong interest in the medical treatment of both male and female sterility.[12] These changes were based on the population policy of the regime, which prolonged the Weimar debates about the nation's loss of potency and the feminization of the German male.[13] The medicalization of reproduction was also reinforced during the late 1930s by the application of new medical laws, with the generalization of premarital medical examinations leading to many new diagnoses of sterility.

Steroid consumption and cancer risk: the diethylstilbestrol connection

The idea that estrogens and other steroids might play a part in the manifestation and development of some forms of cancer preceded this (relatively) widespread use of sex hormones. One can already find early discussions of the topic before World War One, when experimental pathologists working on cancer used the castration of animals as a means to analyse the relationship between endocrine factors and tumour growth.[14] Nevertheless, the link between sex steroids and the incidence of tumors was only used to argue that these hormones may cause cancer in the 1930s. Two types of experimental resource were then introduced into these laboratories: commercially available purified sex hormones, and inbred mice.[15] This conjunction gave rise to the first reports about the formation of tumors in animals following the inoculation of steroids, with a profound effect in the field of cancer research. The work of the French pathologist Antoine Lacassagne was among the most widely cited example of the successful hormonal induction of mammary tumors in mice, first in males and later in females.

Within the KWIB-Schering network, discussions about the possibility that estrogens, and therefore Progynon, could induce cancer started in 1936, when Kaufmann launched a series of experiments which were based on daily inoculation with relatively high doses of the firm's preparation. The question as to whether or not estrogens caused cancer remained, however, a secondary issue when compared to the clinical research on the treatment of sterility and menopause. Two years later, Dodds, working in London, reported that a new synthetic compound prepared with the support of the government's Medical Research Council (MRC), diethylstilbestrol (DES), was a powerful analogue of estrogens.[16] Although it had few structural features in common with the natural sex hormones, this artificial compound was none the less more effective than any other known sex steroid, at least when evaluated using the classical mouse test for estrogen activity.

The MRC did not patent DES, and a few months later IG Farben publicly announced to German doctors that it was ready to supply them with the new drug. For Schering, the commercialization of DES posed a serious threat, as the analogue was easy to produce in large quantities, and was therefore cheaper than Schering's own product Progynon. IG Farben's advertisements provoked a wave of reactions within the Berlin firm.[17] A crisis cell was set up within weeks, including both the biochemist, Butenandt, and Kaufmann in his capacity as gynecological expert, as well as Schering laboratory officials. The first move was to try to persuade the German medical associations and/or the public health administration to take a stand against the artificial substance.

Besides these political interventions, the company's associates pursued an experimental evaluation of DES. Several questions were addressed in this context. Would DES prove as effective a replacement of natural estrogens as announced? Did the artificial compound have toxic side effects at therapeutic dosage? Did it have long-term pathological effects, and in particular, could it cause cancer? The assessment of toxicity was initially conducted both within the physiological laboratory of the firm, and within Kaufmann's service at the Charité hospital. This new topic of research introduced two new features to hormone research in general; first, not only DES but also ovarian hormones and pure estrogens were submitted to increased surveillance and testing. Second, cancer came out of the background and became one of the principal areas to be investigated. The possibility that DES and/or natural estrogens could act as carcinogens had become an important research question to be investigated at the experimental level.[18] Thus, the vision of cancer risk within the Schering network was clearly tied to the company's commercial interests, and more particularly their product line and those of their competitors.

This relationship is clearly illustrated in the correspondence exchanged between Schoeller, Butenandt and W. Cramer, a few weeks before the DES conflict. Cramer was an oncologist performing experiments on rats and mice at the Imperial Cancer Research Fund, who had adopted Lacassagne's view that estrogens could act directly as carcinogens. Cramer had once written to Schoeller that he did "not understand why he (Schoeller) refuses to see the point, which is that a treatment with oestrin prolonged over many years in human beings is a dangerous procedure. Even if it never produces cancer, it will induce pathological changes in the whole endocrine system in 100% of the people treated, and that, surely, is not desirable."[19] To support his views, Cramer sent some male mice that had developed mammary tumours following the administration of estrogens to Schering's *Hauptlaboratorium*. Schoeller strongly opposed this identification of the follicle hormone as a carcinogen, dismissing these experiments with genetically standardized mice as having been performed in an artificial system. His counter argument was that no cancer had ever appeared in normal mice.[20] In addition, he warned Cramer about the consequences of his claims about hormonal cancer genesis. If these were to reach the public sphere, Schoeller argued, they could jeopardize every and any use of the sex steroids.[21]

Following a request from Schoeller for his expert testimony, Butenandt also wrote to Cramer. His letter was more scientific in tone, but did not leave any greater room for doubt: "I have just discussed this point with the finest specialist in estrogen therapy, Prof. Kaufmann. He says that your concerns will disappear if you take into account the question of dosage. If dosage remains in the physiological range, Prof. Kaufmann does not think your view will hold."[22] Cancer risk was thus interpreted as a question of hormone concentrations and in the eyes of the Schering experts current practice was far from being a source of problems, even the hormonal treatment of menopause. The physiological nature of the drugs and their natural origins were critical points in ensuring their safe usage. In addition, Butenandt examined the male mice treated with oestron that Cramer had sent to Schering. His opinion was that tumour cells from these animals contained suspicious microscopic spots, suggesting the presence of a virus. Rather than being a carcinogen, the follicle hormone was in all probability acting as a growth facilitator, enhancing the effects of other carciongenic agents. Given this unambiguous scientific agenda, what kind of modelling practice could the Berlin scientists develop?

Experimentalizing cancer risk: the Schering-Charité-KWIB network

Before the appearance of DES, Kaufmann and his collaborators had based their attempts to produce cancers on the procedures used by Lacassagne. Having selected white rats as their test animals, the Charité gynecologists carried out long-term administrations of estron and estradiol. Their objective in this experiment was not only to wait for the development of visible tumours, but also to carry out complete histological studies of the genital tract in order to follow changes in the appearance of the tissues. Within this context of pathological research, the most important evidence was of a microscopic nature. Reports discussed the status of individual animals and concentrated on microphotographs of the ovaries, uterus and vagina of the animals, although the results were all negative. Just one single tumour was found following the manipulation of a few dozens rats, and as this abnormal growth was not even located in the genital tract, the case was taken as being unrelated to the hormonal treatment.[23] Complementary experiments performed on female rats using a combination of estradiol and progesterone led to observations of enlarged uterus and modified histology, but again no tumour was identified.[24]

Dealing with the DES problem led to several changes in experimental organization, with the main consequence being that Kauffmann's pathological and clinical approach no longer prevailed. First of all, Butenandt's laboratory became directly involved in organizing the testing. The evaluation of the carcinogenic potential of carbohydrates became an independent, significant research topic in its own right, supported by a specific grant from the *Reichsforschungsrat.* This support increased substantially after the beginning of the war. By 1943, the experimentation around cancer supported five scientists within the KWIB, and there are good reasons to think that it was used as a means to have more researchers working at the bench rather than being drafted into the army. Hans Friedrich-Freksa, one of Butenandt's early collaborators, remained at the Dahlem institute as coordinator of a project of national interest.[25]

Second, the transition from a two-partner to a three-partner research community resulted in the introduction of new practices. While Kaufmann had previously obtained the hormones to be tested directly from Schering, with the consequence that these were regular commercial products, one role of the newly integrated KWIB was to prepare the compounds to be evaluated, including new steroids or synthetic analogues like DES and its derivatives. Even more important, however, was the reorganization of how the tests were conducted. The involvement of the biochemists and their biotechnological culture led to a much stronger emphasis on standardization and the implementation of strict experimental protocols.

Echoing the discourse of US experimental researchers, Butenandt and his collaborators advocated the use of mice instead of rats, and more particularly the use of different strains of genetically standardized animals. In their vision, inbred animals were indispensable in order to avoid uncontrolled variability leading to false positives. The target was Lacassagne's early claim that "folliculine" induced mammary tumours, even though his own experiments manifested critical differences between various different genetic backgrounds. Experimentalizing the DES problem and visualizing the putative adverse effects of hormones was seen as a question of scale. Whereas Kaufmann had used a few dozens animals, the KWIB scientists wanted to use much larger numbers, in order to be able to apply statistical methods. A regular supply of inbred mice was finally secured by supplementing local husbandry with the products of a "tumour farm" the *RFR* established in Berlin in order to support experimental cancer research and prepare the creation of a large cancer institute in Posen.[26]

Furthermore, the process of scaling-up redefined the problems to be addressed. As statistically significant numbers started to be assembled, the mode of evaluation changed. The process did not only mean the introduction of some mathematical tests of significance, Friedrich-Freksa and the KWIB workers also redefined the phenomenon to be observed. Pathological images almost vanished, to be replaced by curves on graphs. In studies of carcinogenesis, particularly concerning aromatic compounds like methylcholanthrene, the standard practice was to report the incidence of tumours as a function of the duration of exposition, but this kind of simple dose–effect relationship could only work when the experimental system was producing a sufficient number of relevant events. This did not work very well when the studies were based on a less direct relationship or on long-term manipulation. One innovation of the KWIB-Charité-Schering network was therefore to draw so-called "Tumorerwartungskurven" (tumour expectation curves). These were graphs representing the predicted future evolution of the mouse population under examination. Tumour expectation curves plotted the total proportion of mice that would die from a given type of tumour against time. The juxtaposition of both types of curves thus provided a way to visualize both the risk and the incidence of cancer. Developed at the Charité, the procedure was soon complemented by another one, originating in the KWIB. As the number of compounds tested increased, their effects diversified, including highly toxic phenomena that dramatically modified the life expectancy of the mice. One problematic consequence was that life expectancy became so short that tumours no longer had enough time to develop. Conversely, the hormonal treatment could have favourable effects on general growth and would make the mice live longer, opening new windows of opportunity for tumour formation. Consequently, as Friedrich-Freksa argued, one needed means of comparing tumour formation at a specific age.[27] Scaling-up made the construction of rates on a two-month basis possible.

A report written by Friedrich-Freksa for the *Reichsforschungsrat* in 1943 or 1944, at a time when more than 4,700 mice had been investigated, illustrates the nature of this research program. As their "standard" for what a significant tumour genesis should look like, the KWIB team adopted the sarcoma induced by painting the skin of mice of heterogeneous genetic background with methylcholanthrene. Most compounds tested on this animal–disease model were found to be occasional and indirect carcinogens. The conclusions regarding two compounds in particular, estrogens and DES, are worth mentioning. On the one hand, the Berlin researchers confirmed Lacassagne's results, finding not only that estrogens induced a higher incidence of tumour in some strains, but also that they provoked a second wave of tumour formation analogous to the situation observed in non-breeding animals. The system thus echoed the castration procedure. On the other hand, according to Friedrich-Freksa, this increased incidence of mammary tumours might be related to an increased life expectancy due to the sex steroids. The phenomenon was, however, highly dependent on the genetic background of the test animals and could not be reproduced with all strains. The confusion originating in the multiple effects that one product could have was even more dramatic in the case of the experiments involving DES. The IG-Farben artificial hormone was such a toxic compound that an evaluation of its carcinogenic potency was almost impossible. The mice simply died too quickly from side effects ever to develop mammary or genital tumours.[28]

During the war, the KWIB cancer project was granted the status of "Kriegswichtige Forschung" (research critical to the war effort). The category was not particularly significant as such, as the majority of research projects at the institute received this same label. In the case of the research on cancer and hormones, however, this status was associated with a major change in cancer policy. As recounted by Proctor, the battle against cancer, along with reproductive medicine, became a major issue in national socialist medical policy,[29] leading to a boom in cancer research from 1937 onward.[30] This support and the public interest in the topic of chemical carcinogenesis facilitated the diversification of the research. One direction pursued was to link the cancer project with other research. Local studies of viruses were accordingly reorganized in such a way that an in-house project on the structure of the tobacco mosaic virus (pursued with the support of IG Farben) would be reoriented to look at oncogenic viruses.[31] The selected system was the rabbit papilloma virus, an agent that had been discovered and crystallized at the Rockfeller Institute before the war.[32] This type of research was strongly emphasized within the *Virusforschungsgemeinschaft*, a joint research venture between the *Kaiser Wilhelm Institut für Biochemie* and the *Kaiser Wilhelm Institut für Biologie*.[33]

Somewhere at the boundary between this particular movement of diversification in fundamental research and applied clinical research, Friedrich-Freksa launched an inquiry into the induction of new tumours using liver extracts from cancer patients.[34] In this case, the aim was not to search for transmissible cancer agents, but to test an alternative explanation for the action of sex hormones. Assuming that sex steroids were not directly carcinogenic, the researchers at the KWIB looked for some chemical explanation for their stimulating effects, which would go beyond simply reiterating the fact that sex hormones stimulated growth in general. The basic idea they came up with was to suppose that the weak analogy in chemical structure between the sex steroids and the coal-tar carbohydrates, which did directly cause cancer, was meaningful. Estrogens could thus become carcinogenic agents following a rearrangement of their chemical structure within the body. One favoured possibility was a process of oxidation and ring formation, which could take place as part of the liver catabolism of cholesterol and other natural steroids.[35] This perspective led to the first instance of close collaboration between the KWIB and a cancer clinic. Liver samples from cancer patients with and without liver metastasis were obtained from the Virchow Hospital in Berlin, either post-operatively or post-mortem. Extracts were then dissolved and chemically fractionated, and the resulting preparations inoculated into or painted on the same mice as those used for the hormone project. Many tumours arose in the test animals, but since they were generally not located at the point of application, they were taken to be artifacts. The formation of a sarcoma in the uterus of the test mice was treated as an exception and attributed to the effects of the liver extracts, based on the statistical significance of the occurrence of this particular phenomenon. Once again, a genetic argument for the origin of the sarcoma prevailed. As the uterus tumours affected one of the strains more often than the others, Friedrich-Freksa concluded that "the effect of the liver extract is to activate a pre-existing cancer agent".[36]

The same perspective dominates the public statements concerning this new style of modelling work. In his frequent essays on the relationship between sex hormones and the "cancer problem", Butenandt adopted a twofold argument aimed at undermining the correlation between steroids and tumour formation. The first level of discussion was a plea for a chemical understanding of carcinogenesis. Comparing methylcholanthren and other derivatives that induced local tumours, the director of the KWIB explained that all these molecules contained five aromatic rings, while all the natural steroids had only four. Carcinogens could therefore only arise by means of ring formation, a process that was only possible for cholesterol since all the other sex steroids lacked a lateral chain out of which a new ring could be formed.[37] This point provided the background for the second argument, which was a repetition of the reasoning he had presented in 1938. Sex hormones could stimulate the growth of tissues, and therefore speed up the development of tumours, but they could not induce such cancers on their own. The increased incidence of tumours observed in the experimental systems when relatively high doses were used did not originate in the action of hormones, but in the existence of a carcinogenic agent whose action was facilitated by the sex steroids. In most cases, this agent was of a genetic nature as revealed by the highly heterogeneous patterns of cancer seen in the inbred strains. From this perspective, of course, there was no difference between the natural hormones and DES, which meant that by saving the natural steroids from the accusation of carcinogenesis, Butenandt was unexpectedly clearing the name of IG Farben's product at the same time.[38]

The clinical implications of this perspective were straightforward. In contrast to the warnings arising from previous research, estrogens – especially natural estrogens – were now declared safe. Butenandt repeatedly argued that the KWIB experiments revealed that "the known natural female hormones as well as their esters do not act in ways comparable to the widely discussed chemical carcinogens".[39] His position remained basically unchanged throughout the period of the wartime experiments, despite the increasing documentation about the effects of high doses of estrogens.[40]

Not all observers were convinced that the new KWIB-Schering research strategy of combining large numbers with the genetic control of test animals was the right path to follow. In addition to castration experiments, cancer specialists in various hospitals developed alternative systems, revealing the conditions under which the follicle hormone operated as a carcinogenic agent. Most of these systems were histopathological arrangements focusing on a conjunction of anatomical and microscopic examinations. The example of the Institute of Pathology at the University of Munich led by Max Borst illustrates this point, in particular the work of an *Assistentin* in the laboratory, Hannah Pierson, who persistently investigated the effects of steroid inoculation. From 1939 onwards, she regularly published reports on instances of tumour formation, principally consisting of "clinical" descriptions of isolated cases. This work was not a search for statistically significant figures, but rather a search for clinically significant images. For instance, case KK98 described the fate of a castrated rabbit born in February 1935 that died in March 1938 with an infiltrated tumour of the intestine. What made this case particularly significant was not only the fact that the tumor surfaced after months of hormonal treatment, but also that it presented all the cellular traits of a mammary tumour as illustrated by numerous micrographs.[41] Using a similar approach, other authors also reported on the carcinogenic effects of DES.[42]

The spectre of cancer risk: sex steroids and the sanitary order

From our description of the experimental scene during the 1930s and 1940s, one might be tempted to think that the argument over the carcinogenic nature of steroids had been settled in favour of the safety of the steroids. Experimental systems focusing on standardization and quantitative analysis led their inventors to the conclusion that sex steroids were not the cause of cancer. Under "physiological" or "clinical" conditions of use, the risk was so low that it was practically insignificant. As the head of IG Farben's pharmacology department once put it in a paper on DES, dosage is everything and any drug can become a poison when used in "unsafe" ways.[43] Facing the sophisticated laboratory system developed by the Berlin network, the older "pathology and histology" approach seems to us today rather unsophisticated and unconvincing. Evaluating the discussion on the basis of our modern methodological standards would, however, be misleading. In the 1940s, inbred mice, statistical tests, and molecular synthesis belonged to a world far removed from the clinic, and establishing the link between mice and women was not at all evident. In the eyes of many oncologists, the gap was simply too large to be bridged, and the qualitative histological data from the occasional positive experiments were far more impressive than the reassuring tables of huge amounts of data resulting from low-dose inoculation. In contrast to what Butenandt, Kaufmann and Schoeller might have expected, experimentalizing the cancer and hormone problem and attacking the fundamental issues did not make the situation any easier. The use of estrogens remained an issue of concern, and was considered a medical practice at risk.

This view that there was a danger of cancer associated with the use of hormones could be seen in the medical literature with continued discussions of hypothetical schemes explaining how sex steroids could – under normal physiological or clinical conditions – become carcinogens. We can find eloquent testimony to the variety of resources that could be mobilized to this end by looking at the work of one of Butenandt's long-term associates. During the war, the Berlin pathologist Hermann Druckrey developed an original scheme based on a series of chemical transformations that exploited the recent knowledge of the metabolic pathways of steroids in bacteria.[44] Druckrey then speculated that the same sort of reactions could transform the natural steroids into more potent carcinogens. This transformation process could be of practical clinical significance since the normal intestinal microbial population might react with the estrogens found in food or with the Progynon pills.

The persistence of risk was also visible in debates about the regulation of the use of sex steroids. Up to 1941, the sex steroids were easily available, being initially granted the same status as vitamins based on their classification as natural products. As the medical use of these hormones expanded, physicians in general, and gynecologists in particular, voiced their reservations about this situation. These complaints were occasionally about the putative use of estrogens as means for aborting pregnancy, but most of the published arguments concentrated on the lay, unspecified, and "unprofessional" use of these drugs by women who wanted to alleviate the symptoms accompanying menopause.[45] Many – if not a majority – of the specialists in reproductive medicine claimed that extensive use of steroids for handling menopause was a misuse, if not an abuse, which was too often accepted by general practitioners. Adverse side effects reported in the medical literature concentrated on vascular consequences, most especially uncontrolled bleeding. The introduction of DES intensified this discussion as it implied – if the regulation remained unchanged – easy access to much greater quantities of estrogens. Thus, in June 1940, the President of the *Reichsgesundheitsamt* explained to Schering officials that sooner or later action would be taken on the matter.[46]

Six months later, an annex of the general ordinance that reorganized the supply of drugs in mobilized National-Socialist Germany redefined sex hormones as prescription drugs. This change of legal status appears to have satisfied the medical profession, and at the conference on the evaluation of the uses of sex steroids organized by the Berlin medical society in 1941 the comments on the change were very positive.[47] The chemical treatment of menopause was still recommended as a useful measure for women suffering from severe menopausal symptoms. But estrogen replacement therapy was to be administered under close medical supervision, using low physiological doses, and for only a short duration. Such guidelines and the new legal framework did not, however, succeed in bringing the use of the sex steroids under control. In 1944, Conti, in his capacity as the *Reichsgesundheitsführer*, again raised the issue of hormone use. Citing letters from gynecologists, he argued that the problems German women were experiencing under the war conditions made the increased use of the sex hormones to treat depression, fatigue and psychological disorders understandable. However, the scarcity of the natural steroids made it necessary to enforce tighter control over prescriptions, with the highest priority being given to reproductive disorders of ovarian origin. Conti thus asked the health administration to take new steps like providing special labels and warnings to the physicians.[48]

There is some evidence that the discussion over gynecological misuses was related to the risk of cancer and, although the issue does not surface directly in the archives of the health administration, it is nevertheless suggested by two sorts of elements. First, the medical literature occasionally published clinical reports about women unnecessarily treated with estrogens despite suffering from undetected genital cancers, which consequently enlarged and manifested themselves in the course of the treatment.[49] Second, when the new regulations concerning the hormones were implemented, the cancer issue was of constant concern to Schering's managers. Schoeller's experimental cancer research was then identified as being detrimental to the company's commercial interests.[50]

From gynecology to oncology: the vanishing risk of innovation

In 1949, the *Zeitschrift für Krebsforschung* published a long article on the hormones of follicles and the formation of tumours. Written by researchers from both the Charité and the former KWIB (C. Kaufmann, H. Aurel Müller, A. Butenandt and H. Friedrich-Freksa), this text summarized the experiments performed up until the end of the war.[51] The text did not bring very much new to the table, essentially restating the theory of the indirect contribution of the hormones to the genesis of tumours, although in stronger terms than before. If the therapeutic dosage remained low, the clinical situation remained safe. Thus, the experimental evaluation of the cancer risk supported the same recommendations for professional control over the treatment and appropriate medical training as the previous discussion over the treatment of menopause. Moreover, the question of natural versus artificial compounds had vanished. For Kaufmann and his associates, natural estrogens and DES no longer presented any significant difference in terms of carcinogenic effect.

This paper ended an era, and the German medical press barely raised the issue in the course of the following decade. Kaufmann continued to work on sex steroids and their medical uses, publishing many papers on their application in reproductive medicine, but never discussing the question of the risk of cancer.[52] The experiments at his new women's clinic in Magdeburg focused on the metabolic effects of estrogens and progesterone.[53] Once they had been reassembled in a new biochemical institute in Tübingen, the former KWIB biochemists also chose to pursue other paths of research, only publishing one paper on the cancer problem. This was a biochemical study of a new class of compounds that might possibly play the role of intermediates between cholesterol as a starting product and carcinogenic substances synthesized within the body.[54] The target for this kind of research was always cholesterol, due to its chemical structure, which other participants in the debates that took place in the 1930s and 1940s had already targeted. During the 1950s, German cancer journals as well as general medical periodicals like the *Klinische Wochenschrift* published a very limited number of texts on the problem, and no new experimental research. The issue of hormones as a cause of cancer seems to have vanished from the German medical scene.

One explanation for this situation may be that there was a strong consensus about the results obtained by Kaufmann and Butenandt; at least, this was the case in Germany. However, the debate did not die out everywhere. Cancer specialists in the United States kept working on the issue, particularly at the National Cancer Institute. Michael Shimkin, for instance, a surgeon at the NCI, published some particularly controversial results. Having implanted estrogen pellets in male mice, he claimed that mammary tumours could be elicited using low physiological doses of steroids.[55] Another reason for the abrupt termination of debates in Germany was with the end of the war and the massive destruction in Germany at this period, followed by the post-war reorganization of research. The fate of the KWIB illustrates this situation very well, as, when Butenandt left Berlin in 1944 and relocated in Tübingen, many aspects of the former research system changed as well. First of all, the laboratory's industrial connections were deeply affected, with the exclusive and long-term collaboration with Schering coming to an end.[56] Many projects initiated during the war did not survive these changes, and so limited means and a lack of research material made severe cuts inevitable. Antibiotics, physiological genetics, and hormones controlling the metamorphosis of insects were at the top of the list of priorities, not hormones and cancer.[57] Cancer did not, however, disappear in this context; rather, it was gradually redefined. No longer a topic for bench practice, it became the object of Butenandt's expert testimony.

Although the situation of occupied Germany in the late 1940s certainly contributed to new features in the landscape of biomedical research, it does not – as such – explain why the cancer and hormone issue did not surface later in some form or other. Individual career paths and the circumstances in which various researchers found themselves cannot account for such a general phenomenon, and it may be more useful to look at the post-war professional literature on cancer to try to explain it. Hormones are heavily presented in this literature, but only as therapeutic agents, with the field of hormone therapy dominated by two diseases: prostate cancer and breast cancer.

The hormonal treatment of prostate cancer was initiated in the United States in the early 1940s, when the Chicago surgeon Charles Huggins conducted a series of clinical experiments based on the idea that prostate

cancer depended on male hormones. The therapeutic idea was that reducing
the supply of these compounds would also reduce the tumour growth. Like
many oncologists, Huggins employed castration as a surgical therapy but
with mixed results, and so in parallel, researchers sought to complement this
treatment by using anti-androgen chemicals. The availability of DES transformed this approach into a practice of contra-hormonal therapy. The analogue
of estrogen was first utilized as means of controlling cancer in human
patients after the inoculation of estrogens had apparently slowed down the
development of prostate tumours in dogs, the only animal model spontaneously
affected with this pathology.[58] The procedure crossed the Atlantic in
1945–46 as the centre of gravity of biomedical exchanges shifted to the United
States, and the first reports of hormonal treatment of German patients appeared
in 1948.[59] Protocols featuring the daily injection of up to 100 mg of DES
were strongly advocated as being highly effective. Adverse effects like the
formation of other tumours, particularly breast cancers, could not be avoided,
but this was considered a minor problem that could be resolved by finding
the right dosage. In spite of this optimistic approach, the initial treatments
were followed by reports about feminization associated with the use of
these hormones, as well as a few instances of breast cancer in DES-treated
males.[60]

The prospective therapeutic use of "counter-hormones" was not limited to
tumours associated with the male reproductive organs. Given the widely
acknowledged hormone-dependency of breast tumours, it would have been
surprising if a similar therapeutic approach had not been attempted in
female patients. Indeed, the 1940s also saw the beginning of trials of the
most widely produced male hormone, dehydroandrosterone (DHA), which
served as the industrial precursor of the other sex steroids.[61] Animal models
provided the expected results with the effects of DHA and estrogens understood as simply two opposite poles.[62] Human trials took place in France and
in the United States, with some therapeutic effects and relatively minor
adverse effects. The positive results were, however, so slight that most
German commentators expressed strong reservations. The side effects, on the
other hand, such as a change in the voice, hair growth, etc., became visible
very rapidly, and were considered unacceptable by many clinicians.[63]

A more unexpected outcome of this move toward the hormonal treatment
of cancer was the use of estrogens for the treatment of breast cancer. In 1944,
G. Haddow, a British cancer specialist, reported that DES could be used as
an agent to limit the growth of breast tumours, and he subsequently received
support from other researchers. Tumour reduction could, however, only be
obtained using relatively high doses. In contrast to the consequences of the
use of DHA, adverse effects like increased pigmentation, edema or thin-
ness of the skin did not directly challenge sexual identities, at least in the
view of the doctors. These side-effects were deemed manageable and
the method acceptable, even though it did not "cure" but only "improved"
the situation.[64] Given the long experience of the role of estrogens as a

growth factor, no simple explanation could account for this inhibition of tumour growth. Dosage again provided a means of reconciling conflicting statements in conjunction with the physiological feedback loops linking the pituitary and the ovaries, which had been discovered in the late 1930s. In other words, high doses of estrogens were thought to stimulate the release of pituitary hormones, which in turn had a beneficial effect on breast tissue, but low doses did not do so. In Germany, this interpretation was well received, since it echoed similar trials that had been conducted to investigate the use of Prolan, a pituitary extract sold by IG Farben, to achieve similar reduction of breast tumours.

The development of this "contrasexual" cancer therapy depended directly on the availability of large amounts of sex hormones and their analogues. It could not have emerged before the introduction of the partial synthesis of sex steroids mentioned above, as well as the preparation of DES, although its timing was not exclusively determined by production capabilities. The clinical use of the sex steroids gained legitimacy during the war when the chemotherapy of cancer in general was gradually coming to be accepted as a promising complementary approach to surgery, especially in the treatment of "inoperable" cancers. In addition, the therapeutic fate of sex steroids should be interpreted against the background of the post-war scientific order and the reorganization of research in Europe. In occupied Germany, during the 1940s and the 1950s, establishing shared topics and new links with the US and British researchers was seen as a critical goal for many physicians, who were trying to distance themselves from their recent past. It is tempting to speculate that this situation made the "Western" approach of cancer chemotherapy even more attractive.

The consequences of this therapeutic developement on the status of the sex steroids were far from marginal. Used as therapies in oncology, a medical domain characterized by repeated failures, estrogens and androgens acquired a different aura. Adverse effects had to be balanced against the inescapable fate of patients suffering from a deadly condition. Within this context, the issue was no longer the long-term possibility of inducing new tumours, but the short-term ability to reduce the existing cancer versus the physical and psychological supportability of the development of "countersexual" traits. Adding the therapeutic layer to the issue of "cancer and hormones" changed the global understanding of cancer risk, implying a more central role for a generalized view of the "dosage" framework. Thus, the therapeutic displacement had a knock-on effect on gynecological practice, reinforcing the pharmaceutical normality of the sex hormones, as well as the notion that "low dosage" and professionally controlled use were unproblematic.

Conclusion

During the first two decades after the war, the carcinogenic potential of the sex steroids was no longer a topic for research. This property became a research tool employed in the investigation of the relationship between cell metabolism, endocrine physiology, and the action of "true" cancer agents like methylcholanthren, or cancer viruses. Unsurprisingly, hormonal manipulation of mice and rats was a particularly well developed practice within the laboratories that studied breast cancer. Hormones as a cause of cancer only reappeared on the public scene in the early 1970s when the issue was raised in a very spectacular form by the "DES scandal". This scandal brought the hidden risk of prior hormonal therapy in women to light, as it now became clear that the daughters of women treated with this drug – most commonly for preventing miscarriages – were suffering from an increasing incidence of malformations and genital cancers. The central category used to talk about this issue was now risk,[65] understood as a statistical construction defined by epidemiological surveys that focused on comparisons between controlled populations. This chapter has shown that the genealogy of this "crisis in sex hormones" can be traced back to the 1930s.

Our case study allows us to offer three concluding remarks regarding the nature of biomedical innovation and risk assessment. The first point is simply that the pre-war steroid-related cancer risk was never discussed in terms of risk as we now define it; that is to say it was never related to any form of epidemiological statistical inquiry. Within the clinical culture of the time, risks were adverse or toxic effects; that is to say the – usually short-term – consequences of the administration of drugs. Such effects were defined as a problem of dosage, and the response was to establish the appropriate dose–toxicity curves. These risks were circumvented by defining good therapeutic practice, specifying appropriate indications, and standardizing dosage. Ideally, well-informed physicians would spontaneously implement these measures, although problems often arose when the evaluation of such toxicity gave conflicting results. Overall, toxic side effects rarely challenged the pharmacological paradigm unless they proved to be fatal.[66] During the post-war period major public "crises", like the Thalidomide disaster, the lung cancer and tobacco controversy, or the DES scandal, played a significant role in inducing major changes in the procedures that were intended to make therapeutic risks visible. The sex steroid debate did not link pharmacology with statistical clinical trials, but it was an early element in this same process. The 1938–45 cancer and steroid discussion did displace the time-frame of the adverse effects to be taken into account by focusing on clinically invisible problems, which would become manifest at a later date. In the gynecologists' eyes, the seriousness of the cancer problem was reinforced by the fact that the practices viewed as most problematic and dangerous were associated with attempts to control menopause, then a quite marginal indication lying at the boundary between the normal and the pathological. The years immediately following the war were also dominated by the same pharmacological dynamic of the management of adverse effects, and the issue of "cancer risk" vanished from the German scene once the sex steroids had gained a new status as anti-cancer drugs.

Our second remark concerns the experimental analysis of the correlation between the administration of estrogens and the development of cancer. Since the "risk" to be discussed was clinically invisible, modelling was at the very centre of the hormone and cancer discussion. The pattern of experimentalization followed by the KWIB-Charité-Schering network illustrates typical features of contemporary biomedical research. Modelling practices were deeply affected by patterns reinforcing the standardization and the "molecularization" of medical practices.[67] The model system, which was established at the *Kaiser Wilhelm Institute für Biochemie*, thus combined the biochemical culture of molecular control with the use of inbred mice as research material. This choice reinforced these trends while pushing the system in the direction of a logic of large numbers.

The third and final remark concerns the part played by the "invisible industrialist". Although Schering rarely surfaced in the scientific publications of the KWIB-Charité scientists, the company was nevertheless a prominent actor. The firm's role was – as we have argued elsewhere – to supply essential research materials, to develop in-house research that also delivered results and skills, which could eventually be passed on to external research associates.[68] Schering's intervention also consisted in commissioning reports of expertise, which in the cancer and steroids case proved more important than the company's role as a supplier. Schering did not organize the steroid and cancer studies themselves, and there are even indications that the company's upper management was suspicious of the interest its research director manifested in this issue. The relationship between the firm and its academic partners was, however, close enough to have the latter promptly react to a problem raised by the market, participate in regulatory debates, and invent sophisticated experimental arrangements to confirm the non-existence of the cancer risk. The irony of this story is that this same risk started to become clinically visible when it had already become experimentally invisible.

Notes

1 J.-Y. Nau, "Faut-il traiter la ménopause?", *Le Monde,* Lundi 10 Février 2003, p. 16.
2 L. Marks, *Sexual Chemistry: A History of the Contraceptive Pill,* New Haven: Yale University Press, 2001. N. Pfeffer, *The Stork and the Syringe,* Cambridge: Cambridge University Press, 1993.
3 N. Oudshoorn, *Beyond the Natural Body: An Archeology of Sex Hormones,* London: Routledge, 1994. A. Clarke, *Disciplining Reproduction: Modernity, American Life and the Problems of Sex,* Berkeley: University of California Press, 1998.
4 W. Schoeller, *Tagung der medizinische wissenschaftliche Abteilung,* Schering AG, Dezember 1938, Archiv Scherianum, Bestand 02, Ordner 1585.
5 J.-P. Gaudillière, "Better prepared than purified", *Studies in the History and Philosophy of the Biological and Biomedical Sciences,* in press.
6 *Die ovarielle Hormontherapie mit Progynon, Progynon B oleosum, und Proluton,* Schering-Kahlbaum AG, c. 1936.
7 C. Kaufmann, "Echte Menstruation bei einer kastrierten Frau durch Zufuhr von Ovarialhormonen", *Zentralblatt für Gynäkologie,* 1933, 57: 42–6.

8 C. Kaufmann, "Die Behandlung der Amenorrhoe mit hohen Dosen der Ovarialhormone", *Klinische Wochenschrift* 1933, 12: 1557–62 ; Schering, *Die ovarielle Hormontherapie*, 1936.

9 C. Kaufmann, "Kritische Bewertung der Hormonetherapie", *Archiv der Gynäkologie*, 1938, 166: 113–31.

10 *Progynon and Prolution Reine Ovarial Preparate*, Schering AG, ca. 1940, Archiv Scheringianum.

11 Archiv Scheringianum, Bestand 05, o.361, Verstandsekretariat, 9 Oktober 1945.

12 G. Bock, *Zwangssterilisation im Nationalsozialismus: Studien zur Rassenpolitik und Frauenpolitik*, Westdeutscher Verlag, 1986.

13 F. Vienne, *"Volk ohne Junge" de F. Bürgdörfer, histoire d'un objet de savoir des années 20 à la fin de la seconde guerre mondiale*, Thèse Paris: EHESS, 2000.

14 A. E. C. Lathrop, L. Loeb, "On the Part Played by Internal Secretion in the Spontaneous Development of Tumors", *Journal of Cancer Research*, 1916, 1: 1–16.

15 I. Löwy and J.-P. Gaudillière, "Disciplining Cancer: Mice and the Practice of Genetic Purity", in J.-P. Gaudillière and I. Löwy (eds), *The Invisible Industrialist*, London: Macmillan, 1998, pp. 209–49.

16 N. Pfeffer, "Lessons from History: The Salutary Tale of Stilboestrol", in P. Alderson (ed.), *Consent to Health Treatment and Research: Differing Perspectives*, Report of the Social Science Research Unit Conference, 1992.

17 Archiv der Max Planck Gesellschaft (AMPG), Butenandt Nachlass, III/84, o. 250, Schoeller to Butenandt, 24.7.1938, Butenandt to Schoeller, 27.7.38.

18 AMPG, III/84, o.250, Stalmann to Butenandt, 9.8.38.

19 AMPG, III/84, o.250, Cramer to Neumann, no date.

20 AMPG, III/84, o.250, Schoeller to Cramer, 23.5.1938.

21 AMPG, III/84, o.250, Schoeller to Cramer, 23.5.1938, p. 2.

22 AMPG, III/84, o.250, Butenandt to Cramer, 3.6.1938.

23 C. Kaufmann and E. Steinkamm, "Über die Wirkung fortgesetzter Zufuhr unphysiologischer Mengen Follikelhormon auf das Genitale weiblicher Ratten", *Archiv der Gynaekologie*, 1936, 162: 553–94.

24 C. Kaufmann and E. Steinkamm, "Über die Wirkung unphysiologischer Mengen Keimdrüsenhormon auf das Genitale weiblicher kastrierter Ratten", *Archiv der Gynaekologie*, 1938, 165: 358–73.

25 B. Gausemeier, "An der Heimatfront. 'Kriegswichtige' Forschung am Kaiser-Wilhelm-Institut für Biochemie", in W. Schieder and A. Trunk (Hsg) *Adolf Butenandt und die Kaiser-Wilhelm-Gesellschaft: Wissenschaft, Industrie und Politik im 'Dritten Reich'*, Göttingen: Wallstein, 2004.

26 A. Schwerin, *Tierzucht, Strahlen und Pigmente: Genetik und die Herstellung von Tiermodellen für die Humangenetik. Hans Nachtsheim und die vergleichende und experimentelle Erbpathologie in Deutschland 1920–1945*, Diss. Berlin 2002.

27 H. Friedrich-Freksa, "Sexualhormone und Entstehung bösartiger Geschwülste", *Berichte über der Gynaekologie* 1940, 40: 225–88.

28 AMPG, III/84, o.782, Berichte H. Friedriech-Freksa, o.D.

29 R. Proctor, *The Nazi War on Cancer*, Princeton: Princeton University Press, 1999.

30 J. Steinwachs, *Die Förderung der medizinischen Forschung in Deutschland durch den Reichsforschungsrat während der Jahre 1937 bis 1945 unter besonderer Berücksichtigung der Krebsforschung*, unpublished medical dissertation, Leipzig, 2000.

31 AMPG, III/84, IG-Farben Korrespondenz.

32 A. Creager and J.-P. Gaudillière, "Experimental Arrangements and Technologies of Visualization: Cancer as Viral Epidemic, 1930–1960", in J.-P. Gaudillière and I. Löwy (eds), *Heredity and Infection: A History of Disease Transmission*, London: Routledge, 2001, pp. 203–41.

33 H.-J. Rheinberger, "Virusforschung an den Kaiser-Wilhelm-Instituten für Biochemie und für Biologie", in D. Kaufmann (Hrg.), *Geschichte der Kaiser-Wilhelm-Gesellschaft im*

Nationalsozialismus: Bestandaufnahme und Perspektiven der Forschung, Göttingen: Wallstein, 2000, pp. 667–98.

34 AMPG, III/84, o.407, Versuche zum Nachweis von Stoffen von der Art der cancerogenen Kohlenwasserstoffe in der Leber von Krebskranken, 1943.

35 AMPG, III/84, o.407, Berichte November 1939.

36 H. Friedriech-Freksa, Beuchte 1943.

37 A. Butenandt, "Neue Beiträge der biologischen Chemie zum Krebsprobleme", *Angewandte Chemie*, 1940, 53: 345–52.

38 A. Butenandt, "Neue Beiträge".

39 A. Butenandt, "Neue Beiträge", p. 349.

40 A. Butenandt, A. Dannenberg and H. Friedrich-Freksa, "Experimentelle Beiträge zur Bedeutung der Krebsentstehung", *Angewandte Chemie*, 1953, 56: 221–7.

41 H. Pierson, "Neubildung von mammaähnlichen Bau in den äusseren Magenschichten des Kaninchens bei langdauernder Behandlung mit Follikulin", *Zeitschrift für Krebsforschung*, 1939, 46: 177–82.

42 L. Savnik and V. Premru, "Ein Beitrag zur cancerogenen Wirkung der Stilbenpräparate", *Zeitschrift für Krebsforschung*, 1941, 51: 337–43.

43 D. Huf, "Die Anwendung von Follikelhormonen Distilbenen beim Mann", *Klinische Wochenschrift*, 1942, 21: 1113–21.

44 AMPG, III/84, o. 1359, Druckrey to Butenandt, 29.6.43. H. Druckrey, "Die Pharmakologie krebserregender Substanzen", *Zeitschrift für Krebsforschung*, 1950, 57: 70–85.

45 R. Schröder, "Kritische Besprechung der Sexualhormontherapie", *Deutsche Medizinische Wochenschrift*, 1941, p. 1167.

46 AMPG, III/84, o.250, Schoeller to Butenandt, 21.5.1940

47 "Kritische Bewertung der Sexualhormontherapie", *Klinische Wochenschrift*, 1941, 20: 1037–8.

48 Bundesarchiv Berlin, R86, o.3990, Der Reichsgesundheitsführer an das Reichsgesundheitsamt, 2.11.1944.

49 V. Roth, "Die Bedeutung der veresterten Stilbenpräparate für die Hormontherapie", *Zentralblatt für Gynäkologie*, 1941, 1612–19.

50 C. Kobrack, *National Cultures and International Competition: The Experience of Schering AG*. Cambridge: Cambridge University Press, 2002. Scheringsarchiv, B2/1594, Berckemeyer to Koeppel, 19.4.1943.

51 C. Kaufmann et al., "Experimentelle Beiträge zur Bedeutung des Follikelshormons für die Carcinomentstehung", *Zeitschrift für Krebsforschung*, 1949, 56 : 482–542.

52 C. Kaufmann, "Progesteron, sein Schicksal im Organismus und seine Anwendung in der Therapie", *Klinische Wochenschrift*, 1955, 33: 345–7.

53 J. Zander and J. Schmidt-Thomé, "Über die Auscheidung von Androsteronglukuronid nach Testosteroninjektion", *Klinische Wochenschrift*, 1954, 32: 24–7.

54 H. Dannenberg, "Steranthren, eine neue Beziehung zwischen Steroiden und krebserzeugenden Kohlwasserstoffen", *Zeitschrift für Krebsforschung*, 1957, 62 : 217–29.

55 M. B. Shimkin and R. S. Wyman, "Mammary Tumors in Male Mice Implanted with Estrogen-Cholesterol Pellets", *Journal of the National Cancer Institute*, 1947, pp. 71–5.

56 J.-P. Gaudillière, "Biochemie und Industrie: Der Arbeitskreis Butenandt-Schering im National-Sozialismus", in W. Schieder and A. Trunk (Hsg), *Adolf Butenandt und die Kaiser-Wilhelm-Gesellschaft: Wissenschaft, Industrie und Politik im 'Dritten Reich'*, Göttingen: Wallstein, 2004.

57 P. Karlson, *Adolf Butenandt: Biochemiker, Hormonforscher, Wisschenschaftspolitiker*, Stuttgart: Wissenschaftliche Verlaggesellschaft, 1990.

58 On this clinical research, see C. Huggins, "Hormonabhängige Geschwülste – Klinisch und experimentell", *Klinische Wochenschrift*, 1958, 36: 1102–6.

59 H. Henninger, "Die Hormontherapie des Prostatakarzinoms", *Der Krebsarzt*, 1948, 3: 365–8.

60 J. A. McClure and C. C. Huggins, "Bilateral Carcinoma of Male Breast after Estrogen Therapy", *JAMA*, 146, 1951, 7–9. G. Liebegott, "Mammacarcinom beim Mann nach Follikelhormon Behandlung", *Klinische Wochenschrift*, 1949, 27: 109.

61 J.-P. Gaudillière, "Better prepared than purified", forthcoming in *Studies in History and Philosophy of the Biological and Biomedical Sciences*.

62 C. C. Huggins, 1958.

63 M. Schlemenson, "Die Hormonbehandlung des fortgeschrittenen Brustkreb", *Der Krebsarzt*, 1949, 3: 320–2.

64 H. Tischer, "Kontrollmöglichkeiten kontrasexueller Hormontherapie bei inoperablen Genitalkarzinom", *Der Krebsarzt*, 1953, 8: 224–30.

65 B. Seaman and G. Seaman, *Women and the Crisis in Sex Hormones*, New York: Wyden Books 1977. D. B. Duton, *Worse than the Disease*, Cambridge: Cambridge University Press, 1988.

66 H. Marks, *The Progress of Experiment*, Cambridge: Cambridge University Press, 1997.

67 On the molecularization of twentieth-century biology and medicine: S. de Chadarevian and H. Kamminga (eds), *The Molecularization of Biology and Medicine*, Amsterdam, Harwood, 1998. J.-P. Gaudilliàre, *Inventer la biomédecine*, Paris, La Découverte, 2002.

68 J.-P. Gaudillière and I. Löwy (eds), *The Invisible Industrialist: Manufactures and the Production of Scientific Knowledge*, London: Macmillan, 1998.

10 Risk assessment and medical authority in operative fracture care in the 1960s and 1970s

Thomas Schlich

In this chapter, I will discuss how a specific surgical treatment was perceived and assessed differently according to changing discourses about its risk. I will further show how different views concerning risk were associated with different concepts of medical authority and different power relations, so that taking a particular view of risk also entailed endorsing a particular model of the individual doctor's role in medicine and society.

My example is the case of operative fracture treatment using plates and screws, which in medical terminology is called "osteosynthesis" or "internal fixation". In the late 1950s, this form of treatment was rejected by the majority of surgeons because they thought it was too risky. In fixing a broken bone with screws and plates the surgeon turns a closed fracture into an open wound and creates a point of entry for infectious agents. Bone infection is a very serious complication and can easily result in protracted illness or even the loss of the limb. Other possible complications include delayed healing or a failure of the broken bone to re-unite. In the 1950s, therefore, the tendency was to treat fractures by so-called "conservative methods" such as plaster casts or extensions.[1] Today, by contrast, internal fixation is one of a range of fracture treatments employed on a routine basis.

The procedure was introduced into the repertoire of standard surgical techniques in Europe in the 1960s and in North America in the 1970s, and both proponents and critics of this technique attribute the spread of osteosynthesis to the activities of the Swiss "Association for Osteosynthesis", or the *Arbeitsgemeinschaft für Osteosynthesefragen* (AO/ASIF). The AO was initially founded in 1958 as an association of 13 surgeons who shared the common aim of introducing the systematic use of osteosynthesis into surgical practice. To further this goal, the surgeons brought out a series of textbooks and launched a program of hands-on practical courses. In collaboration with a group of industrial manufacturers, the AO also designed and produced standardized instruments and implants for osteosynthesis. Part of the profits from the sales of these items went to the AO, who then used the money to fund research institutions. The AO ran two institutions itself, one of which functioned as a basic research laboratory while the other was set up as a special documentation centre to study the results of the procedures carried out using the AO's instruments and implants. The combination of preliminary testing and post-operative evaluation enabled the AO surgeons to gain a worldwide position of authority concerning the subject of risk and safety in osteosynthesis. The AO has been able to maintain its prestige, and remains a global player in the business of osteosynthesis, with thousands of members and associates and annual sales worth one billion Swiss Francs.

In the course of this chapter, I would first like to show how the AO succeeded in changing the perception of risk associated with osteosynthesis in a way that permitted the spread of this method of treatment. I will also show how the success of the AO in spreading the method simultaneously served to strengthen its own credibility and authority. In the second section of the paper, I want to point out the limits of the AO's basically successful line of argument. To make this point, I will look at those surgeons who refused to be convinced by the AO. An important point I want to convey is that these critics based their opposition on a different type of medical rationality, one that saw medicine as an art rather than a science, which in turn entails a different concept of the social order and power relations within medicine. The opponents rejected the AO's way of dealing with therapeutic risk, which was based on a scientific concept of surgery. In their view, such an approach undermined the individual surgeon's authority and autonomy, attributes he or she needed to retain in order to decide on and apply the most appropriate fracture treatment in each individual case.

Defusing a discourse about risk

As indicated, the main argument raised against the use of osteosynthesis was the risk of complications. Typically, critics asked whether the benefits associated with this treatment method were "so substantial that the risk inherent in an open procedure is fully justified".[2] Of course, this kind of consideration is not specific to osteosynthesis. Risk and safety are major issues in the acceptance of medical innovations in general,[3] but new operations are subject to particular scrutiny, since in surgery the causal relationship between the doctor's actions and their – possibly fatal – consequences is both more immediate and more evident than in cases involving drug therapy or dietetics.[4]

Discussions about the risks associated with new therapeutic techniques are often controversial, so that one and the same technique can be evaluated very differently by different participants. From an anthropological perspective, Mary Douglas and Aaron Wildavsky have described how risk perception and assessment in general are a matter of focusing on some facts while omitting others. Thus, particular criteria for evaluation are selected and responsibility is attributed in a specific way that depends very much on the worldview and interests of those involved.[5] Seen from this perspective, the testing of novel treatments and the way such tests are documented and analysed are part of the very process of defining risk.[6] In what follows I will describe how the AO participated in such a process and successfully redefined the risk involved in using its technique.

The manageability of danger

The AO adopted two standard approaches in order to lower the level of tension in the debates over the risks associated with their technique.[7] Their first strategy was to demonstrate that, if complications did occur, they could be taken care of. The other line of argument was to show that any complications that did arise were in fact due to errors made by the surgeon in applying the technique rather than being credited to the technique itself.

Right from the beginning and throughout the whole debate over osteosynthesis the main argument against the widespread use of the method lay in the risk of infection and its devastating consequences. Operating on closed fractures was an area of surgery where infection was seen to be the direct consequence of the surgeon's actions, and the AO surgeons knew that the problem of bone infection would determine the fate of osteosynthesis. In their 1963 textbook they noted that even one bone infection in a thousand cases would be a major disaster directly attributable to using osteosynthesis.[8]

One way of assuaging doctors' fears concerning the problem of bone infection due to osteosynthesis was to show that the condition could be successfully treated even if it occurred in a bone that was fixed with a plate and screws.[9] The misconception, according to the AO, was that "it used to be held that an internal fixation device (being a foreign body) in some way, merely by being there, enhanced the chances of wound infection and was absolutely proscribed in the treatment of open fractures".[10] According to this vision, the first thing that had to be done when an infection developed was to remove the metal. On the basis of animal experiments and clinical studies, the AO surgeons showed that internal fixation *per se* did not increase the incidence of bone infection, and, in 1979, AO surgeon Rittmann could write that: "Once infection occurs, the presence of implants is advantageous as long as it provides stability. Indeed the stabilizing effect of implants outweighs the possible harm of their foreign body effect."[11] By the mid-1970s it had become standard practice to leave the device in place in case of a bone infection.[12]

This development also influenced the way bone infection was dealt with after an osteosynthesis operation. One of the leading AO surgeons, Martin Allgöwer, wrote in 1971 that "once an infection has become manifest a clear strategy for how to proceed can prevent a catastrophe".[13] Another author asserted that "a post-operative infection can be disastrous, but if dealt with rapidly and adequately it should be controllable until the bone healing has occurred".[14] Now, the *real* catastrophe was not the infection as such, but its inadequate treatment. Although it was not their primary aim, the AO's emphasis on the manageability of infection led to a change in the discourse over osteosynthesis: attention was diverted away from the procedural risks and redirected towards the surgeons' ability to control the outcome of the treatment. Another effect of the discussion was that a more or less constant, low rate of infection was now considered acceptable,[15] illustrating Ulrich Beck's general point that the very existence of risk management implies a basic willingness to tolerate *some* risk.[16] As two American surgeons concluded as early as 1959, the procedure of internal fixation was viewed as a "calculable risk", and in 1964 Allgöwer was already using statistical material to support his opinion that by employing internal fixation the AO was not irresponsibly subjecting patients to excessively high risks.[17]

Attributing blame

After demonstrating the manageability of complications, the second strategy for defusing the discourse over the risks associated with osteosynthesis was to focus on the individual surgeon's competence or lack of competence. Even before the AO had been established, it had been obvious that the rate of complications in osteosynthesis procedures was closely associated with the skill of the individual surgeon.[18] The AO, however, placed special emphasis on this point, as can be seen in the following passage taken from the introductory chapter of its textbook: "Not every surgeon will achieve equally good results with osteosynthesis. Therefore, we are concerned that everyone should critically check the fractures he has operated upon, not only in order to see the limits of the method in his hands, but also to note his personal limits."[19] The explanation for poor results was to be sought in the incompetence of the individual surgeon and not in the method itself.

The AO surgeons were able to back this argument up empirically using data that showed that the rate of infection varied between 2 and 20 per cent, and that the percentage fell with growing "aseptic and atraumatic discipline" on the part of the surgical team. Statistics further revealed a close correlation between low infection rates and the extent of the individual surgeon's experience. Thus, the way to reduce the danger of bone infection was by systematically improving the skill and discipline exercised in the operation room.[20] As a consequence, infection no longer appeared to be an inevitable side effect of opening up the fracture site, but had instead become "the most important factor over which the treating physician has any influence".[21]

In order to verify the crucial role of surgical skill and experience, outcome studies on the AO technique frequently included an assessment of the competence of the surgeons who performed such osteosynthesis operations.[22] Insufficient pre-operative planning, misplacement of plates and screws, use of plates of the wrong length, incomplete anatomical reconstruction of bone or articular surfaces, and lack of stability are mentioned as typical mistakes made by surgeons.[23] So, many other kinds of complication besides infection could also be attributed to the individual surgeon's incorrect choice of treatment methods, to poor technique or to inappropriate post-operative treatment.[24]

Nevertheless, standards for correct treatment varied, meaning that the very same procedure could be judged as being either correct or faulty. In order to advance their position, it was crucial for the AO surgeons to see their own, very high standards applied.[25]

The risks of osteosynthesis now appeared in a quite different light. The point was no longer that osteosynthesis was a *risky* operation, rather that it was a *difficult* operation. As early as 1966, the AO secretary Robert Schneider wrote in his annual report: "The time has come in which a catastrophe after osteosynthesis is no longer attributed to the method as such but to the surgeon, his incorrect indication and his poor technique."[26]

The majority of surgeons accepted the propositions of the osteosynthesis proponents as the line of argument fit in well with the general tendency of the time to defend medical procedures, arrangements and structures by conceptualizing the individual healthcare worker as a central source of trouble in medical practice.[27] The shift in discourse had an additional effect: any failures in osteosynthesis no longer discredited the AO as the organization advocating the procedure. Instead, since the underlying cause of the failures was now seen as surgical incompetence, the AO's position as a group of competent experts in the field became stronger, not to mention the fact that it was the AO that provided surgeons with the means to become competent in the technique by studying the textbooks or attending courses. Failures could in principle be prevented; what the surgeons had to do was to follow the instructions given by the AO in every detail, and to use the AO's standardized instruments and implants. The AO now had solid grounds for augmenting its various activities concerned with the procedure, including improving the documentation available, and setting up additional courses. On a more general level, Ulrich Beck describes this process in his *Risk Society* as the "transformation of failures and risks into chances for the expansion of science and technology".[28]

Risk assessment: different concepts of science and rationality

Surgery as a science

But the AO's view of risk was not shared by everybody, and there was indeed a minority of surgeons who resisted their line of argument around osteosynthesis. These surgeons also rejected the central goal of turning surgery into a *science* that inevitably shaped the ways in which the AO presented and dealt with risk. Before reviewing the objections raised by these critics, I will first give a brief description of the scientific concept of medicine that lay behind the AO's position.

The most pervasive element of the idea of making medicine a science was the claim that medical innovation should be grounded in scientific discoveries made in the laboratory.[29] But the concept of rendering medicine scientific entailed much more, including the fact that medical practice itself needed to be redescribed as a scientific activity. As the medical historian Harry Marks notes, this project included the claim that "clinical medicine was, or could be, every bit as scientific as the research laboratory, if "scientific method" were directly applied to judging the results of medical treatment".[30] Proponents of this approach felt that, even if the individual doctor was unaware of it, patient care was always a kind of experiment. Practicing medicine was a research activity to which one could apply the same principles as one applied to other areas of experimental research.[31] In the 1950s and 1960s, "clinical researchers aspired to the conditions of the laboratory experiment, where ideally the factors that affected the outcomes were both known and manipulable".[32]

The AO surgeons similarly formulated their practical aims in the language of laboratory science. They defined their research activities not as an effort to propagate osteosynthesis but as a scientific project whose aim was to "prove or disprove" the "hypothesis" that osteosynthesis enabled the successful treatment of fractures.[33] Fracture care, they claimed, should no longer be "empirical" but "rational". Like a well devised and well performed laboratory experiment, the outcome of every single surgical intervention should be reproducible and independent of the individual who actually performed it.[34] The boundaries became increasingly blurred between therapy and research, as well as between medicine and science. Every single case of fracture had to be dealt with in the manner of a standardized scientific experiment, each surgical intervention being performed and documented according to a standardized protocol. In this way, potential sources of failure could be detected and kept under control. According to Allgöwer, the AO's goal was "to increase the reliability and reproducibility of good results by the average trauma surgeon".[35] In the same way that a particular experimental result can only be reliably reproduced if the experimenter respects all the details of the experimental setting and procedure, standardization became the indispensable precondition for the reliable application of osteosynthesis. The AO surgeons came to believe that perfect reproducibility could only be achieved if every movement, every instrument and every implant was strictly standardized.

Surgery was particularly suitable for being reconceived as a scientific activity, since, in the words of medical historian Christopher Lawrence, "in surgery the fiction that medicine had nothing to do with politics reached its purest expression. Surgical intervention could be represented as the inevitable, scientific solution to disease, in comparison to which the alternative solutions seemed inferior".[36] Surgical intervention also aims at controlling the phenomena of life, just like a scientific experiment, making experimentalism an appropriate approach for surgeons. Robert Danis, a Belgian surgeon who was not only a pioneer in osteosynthesis but also a role model for the AO surgeons, thought that the success of an osteosynthesis operation was guaranteed as long as the basic laws of bone healing were respected, just as the laws of nature determined the result of any particular experiment. In 1939, he wrote that he made every effort to give his surgical operations the character of well-performed experiments.[37]

Individualization and risk

This idea of thoroughly standardizing surgical care was exactly what opponents criticised. In particular they objected to the procedure of collecting outcome data and using it as a basis for balancing potential benefits against potential dangers with the aim of calculating and justifying risk at an abstract, generalized level. For them, the deleterious effects of a complication on the individual concerned were reason enough to reject this sort of treatment outright. The potential benefits simply did not outweigh the possible harm in the case of complications. Statistical data, they stressed, could neither predict the outcome in any individual case nor appropriately take into account the individual tragedy of a complication for the patients concerned.[38]

This kind of opposition was often accompanied by a more general critique of a generalizing approach to medical practice. In his rejection of statistical rationality the Head Surgeon at Zurich University and AO opponent Hans-Ulrich Buff even went so far as to deny statistics any practical value at all. In a 1971 article, Buff thought it legitimate to express his opinion concerning treatment methods based exclusively on his "personal experience and impressions of thirty years of practice", abstaining from "giving any figures, statistical arrangements and comparisons".[39] Though not many surgeons would have agreed with such an extreme standpoint, surgery was nevertheless considered a particularly difficult field for the application of the sophisticated methods of clinical research such as randomized clinical trials, because "every patient presented a unique challenge, every surgeon had different skills, and each operation could utilize a bewildering range of procedures".[40] This observation applied to fracture treatment and orthopedic surgery in particular. In 1939, while interrogating the possibility of establishing general fracture descriptions, Willis Campbell had already asked whether any "classification of orthopedic affections can be entirely satisfactory". Thus, when it came to surgery there were "so many factors involved in any one condition that a survey of end results can be of only questionable value unless the minute details of each case are considered".[41] Another Swiss critic of AO, Max Geiser, went so far as to doubt that objective assessment was possible at all. For him, the character and location of the fracture, the blood supply to the affected area, the condition of the bone before the fracture, and the technical details of the treatment performed varied so much that coming up with reliable comparative statistics was impossible.[42] This skeptical perspective could also be applied to well-planned clinical trials, despite their "randomization, replication, and unbiased assessment of results". Two American surgeons wrote in 1979 that "[e]ven if all future studies were both complete and standardized, comparisons between results obtained with different methods at different institutions would still be inaccurate" because of the many variables involved.[43] Trying to compensate for relevant differences was an open-ended task.

Even the most advanced methods of clinical research cannot overcome this sort of resistance, where those who are not interested in this type of generalized information refuse to be convinced by statistical reasoning. This fundamental difference in worldviews is part of an "ethical clash" that historians of medicine have identified as taking place in the twentieth century between those doctors who endorsed "professional values centered on the individual" and others who advocated "the statistical necessity of taking averages".[44] Its critics charged scientific medicine with neglecting the individual nature of medical problems, and it is easy to see where this criticism came from: if patient care is viewed as a controlled, reproducible experiment, then treatment procedures, like any other experimental procedures, must be standardized and treatment results handled in the same way as data generated by any experiment in the physical sciences. This means that, as in experimental science, a few precisely defined parameters are brought into focus and measured in a way that makes them comparable. At the same time, the differences between the individual cases must be played down. As a consequence, the similarities between body parts and injuries are emphasized and the particularities of any patient's individual problems recede into the background.[45]

Those surgeons who opposed the de-individualizing aspects of the scientific approach to surgery in general were often also wary of the AO's systematic application of treatment methods and stressed that each injury was unique and should be treated in an individual way.[46] In a typical statement, the British surgeon Ernest Alexander Nicoll argued that it was not justifiable to operate on 100 patients in order to find those five patients who would actually benefit from osteosynthesis. As he described it: "That would be equivalent to sending 100 people to prison because five of them might be criminals."[47] These surgeons, who preferred referring to medicine as an "art" rather than as a "science", rejected the idea that medical decisions can be based on universal scientific principles, seeing them instead as fundamentally personal and individual.[48]

In his study of early-twentieth-century American medicine, Joel Howell identified a general "deep-seated cultural bias in favor of an individual clinician's judgment ... a fundamental belief that individual clinicians make decisions using information and modes of analysis which simply cannot be captured by any set of formal rules or procedures".[49] Critics warned that medical practice governed by this sort of standardized procedure would turn medical treatment into a mere technology, performed by "unthinking physicians". In their view, the art of medicine required diligence, experience, skill, individual attention, sound clinical judgment and common sense – all instances of "tacit knowledge" that cannot be passed on in an explicit and systematic manner but have to be acquired through individual experience.[50] At a general level, Howell correctly remarks that "the tension between seeing medical decisions as fundamentally personal and individual and seeing medical decisions as fundamentally based on universal scientific principles has existed throughout the twentieth century. Although many physicians perceive clinical practice guidelines as providing useful advice, a sizable group sees them as 'oversimplified' and 'too rigid to apply to individual patients'."[51]

Much of the disagreement concerning the strategy adopted by the AO has its roots in the conflict between these two opposed worldviews. In the sphere of instruction, critics typically rejected the AO's efforts at systematic training and emphasized the personal, tacit dimension of surgical and diagnostic skill which could not be learned from a manual or a course. In the sphere of treatment, they opposed the AO's goal of systematization and standardization as it prevented the surgeons from dealing with patients on an individual basis. Buff, for instance, criticised the AO for doing everything systematically and ignoring the circumstances of the individual case.[52] For Geiser such a practice constituted an instance of inappropriate "absolutism" or "schematism". The choice of treatment had to be made individually, according not only to the type and location of the fracture, but also to the patient's personality, age, occupation, physical and mental health, not to mention the hospital's technological and hygienic status and the surgeon's familiarity with the treatment methods. Apart from bone biology, functional anatomy and pathology, the decision should also be informed by "a good dose of common sense".[53] In the same vein, Nicoll accused the AO of adopting a "totalitarian approach". In a sideswipe at the AO courses he remarked that the "high degree of clinical judgment" necessary for individualized fracture care was "harder to acquire, or to impart, than technical virtuosity in the operating theatre".[54]

Even though the AO surgeons did stress the individual nature of the cases as well as the specificity and uniqueness of each surgical intervention,[55] it was nevertheless clear that they placed more confidence in explicit instruction than in individual judgment. In a typical comment on the treatment of bone infection, for example, Allgöwer stated that surgeons should not rely on intuition but on clear, well-tested rules.[56]

Both sides knew that the AO's strategy of turning surgery into a science was part of a wider trend evident in the medical profession. Allgöwer himself drew a parallel between the new way of treating fractures and the modern *zeitgeist* and its associated accelerated lifestyle.[57] But while the AO surgeons were in favour of this modern style, their critics took a more conservative stance. Buff castigated modern man's excessive belief in the capacities of contemporary science and technology, calling it "Wissenschaftsaberglaube" – "science-superstition". He argued that medicine was often described as being a combination of art and science, and the error made by the adherents of modern science was to believe that medical progress consisted in steadily increasing the science portion.[58] Similarly, Geiser interpreted the image of cool technological elegance associated with osteosynthesis as being seductive,[59] and the leading British orthopedic surgeon John Charnley warned of the "superficial impression of precision presented by operative techniques", and their appearance of "operative simplicity" and "modernity".[60] Charnley was also suspicious of the modern scientific means of obtaining knowledge and their apparent plausibility. He complained of the "tendency to imagine that serious research can now-a-days only come out of the laboratory". Charnley reflected that "today our credulity lies in the accuracy which we attribute to our special research tools, such as the electron microscope", and warned that "we must not forget that sight and touch together make the greatest clinical faculty of all, namely, common sense."[61]

Authority and power

Beyond these conceptual and practical considerations, however, there was also a social dimension to the opposition raised against turning surgery into a science. The two models of medical practice also implied different roles for the practitioners associated with different conceptions of their authority and power.[62] First of all, scientific surgery embodied a democratic idea of expertise, following the principle that if surgery was really a science, then by pursuing appropriate training every surgeon could eventually achieve good treatment results.[63] Deborah Gordon has noted that, as a form of knowledge, "clinical science is characteristically explicit, universal, abstract and public". Criteria for practice can be scrutinized and judged by "peers, junior physicians, external agencies, and patients".[64] In a scientific framework, clinical skill and knowledge are generally attainable independently of the surgeon's personality or natural gifts, following the principle that anyone who adheres to the rules can achieve good operative results. Expertise thus becomes a depersonalized "technique to be mastered" instead of a personal "experience to be amassed".[65]

On the other hand, if surgery is considered to be an art, hierarchy and personal authority become of central importance. According to Buff, good medical practice depends on the doctor's own personality and cannot be achieved simply by receiving the right kind of instruction.[66] From this perspective, medical expertise can only be passed on by "apprenticeship, oral culture, and the case method". Being "implicit, ineffable and tacit, clinical knowledge is less open to public scrutiny and outside surveillance". It is easy to imagine how such a concept "supports a hierarchy based on expertise".[67]

Generally, becoming scientific was a very successful professional strategy for medicine on its rise to social and cultural dominance starting in the nineteenth century. On the individual level, however, this strategy threatened the doctor's personal authority. For this reason there was always a counter-current within the medical profession that sought to protect the individual practitioner's autonomy by interpreting medicine as an "inexplicable art".[68] As part of this counter-current, the opponents of the AO considered that the organization's concept of expertise threatened their professional autonomy. For Buff, the AO's concept reduced the individual doctor's role to that of a mediator between the patient on one side and the AO as a central agency issuing the directions for treatment on the other. He argued that this situation was detrimental to good medical practice, which consisted in the interpretation of medical knowledge in the context of the individual case, something that depended on the surgeon's autonomy and his mature and morally sound character.[69] Buff should, therefore, be understood as a similar figure to the Victorian gentleman doctor described by Christopher Lawrence,[70] or an orthopedist in the post-war period like Harry Platt – Charnley's teacher – portrayed by Roger Cooter in his study on orthopedics and the organization of modern medicine.[71]

Many critics of the AO also considered that the popularity of osteosynthesis among patients constituted a supplementary threat to surgeon's authority. Thus, for example, Charnley appealed to the academically trained doctor's awareness of his superiority as a means to resist such pressure from outside the profession. "Learned professions must guard against the insidious danger of being influenced by advertisements of the popular press", he wrote, complaining that "sound biological facts never have publicity value, but unfortunately methods which are unsound often possess news value because they appeal to a public which understands mechanical engineering but not surgery. The thinking surgeon cannot share his patient's pleasure in a perfect radiological reduction."[72]

According to Buff, the exemplary moral character of the experienced and learned surgeon was the best antidote to fads like osteosynthesis. In order to develop the required strength of character, doctors had to avoid technical over-specialization, acquiring instead a broad general education in the sense of the German term "Bildung," which includes forming one's character. Such general training would provide them with a basis for their personal freedom and autonomy, allowing them to withstand pressure from patients and resist the popular error of seeing medicine as a science-driven enterprise. Buff believed that, despite the popularity of osteosynthesis, conservative treatment was generally the best approach for the patient, and that the surgeon's primary task was to use his authority to guide the misinformed patient through the lengthy process of conservative treatment. Moral integrity and a stable personality would enable him to protect his patients' interests and earn the trust that they placed in him.

Buff believed that this whole process was being threatened by a subversive tendency that led towards mechanization and teamwork, and he attributed this general development to the international growth of American cultural hegemony that imposed the values embodied by the industrialist Henry Ford.[73] According to Buff's line of argument, good medicine could only operate within the framework of a liberal profession, in which the doctor could assume responsibility for his actions as a free human being. Only the autonomous doctor would be able to resist the trend towards growing dehumanization and depersonalization of medical care and protect himself against the explosion in the cost of modern medicine. This position allows us to locate the Zurich professor as a rather radical, but none the less typical, exponent of the modern tradition of defending what Sturdy and Cooter have characterized as the "individualized" against the "administrative" way of knowing.[74]

It is obvious that both concepts of medicine embody particular values and specific ideas about the doctor's role in society. Importantly, the scientific view of medicine endorsed by the AO is only a partial view of reality, as also is its counterpart that holds medicine up as an art. The observation made by Deborah Gordon is quite relevant in this context: "Although scientific rationality is assumed to be unbiased, it too is a particular approach to reality, albeit a particularly powerful one, that is as committed to a particular set of values as any other approach. The demand for precision and predictability, the hallmarks of science, are not neutral because certain specific measurements are selected for while other types of information are rendered unimportant or irrelevant."[75]

Conclusion

Thus, the example of osteosynthesis provides us with two contrasting concepts of rationality in medicine and, associated with these, two contrasting views of risk. On the one side was the AO with its goal of managing risk by standardizing the rules for indication and performance of the operations. They aimed to make the achievement of good results largely independent of the particularities of the individual case and the idiosyncrasies of the surgeon. If this can be done, then it makes sense to calculate whether the risk involved in a certain operation is worth taking or not on a general and abstract level. On the other side were those surgeons who emphasized the specific nature of each individual case at hand and saw medical practice as being completely determined by the individual doctor, his experience, his skill and even his character. As far as the issue of risk was concerned, these two points of view were seen as being incompatible. The AO's opponents essentially rejected the strategy of framing dangers as calculable and manageable risks. They refused to consider the issue at the level of populations and probabilities and wanted to discuss the problem at the level of individuals. However, both attitudes were rational in their own way. It has to be born in mind that these two positions were based on very different understandings of the surgeon's power and authority, and so the acceptance or rejection of the AO's "scientific" way of dealing with risk also entailed the acceptance or rejection of a certain conception of the role of the individual doctor in medicine and even in society at large.

Notes

1   See my book, T. Schlich, *Surgery, Science and Industry: A Revolution in Fracture Care, 1950s–1990s*, Houndsmill, Basingstoke: Palgrave 2002 (Series: Science, Technology and Medicine in Modern History).

182   *Thomas Schlich*

2 Quote: G. W. Bagby, "Compression Bone-Plating: Historical Considerations", *Journal of Bone and Joint Surgery* 59-A, 1977, 625–31; see also J. Pettavel, "Considérations sur le traitement des fractures transverses du tibia", *Helvetica Chirurgica Acta* 22, 1955, 435–6; G. Maurer and F. Lechner, "Allgemeines über Knochen und Gelenke sowie Frakturen und Luxationen", in *Handbuch der gesamten Unfallheilkunde*, H. Bürkle de la Camp and M. Schwaiger (eds), 3 vols, 3rd edn. Stuttgart: Ferdinand Enke, vol.1, 1963, 482–579; see p. 505; H. U. Buff, "Bemerkungen zur Behandlung der Unterschenkelfrakturen bei Erwachsenen", *Praxis. Schweizerische Rundschau für Medizin* 60, 1971, 1193–6; see p. 1194.

3 R. C. Fox and J. P. Swazey, *Spare Parts: Organ Replacement in American Society*, New York, Oxford: Oxford University Press, 1992, p. 2.

4 J. Liebenau, "Medicine and Technology", *Perspectives in Biology and Medicine* 27, 1983, 76–92; see p. 82; U. Tröhler, " 'To Operate or Not to Operate?' Scientific and Extraneous Factors in Therapeutical Controversies within the Swiss Society of Surgery 1913–1988", *Clio Medica* 22, 1991, 89–113; see p. 90; B. Elkeles, *Der moralische Diskurs über das Menschenexperiment im 19. Jahrhundert*, Stuttgart: Gustav Fischer, 1996, p. 68; on the importance of attribution of cause in discussions about risk, see U. Beck, *Risikogesellschaft: Auf dem Weg in eine andere Moderne*, Frankfurt: Suhrkamp Verlag, 1986, p. 83.

5 M. Douglas and A. Wildavsky, *Risk and Culture: An Essay on the Selection of Technological and Environmental Dangers*. Berkeley, Los Angeles, London: University of California Press, 1982.

6 Beck, *Risikogesellschaft*, p. 292; see also pp. 62, 76–7, 95, 289; G. Gigerenzer *et al.*, *The Empire of Chance: How Probability Changed Science and Everyday Life*, Cambridge: Cambridge University Press, 1989, p. 266; on the normative and political character of all therapeutic evaluation and risk assessment, see E. Richards, "The Politics of Therapeutic Evaluation: The Vitamin C and Cancer Controversy", *Social Studies of Science* 18, 1988, 653–701.

7 The AO surgeons in no way denied the dangers of osteosynthesis, an attitude that earned them much credibility in the field. As described in Schlich, *Surgery*, they tried to lower the rate of complications by controlling and improving the competence of those surgeons who used their technique. However, control became increasingly difficult as more and more surgeons started to use the AO technique.

8 M. E. Müller, M. Allgöwer and H. Willenegger, *Technik der operativen Frakturenbehandlung*, Berlin: Springer-Verlag, 1963, p. 21. The subject was frequently discussed and taken very seriously; for the numerous contributions to this discussion, see Schlich, *Surgery*, chapter 6.

9 See, e.g., C. R. Berkin and D. V. Marshall, "Three-Sided Plate Fixation for Fractures of the Tibial and Fermoral Shafts", *Journal of Bone and Joint Surgery* 54-A, 1972, 1105–13; see p. 1112; T. Rüedi, J. K. Webb and M. Allgöwer, "Experience with the Dynamic Compression Plate (DCP) in 418 Recent Fractures of the Tibial Shaft", *Injury* 7, 1975, 252–7; see p. 254; W. Van der Linden and K. Larson, "Plate Fixation versus Conservative Treatment of Tibial Shaft Fractures", *Journal of Bone and Joint Surgery* 61-A, 1979, 873–8; see p. 877.

10 C. A. Rockwood, and D. P. Green, *Fractures*, 2 vols, Philadelphia and Toronto: J. B. Lippincott Company, 1975, p. 77.

11 W. W. Rittmann *et al.*, "Open Fractures: Long-term Results in 200 Consecutive Cases", *Clinical Orthopaedics and Related Research* 138, 1979, 132–40; see p. 138; see also J. Schatzker, "Compression in the Surgical Treatment of Fractures in of the Tibia", *Clinical Orthopaedics and Related Research* 105, 1974, 220–39; see pp. 203–1; W. W. Rittmann and S. M. Perren, *Corticale Knochenheilung nach Osteosynthese und Infektion: Biomechanik und Biologie*, Berlin: Springer-Verlag, 1974.

12 J. H. Hicks, "Internal Fixation of Fractures", in R. Clarke, F. G. Badger and S. Sevitt (eds) *Modern Trends in Accident Surgery and Medicine*, London: Butterworth 1959, 196–213; see p. 205; J. C. McNeur, "The Management of Open Skeletal Trauma with Particular

Reference to Internal Fixation", *Journal of Bone and Joint Surgery* 52-B, 1970, 54–60; see pp. 59–60; Rockwood and Green, *Fractures*, p. 77.

13 M. Allgöwer, "Weichteilprobleme und Infektionsrisiko der Osteosynthese", *Langenbecks Archiv für Chirurgie* 329, 1971, 1127–36; see p. 1131.

14 S. Olerud, "Operative Treatment of Supracondylar-Condylar Fractures of the Femur. Technique and Results in Fifteen Cases", *Journal of Bone and Joint Surgery* 54-A, 1972, 1015–32; see p. 1031.

15 "We believe that incidence of infections can be kept at an acceptable level by meticulous technique", in Berkin and Marshall, *Three-Sided Plate*, p. 1112; according to Allgöwer a one per cent infection rate was acceptable, three per cent disquieting and more than three per cent alarming: Allgöwer, *Weichteilprobleme*, p. 1131.

16 Beck, *Risikogesellschaft*, p. 86.

17 O. P. Hampton and W. T. Fitts, *Open Reduction of Common Fractures*, New York/London: Grune and Stratton, 1959, p. 4; M. Allgöwer, "Osteosynthese und primäre Knochenheilung", *Langenbecks Archiv für Chirurgie* 308, 1964, 423–34; see p. 433.

18 Pettavel, *Considérations*, p. 453.

19 Müller, Allgöwer and Willenegger, *Technik*, p. 7 (my translation); similarly: G. S. Laros and P. G. Spiegel, "Editorial Comments. Rigid Internal Fixation of Fractures", *Clinical Orthopaedics and Related Research* 138, 1979, 2–22; see p. 3; J. Schatzker and D. C. Lambert, "Supracondylar Fractures of the Femur", *Clinical Orthopaedics and Related Research* 138, 179, 77–83; see p. 82.

20 Müller, Allgöwer and Willenegger, *Technik*, p. 7; Minutes of the AO Meetings (abbreviated AO), Archives of the AO Centre, Davos, Switzerland 22–23 Nov. 1968; AO 7–8 May 1971, scientific session, pp. 14–5, 27; Allgöwer, *Weichteilprobleme*, pp. 1130–1; AO 28–30 Apr. 1972, scientific session, p. 15; AO 16–17 Nov. 1973, adm. session, pp. 2–7, scientific session, p. 12; Rüedi *et al.*, Experience, 1975, p. 256; M. Allgöwer and P. G. Spiegel, "Internal Fixation of Fractures: Evolution of Concepts", *Clinical Orthopaedics and Related Research* 138, 1979, 26–9; see p. 28.

21 G. J. Clance and S. T. Hansen, "Open Fractures of the Tibia: A Review of One Hundred and Two Cases", *Journal of Bone and Joint Surgery* 60-A, 1978, 118–22; see p. 120.

22 S. Olerud and G. Karlström, "Tibial Fractures Treated by AO Compression Osteosynthesis: Experiences from a Five Year Material", *Acta Orthopaedica Scandinavica*, suppl. 144, 1972, p. 15; see also J. Müller, U. Plaas and H. Willenegger, "Spätergebnisse nach operativ behandelten Malleolarfrakturen", *Helvetica Chirurgica Acta* 38, 1971, 329–37; H. S. Dodge and G. W. Cady, "Treatment of Fractures of the Radius and Ulna with Compression Plates", *Journal of Bone and Joint Surgery* 54-A, 1972, 1167–76; see p. 1167; L. D. Anderson *et al.*, "Compression-Plate Fixation in Acute Diaphyseal Fractures of the Radius and Ulna", *Journal of Bone and Joint Surgery* 57-A, 1975, 287–97; see p. 295; C. Burri *et al.*, "Fractures of the Tibial Plateau", *Clinical Orthopaedics and Related Research* 138, 1979, 84–93; Van der Linden and Larsson, *Plate*, p. 873; T. P. Rüedi and M. Allgöwer, "The Operative Treatment of Intra-articular Fractures of the Lower End of the Tibia", *Clinical Orthopaedics and Related Research* 138, 1979, 105–10; see pp. 109–10; Laros and Spiegel, *Rigid*, p. 12; R. Ganz, R. J. Thomas and C. P. Hammerle, "Trochanteric Fractures of the Femur: Treatment and Results", *Clinical Orthopaedics and Related Research* 138, 1979, 30–40; see p. 38.

23 P. T. Naiman, A. J. Schein and R. S. Siffert, "Use of ASIF Compression Plates in Selected Shaft Fractures of the Upper Extremity: A Preliminary Report", *Clinical Orthopaedics and Related Research* 71, 1970, 208–16; see pp. 212–15; Olerud and Karlström, *Tibial*, pp. 41–2, Rüedi and Allgöwer, *Operative*, p. 105; Ganz *et al.*, *Trochanteric*, p. 37.

24 M. E. Müller, *Principes d'ostéosynthèse*, Helvetica Chirurgica Acta 28: 1961 198–206; M. Allgöwer, "Cinderella of Surgery – Fractures?", *Surgical Clinics of North America* 58, 1978, 1071–93; see p. 1091; Allgöwer and Spiegel, *Internal*, p. 28, Laros and Spiegel, *Rigid*, p. 10.

25 Schatzker and Lambert, *Supracondylar*, p. 81.

26 AO 29–30 Apr. 1966, annual report 1965, p. 1.

27 M. Berg, *Rationalizing Medical Work. Decision Support Techniques and Medical Practices*, Cambridge, MA and London: The MIT Press, 1997, p. 22.

28 Beck, *Risikogesellschaft*, p. 260.

29 See chapter 5 in Schlich, *Surgery*.

30 H. M. Marks, *The Progress of Experiment. Science and Therapeutic Reform in the United States, 1900–1990*. Cambridge, New York: Cambridge University Press, 1997, see p. 2.

31 M. Berg, "Turning a Practice into a Science: Reconceptualizing Postwar Medical Practice", *Social Studies of Science* 25, 1995, 437–76; p. 449; M. Berg, *Rationalizing Medical Work. Decision Support Techniques and Medical Practices*, Cambridge, MA and London: The MIT Press, 1997, p. 22.

32 Marks, *Progress*, p. 2.

33 Allgöwer, *Cinderella*, p. 1073.

34 M. E. Müller, M. Allgöwer and H. Willenegger, *Manual der Osteosynthese: AO-Technik*, Berlin: Springer-Verlag, 1969, p. 16.

35 Allgöwer, *Cinderella*.

36 C. Lawrence, "Democratic, Divine and Heroic: The History and Historiography of Surgery", in C. Lawrence (ed.) *Medical Theory, Surgical Practice: Studies in the History of Surgery*, London, New York: Routledge, 1992, 1–47; see p. 32

37 R. Danis, *Théorie et pratique de l'ostéosynthèse*, Paris: Masson, 1949, pp. 5–6.

38 E. Gögler, *Unfallopfer im Straßenverkehr*. Basel: J. R. Geigy S.A. 1962, p. 58, cites the eminent Heidelberg surgeon K. H. Bauer who noted that one grave failure could not be balanced by fifty excellent results; M. Geiser, "Beiträge zur Biologie der Knochenbruchheilung", *Zeitschrift für Orthopädie* 97, suppl. 2, 1963, pp. 96–7, speaks of one osteomyelitis against 99 excellent cases; P. Groh, *Die Behandlung von Frakturen langer Röhrenknochen mit der AO-Osteosynthesemethode und ihre Ergebnisse*, MD thesis, University of Saarland, 1968, pp. 79–80; the limits of statistical statements for evaluating the individual case were also acknowledged by the AO surgeons; see, for example, Allgöwer's preface to Rittmann and Perren, *Corticale*, p. v.

39 Buff, *Bemerkungen*, p. 3.

40 D. S. Jones, "Visions of a Cure: Visualization, Clinical Trials, and Controversies in Cardiac Therapeutics, 1968–1998", *Isis* 91, 2000, 504–41; see p. 3.

41 Willis C. Campbell, "Preface to the first edition", in A. H. Crenshaw (ed.) *Campbell's Operative Orthopaedics*, 2 vols, 4th edn, St. Louis: The C. V. Mosby Company, 1963, pp. xiii–xiv.

42 Geiser, *Beiträge*, pp. 87–8; on the problem in general, see I. Löwy, *Between Bench and Bedside: Science, Healing, and Interleukin-2 in a Cancer Ward*, Cambridge, MA: Harvard University Press, 1996, pp. 48–54.

43 Van der Linden and Larsson, *Plate*, pp. 874–7.

44 Gigerenzer *et al.*, *Empire*, p. 261; on the conflict between the principle of the controlled trial and clinical tradition, see Löwy, *Bench*, pp. 48–54.

45 J. D. Howell, *Technology in the Hospital: Transforming Patient Care in the Early Twentieth Century*, Baltimore and London: The Johns Hopkins University Press, 1995, p. 131; according to critics, randomized clinical trials are centred on disease and disease-related variables rather than on patients and patient-related variables, Löwy, *Bench*, p. 50.

46 F. G. Badger, "Principles of the Treatment of Fractures", in R. Clarke, F. G. Badger and S. Sevitt (eds), *Modern Trends in Accident Surgery and Medicine*, London: Butterworth, 1959, 123–39; see p. 123.

47 E. A. Nicoll, "Closed and Open Treatment of Tibial Fractures", *Clinical Orthopaedics and Related Research* 105, 1974, 144–53; see p. 149; Nicoll was a general surgeon who in the 1930s founded a specialized fracture and rehabilitation center at Berry Hill, Nottinghamshire. See R. Cooter, *Surgery and Society in Peace and War: Orthopaedics and the Organization of Modern Medicine, 1880–1948*, Houndsmill, Basingstoke: Macmillan, 1993, pp. 208–11.

48 Howell, *Technology*, p. 245. However, as D. R. Gordon ("Clinical Science and Clinical Expertise: Changing Boundaries between Art and Science in Medicine", in M. Lock and D. Gordon (eds) *Biomedicine Examined*, Dordrecht: Kluwer, 1988, p. 258) correctly points out, "the symbols 'art' and 'science' have been large protective shields in medicine, hiding much that is not very scientific or artful". "The term science can have different meanings in the first place; in the same way that medical practice has many faces, so does its 'scientific nature' ", Berg, *Turning*, p. 458. Some AO critics who advocated individualization claimed that their approach was the one that was truly scientific, Nicoll, *Closed*, p. 150.

49 Howell, *Technology*, p. 246.

50 H. M. Marks, "Medical Technologies: Social Contexts and Consequences", in W. F. Bynum and R. Porter (eds) *Companion Encyclopedia of the History of Medicine*, vol. 2, 1993, 1592–1618, London, New York: Routledge; Berg, *Turning*, p. 442; on the medical diagnostician's skill as tacit knowledge, see M. Polanyi, *Personal Knowledge: Toward a Post-Critical Philosophy*, London: Routledge and Kegan Paul, 1973 (first published in 1958, p. 54); see also chapter 4 of Schlich, *Surgery*.

51 Howell, *Technology*, p. 245.

52 H. U. Buff, "Der Arzt als freier Beruf", in B. Staehlin, S. Jenny and S. Geroulanos (eds) *Freiheit: Aktuelle Hinweise und Beiträge aus verschiedenen Gebieten zum Problem der Freiheit*, Zurich: Editio Academica, 1975, pp. 185–98; see p. 186; Interview H. U. Buff, Zurich 31 Jan 1999.

53 Geiser, *Beiträge*, pp. 87–97.

54 Nicoll, *Closed*, p. 144.

55 Allgöwer, *Cinderella*, p. 1091; Allgöwer and Spiegel, *Internal*, p. 28.

56 "Preface" to Rittmann and Perren, *Corticale*, p. v.

57 Allgöwer, *Osteosynthese*, p. 425.

58 Buff, *Arzt*, pp. 186–91.

59 Geiser, *Beiträge*, p. 95.

60 J. Charnley, *The Closed Treatment of Common Fractures*. Edinburgh and London: E. and S. Livingstone Ltd, 1957, p. vii. Charnley was, however, a leading proponent of a new generation in post-WW2 British orthopedics which was operative and scientifically oriented and keen to abandon the conservative, holistic philosophy that had dominated the field; Cooter, *Surgery*, p. 238. Perhaps one has to consider here the background of Charnley's long-standing dispute about internal fixation with William Gissane of the Birmingham Accident Hospital, see W. Waugh, *John Charnley: The Man and the Hip*, Berlin: Springer-Verlag, 1990, pp. 57–60, 68–71.

61 Quoted after Waugh, *Man*, p. 71; see also J. Charnley, *Die konservative Therapie der Extremitätenfrakturen. Ihre wissenschaftlichen Grundlagen und ihre Technik*, translated and revised edn of the third English edn by Rudolf Bimler, Berlin: Springer-Verlag, 1968, p. vii.

62 S. Sturdy and R. Cooter, "Science, Scientific Management, and the Transformation of Medicine in Britain c. 1870–1950", *History of Science* 36, 1998, 421–66; p. 447.

63 Gigerenzer *et al.*, *Empire*, p. 265; T. M. Porter, *Trust in Numbers: The Pursuit of Objectivity in Science and Public Life*, Princeton, NJ: Princeton University Press, 1995, p. 204.

64 Gordon, *Clinical*, pp. 259–60; see also Gigerenzer *et al.*, *Empire*, 1989, p. 236, for the general tendency, and Marks, *Progress*, p. 3, for medicine.

65 See Gigerenzer *et al.*, *Empire*, p. 265, with regard to the statistical mode of thinking. In a similar way, "any vestiges of personalized judgement from the assessment of the effect of drugs" were to be eliminated by the introduction of the clinical trial in drug therapy, Sturdy and Cooter, *Science*, p. 446.

66 Buff, *Arzt*, p. 186.

67 Gordon, *Clinical*, pp. 259–60.

68 On the gentleman doctor of late Victorian Britain, see C. Lawrence, "Incommunicable Knowledge: Science, Technology and the Clinical Art in Britain 1850–1914", *Journal of*

Contemporary History 20, 1985, 503–20; in inter-war Britain, C. Lawrence, "Still Incommunicable: Clinical Holists and Medical Knowledge in Interwar Britain", in C. Lawrence and G. Weisz (eds) *Greater than the Parts: Holism in Biomedicine, 1920–1950*, New York, Oxford: Oxford University Press, 1998; on anti-specialist tendencies in British orthopedics, see Cooter, *Surgery*, pp. 245–7; on the conflicting approaches to medicine between 1870 and 1950, see Sturdy and Cooter, *Science*, pp. 435–9; for the 1970s, see Gordon, *Clinical*, pp. 257–9.

69 Buff, *Arzt*, 1975, p. 186; Interview H. U. Buff, Zurich, 31 Jan 1999.

70 Lawrence, *Incommunicable*.

71 Cooter, *Surgery*, pp. 245–7.

72 Charnley, *Closed*, p. viii.

73 Buff, *Bemerkungen*, p. 119; Buff, *Arzt*, pp. 186–95; interview H. U. Buff, Zurich, 31 Mar, 1999; cf. the similar arguments of doctors in inter-war Britain, Lawrence, *Still Incommunicable*, pp. 104–6.

74 Sturdy and Cooter, *Science*, pp. 435–9.

75 Gordon, *Clinical*, p. 283.

11 Assessing the risk and safety of the pill

Maternal mortality and the pill

Lara Marks[1]

Since 1954, when the oral contraceptive was first tested in clinical trials, nearly 200 million women have swallowed the pill. By 1966, within six years of the initial marketing of the drug in the United States, the number of pills sold worldwide exceeded any other single pharmaceutical product of an ethical nature and in some cases outsold many proprietary items such as aspirin.[2] By end of the twentieth century, the oral contraceptive had become a feature of everyday life with over 70 million women reaching for it on a daily basis around the globe.[3]

Like Librium and Thalidomide, the pill remains one of several revolutionary new drugs introduced in the 1960s, which reshaped pharmacology, social perceptions of medication and risk, and the regulatory process for new drugs during the second half of the twentieth century. Although not identified as such at the time it was created, the pill can be called the first "designer" or "lifestyle" drug of the twentieth century. Most drugs are intended for the treatment of organic diseases. By contrast the pill is aimed at preventing pregnancy, a condition not commonly considered pathological. Taken by healthy women of reproductive age for long periods of time, the drug raises questions about its potential for harm in terms of fertility as well as long-term health. Unlike previous forms of contraception, the pill was considered revolutionary in the late 1950s because it could be taken orally and at a time separate from intercourse. Moreover, in contrast to most other forms of contraception at the time, the pill had a physiological effect on the body.

From the time that it was first marketed as a contraceptive, the pill aroused great debate about its safety. Some physicians were deeply concerned about the long-term risks it posed to women's health. For some, the drug seemed to go against nature and the way that the body worked. As one British doctor asked in 1961:

[a]re none of my colleagues as apprehensive as I am about the threatened advent of oral contraceptive therapy? The prime function of the human race was to reproduce itself, and we are threatening to strike a blow at the very heart of the process which is responsible for the miracle of life itself. Will Nature let this indignity go unchallenged? Will she allow

the creatures to whom she has given the privilege of existence to interfere with the process that gave them the existence?

To prevent contraception by mechanical barriers is a different thing altogether – this is merely controlling the end product of a natural process, not interfering with the process itself. If Nature decides that science has invaded the very heart of her domain, what terrible penalties may she inflict upon the female of the species. Sterility? Ovarian atrophy? Malignant disease?[4]

Fears about the dangers of the pill were first raised when in November 1961, within months of its introduction to the British market, a British family doctor from Suffolk wrote to the *Lancet* of a woman who had developed thrombotic (blood clot) complications after taking the drug.[5] Although she returned to normal health after three months, this woman was the first of many such cases to be reported in Britain and the United States in the months that followed. By August 1962, the American Food and Drug Administration (FDA) had received reports of 26 women who had suffered blood clots in their veins (thrombophlebitis), six of whom had died.[6] Two years later further concerns were voiced about the contraceptive when a team of researchers at the University of Oregon demonstrated that certain hormones, such as the progestogen and oestrogen contained in the first marketed pill, Enovid, promoted the growth of cancers in animals such as rats.[7]

The anxieties of the early 1960s were not alleviated in the coming years. Lingering suspicions about the pill's safety have made it one of the most heavily scrutinized drugs in the world. Moreover, serious concerns about the implications of its long-term use by healthy women has led to the implementation of novel and innovative medical approaches for tracking patients for long periods of time, and for detecting and reporting serious adverse reactions to drugs.

Focusing on Britain and America in the late twentieth century this chapter examines the different ways in which the notion of risk was assessed in relation to the pill. Central to the paper is how the association between the contraceptive and risk changed over time and how this varied between those involved in the pharmaceutical industry, medical profession, government, media and women themselves. Among the issues considered is how the risk and safety of the drug was historically viewed in relation to the hazards of pregnancy and childbirth, thrombosis and cancer. The chapter also explores how the pill shifted from being seen merely as a tool for contraception to a weapon to fight cancer, and what implications this had for understanding its risk.

The risk of pregnancy and childbirth

From its earliest days many within the medical profession justified prescribing the oral contraceptive on the basis that it protected women from pregnancy and childbirth. As one American doctor arguing in favour of the pill put it, pregnancy could not be regarded as completely "benign".[8] Many physicians saw the risk of dying as a result of pregnancy as greater than the potential hazards the pill could cause.[9] Much of their argument was based on the notion that many pregnancies, particularly those that were unwanted, resulted in maternal deaths, either because of ill-performed abortions or inadequate access to good obstetric care. The high incidence of maternal mortality, especially among underprivileged women, gave strong credence to this assertion.

A powerful proponent of such a view was Dr Joseph Goldzieher who had strong connections with the first pharmaceutical companies to market the pill.[10] He showed that, in America in the late 1960s, underprivileged women faced a five times greater risk of dying in childbirth from complications during delivery than economically privileged women whose maternal mortality rate was 250 per million. In developing countries the maternal mortality rate was often much higher. In Ceylon, for instance, the death rate in 1969 was reported to be between 6,000 and 7,000 per million pregnant women.[11]

Goldzieher and other medical professionals argued that all women were potentially at risk of dying even if taking contraceptive precautions other than the pill. This they justified on the grounds that other forms of contraception were far less effective in guarding women from pregnancy and possible death than the pill. Even when the pill began to be linked with thrombosis such claims did not diminish in the early 1970s. Women were still considered to be at greater risk of mortality if they used other forms of contraception than dying from complications such as thrombosis from the pill. In 1970 one medical expert estimated that the number of women who would die as a result of taking oral contraceptives would only be between 15 and 40 deaths per million women taking the pill. By contrast the number of deaths was estimated to be between three and 300 amongst women using other methods of contraception.[12]

In this context pregnancy and childbirth were viewed not as a natural process but rather as a pathological one that required medical intervention such as the taking of a contraceptive pill. Such ideas were not new. During the inter-war years a number of physicians, driven by concern about rising rates of maternal mortality, had advocated greater medical intervention, such as prophylactic episiotomies and instrumental deliveries, to shield women from the fatal consequences of childbirth. Some physicians argued such intervention was necessary because they claimed women's bodies had been weakened by the process of civilization and could not withstand the difficulties of labour.[13]

Not all medical practitioners, however, were confident that the risks of pregnancy and childbirth necessitated the prescription of the pill. As one American obstetrician and gynaecologist, Dr Hugh Davis (director of a contraceptive clinic and assistant professor of obstetrics and gynaecology at

Johns Hopkins Medical School) pointed out, while the pill might be more effective than other contraceptives, it produced systemic changes in the body that other contraceptives did not.[14] Similar arguments were made in an editorial published in the British journal the *Lancet* which, in listing 50 metabolic side-effects from the pill, stated:

> These changes are unnecessary for contraception and their ultimate effect on the health of the user is unknown. But clearly they cannot be ignored, since they raise the possibility of irreversible structural changes, such as arteriosclerosis, after 10 or 20 years. In view of these doubts, the wisdom of administering such compounds to healthy women for many years must be seriously questioned.[15]

Dr William Inman, who undertook pioneering research in Britain on the thromboembolic effects of the pill for the British Committee on the Safety of Drugs in the 1960s and 1970s, also argued:

> Many comparisons with the risks of pregnancy have ignored the obvious fact that a woman has to become pregnant before she can run any risk of dying as a result of this pregnancy. If, for example, mechanical methods of contraception had a failure rate of 10% per annum, as against nil for oral contraception, the mortality due to the latter should be compared with one-tenth of the mortality associated with one pregnancy.[16]

Inman warned that any evaluation of the risks of the pill against maternal mortality should take into account the fact that many of the women who died in childbirth had not died as a result of their pregnancy. A report from the British Department of Health and Social Security in the early 1960s showed that, with the exception of abortion, at least 30 per cent of the women dying during pregnancy, delivery or the periperium, died of underlying medical or surgical complications they had suffered before becoming pregnant.[17] This indicated the fallacy of regarding all pregnancies as pathological and posing a greater risk than the pill.

What was at stake in the debate was whether unwanted pregnancies constituted a "pre-existing pathological state". As Dr Roy Hertz, associate medical director of the biomedical division at the Population Council in America,[18] put it in 1970:

> The view we have to take, I think ... is that we are now seeing the emergence of a new preventive public health practice; namely the prevention of births. We have not yet socially agreed what extremes we have to go in order to protect ourselves in terms of survival.
>
> For these reasons the degree of risk involved in averting an unwanted pregnancy remains a tremendously undefined term, both in social as well as medical terms.[19]

The pill as "normal hormone"

In many cases doctors dismissed the risks associated with the pill on the grounds that it induced a "natural state" for women, merely mimicking the natural hormones of a menstrual cycle or pregnancy. Such thinking can partly be attributed to one of the original clinical testers of the pill, the Catholic obstetrician-gynaecologist Dr John Rock who was a key advocate for the acceptance of the pill by the Vatican. He argued that the pill merely provided "a natural means of fertility control such as nature uses after ovulation and during pregnancy".[20] Explanations given to doctors and patients replicated this model in explaining how the pill worked and its side effects.[21] Thus minor symptoms such as nausea, breast changes, fluid retention, headaches, depression, abdominal cramp, weight increase and glucose intolerance were initially rejected on the basis that they also occurred during the menstrual cycle and pregnancy.[22]

Comparable arguments were also made in relation to the possible long-term hazards of the pill. In 1963, for instance, Dr A. S. Parkes, a British scientist closely involved in the initiation of the first clinical trials in Britain, claimed that the pill would not have a detrimental effect on the anterior pituitary gland. As he declared:

> In fairness it should be pointed out that the ovulation-producing activity of the human-pituitary gland is inhibited for a year of more during pregnancy and lactation; so in this respect the continued use of the pill may be likened to a rapid succession of pregnancies. However undesirable in other ways, a succession of pregnancies is not usually regarded as carcinogenic or endocrinologically catastrophic.[23]

Not everyone was happy with such thinking. Many, for example, feared that interference with the pituitary gland might cause cancer. Dr Hilton Salhanick, professor of obstetrics and gynecology at Harvard University, for instance, stressed that contraceptive steroids were not equal to natural hormones. They differed substantially both in their chemical structure and in their biological function.[24] This was a view also promoted by Dr Hugh Davis, who argued that to think of contraceptives "as natural is comforting but quite false". He went on to warn: "In using these agents, we are in fact embarking on a massive endocrinologic experiment with millions of healthy women."[25]

The risk of thrombosis compared with pregnancy

The debate over whether the oral contraceptive was "natural" and merely mimicked pregnancy became especially important in the wake of reports linking the pill with thrombosis. One of the most interesting features of this discussion was the subtle ways in which the concept of the dangers of pregnancy was used to understand and even justify the thrombotic effects of the pill. The pill was regarded as carrying no more danger of causing thrombotic disease, particularly thrombophlebitis, than a normal pregnancy. It was on these grounds that pharmaceutical companies initially dismissed the need to issue any warnings about thrombotic complications.[26]

By the late 1960s, however, a number of British studies were showing clear connections between the pill and life-threatening thromboembolic disorders. The most famous was that published by Drs William Inman and Martin Vessey in 1968. They concluded that "irrespective of age, the risk of death from pulmonary embolism or cerebral thrombosis was increased seven to eight times in users of oral contraceptives". The danger was greater for those women aged 35–44 than those aged 20–34, with the mortality being respectively 3.4 and 1.3 per 100,000 users per annum.[27]

When weighing up the overall safety of the pill, Inman and Vessey, like other medical professionals, framed it within the context of the dangers of pregnancy. They argued: "On balance, it seems reasonable to conclude that the risk of death from pulmonary embolism during one year's treatment with oral contraceptives is of the same order as the comparable risk of bearing one child." Unlike many other medical professionals however, they pointed out that,

> [I]n assessing the risks ... it is important to remember that women in the United Kingdom give birth, on average, to only two or three children in their lifetime, and that other methods of contraception are reasonably effective, and that birth control may be practised during most of a woman's child-bearing years.[28]

Any assessment of the thrombotic complications with the pill, however, had to take into account the different levels of maternal mortality across the world. One study published in 1977 by Dr Vessey and Professor Richard Doll highlighted the fact that, while those using oral contraceptives had a two to ten times greater risk of mortality than intrauterine devices and diaphragms, this risk diminished when put in the context of other countries where maternal mortality rates were high and the population less susceptible to vascular disease.[29]

The hazards of pregnancy and childbirth continued to inform the debate on the safety of the pill in the coming decades. In 1995, when the British government decided to withdraw six brands of oral contraceptive because of their links to venous thrombosis, women were told: "It should be understood that health risks from pills containing the progestogens desogestrel or gestodene are very low. The risks from an unplanned or unwanted pregnancy are far greater in comparison."[30]

Lifestyle risks

For some doctors the hazards associated with oral contraceptives were minimal compared with other activities such as travelling by air, by car, by motorbike, rock climbing, smoking, domestic accidents, or playing soccer. As two medical experts pointed out in a contraceptive textbook in 1969:

> There are a large number of recreational activities which are more dangerous than taking the Pill. In the U.S.A. there are over 5,000 boating and swimming fatalities a year and there is ten times the likelihood of a death in the family if father buys an outboard motor boat than if a mother uses oral contraceptives. It is probable that the amateur cricketer or footballer (activities which caused twenty-seven deaths in the UK, 1955–8) is more likely to die playing sports at the weekend than his wife is to die from using oral contraceptives.[31]

Such a comment is particularly interesting for understanding the ways in which questions of gender informed the debate about the risks of the pill. What is most noteworthy is that it was primarily male recreational pursuits that were used as the comparative tool for assessing the risks women faced when taking the oral contraceptive. The words also indicate the ways in which some doctors viewed the use of the pill as merely a matter of recreation. It would be a mistake, however, to equate the choice of men to sail a boat, swim, or even to play football or cricket with that made by women when engaging in sexual intercourse and the possibility of pregnancy.

In addition to sporting pursuits, the safety of the pill was viewed within the context of other lifestyle decisions. As the writers of the contraceptive textbook of 1969 emphasized:

> Almost without exception the consequences of contraception are beneficial and contribute significantly to the health and well-being of the community. In contrast, many societies permit drugs and other practices which are of questionable value or are demonstrably harmful. The ill-effects of alcohol and tobacco, which are tolerated for no better reason than that they provide comfort and pleasure, add appreciably to the mortality and morbidity rates of many societies, but they are inadequately regulated by civil law and social custom and do not fall within the sphere of medical prescription at all.[32]

Many went further to argue that oral contraceptives brought "an inestimable benefit to mankind".[33] In this situation, the choice of an individual woman and her health was pushed to one side in favour of the good of society as a whole.

Notions of risk and lifestyle choices were important in discussions about the dangers of the pill in other ways. While in the 1960s women were depicted as pursuing risky behaviour if they did not take the pill on account of the threat of pregnancy, by the 1970s those considered to be behaving dangerously were those who took the pill who were over the age of 35 and smoked, as this was thought to increase the risk of myocardial infarction (heart disease).[34] Those most at risk were heavy smokers who took the pill with the highest dose of oestrogen. Heavy smokers who took the pill aged over 35 years old were two to three times more likely to die of myocardial infarction than women who took the pill and did not smoke.[35]

The risk of cancer

From the time of its first development many medical practitioners were concerned about the risk the pill posed for cancer. The importance of uncovering the potential carcinogenic effects of the pill was considered particularly great given that both breast and cervical cancers appeared to be increasing just at the moment that consumption of the drug was rising. One of the main concerns troubling both medical practitioners and government officials was that the carcinogenic repercussions of the pill would not become apparent for many years. As one cancer expert advising those running British clinical trials of the pill stated in 1960: "The induction period of all cancers in man is long (15–25 years) and therefore the effects of these compounds in cancer induction will not be seen for many years to come."[36]

The earliest public alarms about cancer and oral contraceptives occurred in 1964 when a team of researchers at the University of Oregon demonstrated that certain hormones, such as the progestogen and oestrogen contained in the first oral contraceptive, Enovid, promoted the growth of cancers in animals such as rats. While the American Medical Association advised women that the pill carried no risk, fears were heightened in the late 1960s and 1970s when reports showed that female dogs developed breast cancer when given certain oral contraceptives, and evidence linked oral contraceptives with non-malignant tumours in the livers of some women, an extremely rare condition which can prove fatal should the tumour rupture and cause internal bleeding.[37] Anxieties were not eased by the fact that in 1975 sequential pills were withdrawn from the American market for fear that they increased the risk of endometrial cancer.[38]

During the 1970s suspicion about the carcinogenic effects of the pill was reinforced when news broke that stilboestrol, a steroid drug containing high oestrogen, had caused vaginal cancer (an extremely rare disease) in the daughters of mothers who, from the 1940s, had taken the drug to prevent miscarriage. The same drug was then being explored for its properties as a morning-after contraceptive.[39] By 1984, some women who had been given stilboestrol 20 years earlier were discovered to have breast cancer.[40] With the possible links between stilboestrol and cancer having taken years to emerge, many people wondered about the long-term safety of the oral contraceptive.[41]

Not all the news about the pill was so troubling. As early as 1961 Gregory Pincus, one of the early developers of Enovid, announced that it could potentially prevent breast and cervical cancer. His declaration offered an important glimmer of hope for the 15,000 American women dying from cervical cancer in these years.[42] Not everyone, however, was convinced by

Pincus's evidence. Indeed, by the early 1960s a number of medical practitioners were becoming increasingly uneasy about the potential carcinogenic effects of the pill. One of the prominent figures to sound a note of caution was Dr Roy Hertz, who advised the FDA's Advisory Committee on Obstetrics and Gynecology from the mid-1960s. He played a key role in cautioning against the mass use of contraceptives before their carcinogenic risks had been assessed. Summing up the potential carcinogenic risk, he pointed out:

> Our inadequate knowledge concerning the relationship of estrogens to cancer in women is comparable with what is known about the association between lung cancer and cigarette smoking before extensive epidemiological studies delineated this overwhelming significant statistical relationship.[43]

None the less, by the early 1970s a number of studies began to confirm Pincus's theory that the pill might have some anti-cancer benefits, indicating that the pill could prevent breast, ovarian and endometrial cancer.[44] Such findings were particularly welcome given the rising incidence of ovarian cancer in Britain and America since the 1950s. It was also heartening because ovarian and endometrial tumours are difficult to detect in their early stages and are frequently fatal. In this context many medical practitioners looked to the pill as a preventative tool.

In 1983 optimism about the pill's benefits was shattered when a number of investigations suggested that it could increase the risk of breast and cervical cancer among women in later life. Those most at danger were young women who had taken the pill for many years before the age of 25.[45] Such revelations were particularly discomforting given the recent increase of younger women taking the pill and the rising incidence of breast and cervical cancer since the 1950s.[46] The most disquieting aspect of the news was that progestogens might be implicated in the cancer. This was unlike previous scares where oestrogen had been blamed for side effects such as thrombosis. Many women who had been switched to low-dose pills in the wake of the cardiovascular troubles of the late 1960s were now surprised to discover that their drug was not as safe as presumed. Pills with high doses of progestogen were now regarded as dangerous.[47]

Many within the medical community, however, felt the new evidence was inconclusive, and bitter tensions emerged between epidemiologists on this question. Professional reputations were not the only issue at stake: so were women's lives. What concerned many was that the danger of breast cancer, thought to be increased in younger women taking the pill, might persist into their middle age. Should this happen, medical experts feared they would witness an unprecedented rise in breast cancer in years to come. By 1988 over 30 epidemiological studies had been undertaken to investigate the links between oral contraceptive use and breast cancer; not a single study had provided a statistically significant answer.[48]

In 1993, however, the epidemiologist professor Valerie Beral and her team appeared to solve the problem when they announced the results of a study which had analysed the evidence of 53,297 women with breast cancer and 100,239 controls. Using data from 54 investigations in 25 countries around the world, which represented about 90 per cent of the epidemiological information collected on breast cancer risk and use of hormonal contraceptive in the past two decades, Beral and her colleagues revealed what no one had seen before: that the carcinogenic effect of the pill on the breast was related to its recent use. They also showed that tumours that were diagnosed in women taking oral contraceptives tended to be localized to the breast and were less clinically advanced. This contrasted with women who had never used oral contraceptives, where the cancer was more likely to spread to other parts of the body. The tumours diagnosed in women taking the pill were therefore potentially easier to treat. A woman's family history of breast cancer made no impact on the results. The data also indicated that the risk was unrelated to any particular oestrogen or progestogen. Interestingly, the higher doses of hormones were seen to be associated with less risk.[49]

Many within the medical profession greeted Beral's study with relief. One of the most reassuring aspects of the study was the fact that it seemed that the carcinogenic effect of the pill on the breast diminished after ten years of stopping the pill. It was therefore unlikely that the medical profession would witness an epidemic of breast cancer in future years among older women who had taken the pill. Physicians were once again comforted in January 1999 when a twenty-five-year follow-up of 46,000 women by the British Royal College of General Practitioners confirmed the earlier findings of Beral's collaborative study.[50]

For the moment Beral's study put to rest one of the major concerns that had weighed on people's minds for years. Breast cancer was the one factor that many had feared might tip the odds against the safety of the pill overall. The extent to which it was of major public concern was highlighted by data from France and the United States in the 1990s which showed that breast cancer reduced women's life expectancy by ten years. As one epidemiologist pointed out in 1991, shortly before Beral's collaborative study was launched, breast cancer was so common that "any increase in risk associated with a widely used method of contraception would be a serious concern". He went on to point out that: "Breast cancer also happens to be a disease that women and their families particularly fear, so any increase in risk might carry a disproportionate weight when choices of contraception are being made."[51]

Women's attitude to the risk of the pill

Just as medical experts have debated and changed their views about the safety of the pill over time, so women have formed different opinions about

its risk. Some women who took the drug in its earliest days were aware of
the potential risks they were taking, but weighed them against other factors.
The reasoning of such women is exemplified by the case of Mrs J. S., who
took the pill as part of a British trial in the early 1960s. She dismissed
people who saw the pill as something unnatural and dangerous. As she
commented,

> [P]erhaps I was naive but I don't think I was, I thought well people –
> my mother-in-law had eleven pregnancies, and nine children came out
> of that, and if you were sort of artificially pregnant it's only what you
> would have been if you hadn't been on the pill, wasn't it? And that's the
> way I looked at [it, and] people said to me, "it isn't natural", but what is
> natural? To have a baby every year, isn't [is] it? [52]

Such reactions were not uncommon. Many women were prepared to put up
with very debilitating side effects because of the benefits that the pill
promised. This is captured by the attitude of one British woman, Betty
Vincent, who started taking the pill on a trial basis after she was forced to
abandon nurse training because of conceiving four children in quick succes-
sion. After the trial she had continued to take one of the earliest and
strongest oral contraceptives for 17 years with no ill effects. She was willing
to take the drug whatever the costs were to her health. As she put it, "I
wouldn't have cared if I had [had problems]. I would have put up with
headaches and things like that because the alternative was to keep getting
pregnant every year."[53] Such a response was not unique. One American
woman, when asked by a doctor in the late 1960s to stop using the pill
because of the possibility of cancer, retorted:

> Look, I don't care if you *promise* me cancer in five years, I'm staying on
> the pill. At least I'll enjoy five years I have left. For the first time in
> eighteen years of married life I can put my feet up for an hour and read a
> magazine. I can watch my favorite TV program without having to catch
> up on my ironing at the same time. I can usually get a full night's sleep
> because there is no baby to feed or toddler to take to the toilet. If you
> refuse to give me the pill, I'll go get it from someone else.[54]

Even where some women suffered side effects, they continued the medication. Some American women interviewed in the late 1960s, for instance,
who experienced such side effects as bloated breasts, were reluctant to give
up the pill because they saw the enhanced breast size as enhancing their
feminine attractiveness. Others were also keen on the pill because it had
improved their complexion.[55]

Not all women, however, were content with the side reactions caused by
the pill, and relinquished it quickly. In some cases the adverse reactions
had a dramatic and long-lasting impact on the women's lives. This was

particularly the case for those who suffered cardiovascular complications from taking the high oestrogen pills in the early 1960s. While some died, others were left maimed and incapacitated, the most unfortunate having to have one of their limbs amputated. In many cases these effects led not just to poor health, but to social isolation and complications in carrying on a normal life.

As time went on, women became increasing concerned about the long-term impact the pill could have on their health. A survey undertaken in Britain between 1967 and 1971 indicates how married mothers became increasingly aware of the health hazards associated with the contraceptive. The survey is particularly interesting because it began the moment that thrombosis associated with the pill hit the media headlines and ended when the British government called on doctors to cease prescribing high-oestrogen pills associated with the problem. In 1967, 37 per cent of the women interviewed for the survey spontaneously mentioned the possibility that the pill might cause heart disease, thrombosis or even result in death. By 1970 the proportion had gone up to 58 per cent. Similarly, the numbers of mothers who perceived a definite risk of thrombosis or heart attack also increased from 25 to 58 per cent in these years.[56]

What effect the increasing awareness of the dangers of the pill had on women's decision to take the pill is hard to measure. Much depended on how women were alerted to its risks and how these were presented against other factors in their lives.[57] Clearly this was a very individual decision, based on the kind of relationship a woman had, her family circumstances, her medical history and the alternative contraceptives available to her. Yet where she lived was also an important factor in her decision. From the early 1970s, for example, American women dropped the contraceptive much more rapidly and consistently than did women in Britain. American women first stopped taking the pill in the light of the news about thrombosis and the pill in the late 1960s, and relinquished its use even further with revelations that it could cause cancer. A survey conducted in the United States in 1985 indicated that at least 76 per cent of American women believed there were substantial risks associated with the pill.[58] While British women exhibited similar patterns, the decline was less dramatic, and in fact the percentage taking the pill continued to rise overall despite publicized risks.

The slowness among British women to discontinue the contraceptive, given the prominence of British medical scientists in reporting the risks of both thrombosis and cancer, is particularly interesting when contrasted with the United States, where scientists were slower to connect adverse reactions with the pill. Yet American women tended to be more vocal and protested much more publicly about the side effects of the pill and led an effective campaign in the 1970s to have them included on the products' labels. Their actions might therefore have been instrumental in swaying public opinion. In Britain, protests by women were virtually non-existent, partially reflecting the relative weakness of the women's movement in the country and the absence of a strong consumer lobby in the National Health Service.[59] Another explanation for the quicker response in the United States is that the American public tend to be quicker overall than the British to adopt technological innovation as well as quicker to absorb scientific information about its risks. Studies in the United States during the 1970s and 1980s indicated that much of the discontinuation of the pill in these years was strongly correlated with media reports of the drug's adverse effects.[60]

Conclusion

The history of the contraceptive pill reveals many of the twists and turns that debates can take about the risk of medication. Regarded with suspicion by many medical practitioners when first introduced to the market, the pill rapidly became accepted as a safe and important feature of life. Moreover, any risks associated with its use were quickly dismissed in the light of the greater hazards posed by an unplanned and unwanted pregnancy and potential maternal mortality, and were also regarded as irrelevant when seen in the context of other hazards in life.

Yet, as this paper has shown, not all medical practitioners weighed up the dangers posed by the pill in the same way as pregnancy or childbirth or recreational pursuits. Furthermore the debate about the safety of the pill changed as more research examined the links between the drug and the complications of thrombosis and cancer. While in the early years much of the concern of the medical profession and governments focused on the potential cardiovascular problems that could be associated with the contraceptive, by the 1970s some medical experts began to see it in a new light when investigations revealed its potential to prevent ovarian and endometrial cancer. Within this context some medical practitioners began to see the pill as more than just a contraceptive and to embrace it as a weapon to fight cancer and a means of increasing life expectancy.[61] Dr Joseph Goldzieher, who has strong attachments with pharmaceutical companies making oral contraceptives, argued in the 1990s that all women of reproductive age and even older should be using oral contraceptives for at least two years of their lives because of their "anticancer effect".[62]

Not all medical professionals, however, were as confident about the pill as Goldzieher. During the 1980s and early 1990s many medical experts were very concerned about the potential carcinogenic effect of the drug on the breast and cervix. Some of the concern about breast cancer was put to rest in the early 1990s with the large collaborative study led by Professor Beral. It is unlikely, however, that the arguments about the safety of the pill are over. To date, most of the research has been conducted on the effects of the earlier formulations of oral contraceptives, but little has been done on the newer ones. One of the questions currently being asked is whether the older and higher doses of oral contraceptives might be better protectors against cancer than the newer low-dose ones. Given the need for a long period to pass before carcinogenic effects might be observed, the carcinogenic risks of the pill will continue to be debated for many years to come.

While medical experts have debated and tried to define the statistical dangers posed by the pill, women have faced different questions. Initially held up as a miraculous and convenient means of contraception in the early 1960s, the decision to take the pill has become a complex issue that cannot be easily assessed. One American woman who gave up the pill in the late 1960s sums up the dilemma women faced on taking the pill:

> We're all doing so many terrible things to our bodies. Up to a point, medicine and science made great advances. But now things are getting all mixed up. What can you do when you're caught up in this swirl of convenience-and-pollution? Air pollution. Water pollution. Body pollution. Additives to foods that may by poisonous. What do you do? Move to Tahiti? Grow your own vegetables in the backyard or on the roof? The pill is part of the whole picture. Once you agree to live in a civilized, "convenient" life, where do you draw the line?[63]

Notes

1 Material for this paper is drawn from my book *Sexual Chemistry: A History of the Contraceptive Pill*, Yale: Yale University Press, 2001. Many thanks go to the Wellcome Trust for supporting the research that went into the book and this paper.

2 H. Lewin to A. Guttmacher, 22 July 1966, Population Council Papers, Box 124, Rockefeller Archive.

3 G. Guillebaud, "Introduction", in J. Guillebaud, *The Pill*, Oxford: Oxford Paperbacks, 1980, new edition 1991, p. 3.

4 *British Medical Journal*, vol. 1, 1961, 432.

5 W. M. Jordan (Suffolk) letter to editor, *Lancet*, 18 Nov 1961, 1146–7.

6 Memo from G. D. Searle to Shareowners, 9 Aug 1962, Smithsonian Papers, National Museum of American History, Washington DC; *New York Times*, 9 Aug. 1962; Memo to PPFA Affiliates from M. S. Calderone, 6 Aug. 1962, Schlesinger Library, Calderone's Papers, Box 12, fo.216; *British Medical Journal* 11 Aug 1962, 426; J. Davey, "How Safe are the Birth Control Pills", *Redbook* (Feb 1963), Gregory Pincus's Papers, Library of Congress (GP-LC), Box 60.

7 *Time*, vol. 84, 3 July 1964, 46. See also E. Watkins, *On the Pill: A Social History of Oral Contraceptives, 1950–1970*, Baltimore: Johns Hopkins University Press, 1998, 43–4, 83.

8 Dr David B. Clark, professor of neurology at the Kentucky University Medical Center, evidence to Competitive Problems in the Drug Industry: Hearings before the Subcommittee on Monopoly of the Select Committee on Small Business: US Senate 91st Congress Second Session on Present Status of Competition in the Pharmaceutical Industry (henceforth *Nelson Hearings*), Part 15, Jan 1970, 6136.

9 Hilary Hill, "Risks of the Pill", FPA release c.1960s, SA/FPA/A5/160/2, Box 250. Henceforth all references SA/FPA indicates British Family Planning Association papers, Contemporary Medical Archives Collection, Wellcome Library for the History and Understanding of Medicine.

10 Goldzieher was formally the director of the division of Clinical Sciences for the South West Foundation for Research and Education in San Antonio.

11 *Nelson Hearings*, Part 15, 6353–4. A similar argument is made in C. Wood, *Birth Control Now and Tomorrow*, Gateshead, 1969, 156–8.

12 *Nelson Hearings*, Part 15, 6354. See also D. F. Hawkins, "Thromboembolic Risks in Contraception", *Spectrum*, 1, 1973.

13 I. Loudon, *Deaths in Childbirth: An International Study of Maternal Care and Maternal Mortality 1800–1950*, Oxford: Oxford University Press, 1992, 352–7, and J. Leavitt, "Joseph DeLee and the Practice of Preventive Obstetrics", *American Journal of Public Health*, vol.78, No. 10, 1988, 1353–9.

14 *Nelson Hearings*, Part 15, 5933. See also L. Grant, *Sexing the Millennium*, London: New York Grove Press, 1993, 184–5. Davis had a vested interest promoting intrauterine devices in place of oral contraceptives. For more on Davis and the Dalkon Shield see N. J. Grant, *The Selling of Contraception: The Dalkon Shield Case, Sexuality, and Women's Autonomy*, Ohio: Ohio State University Press, 1992, 31–2, 37, 43–51.

15 *Lancet*, 11 Oct 1970, cited in *Nelson Hearings*, Part 15, 5927.

16 W. H. W. Inman, "Role of Drug-Reaction Monitoring in the Investigation of Thrombosis and 'The Pill' ", *British Medical Bulletin*, vol. 26, No. 3, 1970, 248–56; pp. 252–3.

17 Cited in Inman, "Role of Drug-Reaction Monitoring".

18 Hertz also worked in various capacities for the National Institute of Health.

19 *Nelson Hearings*, Part 15, 6041.

20 J. Rock, *The Time has Come: A Catholic Doctor's Proposals to End the Battle over Birth Control*, New York: Alfred Knopf, 1963, p. 167. For more information on Rock's fight for the Vatican's approval of the pill see Marks, *Sexual Chemistry*, chapter 9.

21 Physicians' booklet, Conovid (Searle, July 1960), SA/FPA/A5/161/3, Box 251. Information for volunteers, no date SA/FPA/A5/162.3, Box 252; also Information for Volunteers, no date, SA/FPA/A5/157/1, Box 249.

22 G. Venning, Letter to Editor of *British Medical Journal*, 8 Aug 1962.

23 A. S. Parkes, *Lancet*, 16 Jan 1963, SA\FPA\A5\126, Box 245.

24 *Nelson Hearings*, Part 15, 6382.

25 *Nelson Hearings*, Part 15, 5925.

26 Venning, Letter to Editor. See also G. I. M. Swyer, "Fertility Control: Achievements and Prospects", lecture given 2 Feb 1967, London School of Hygiene and Tropical Medicine, SA/FPA/A5/135 Box 246.

27 W. H. W. Inman and M. P. Vessey, "Investigation of deaths from pulmonary, coronary, and cerebral thrombosis and embolism in women of childbearing age", *British Medical Journal*, 27 April 1968, 193–9; p. 194.

28 Inman and Vessey, "Investigation of deaths", p. 198.

29 *Lancet*, 8 Oct 1977, 747–8.

30 Dr Olav Meirik, Chief of the HRP Task Force for Epidemiological Research in Reproductive Health, 1996, Press Release WHO/77 – 20 Oct 1995.

31 J. Peel and D. M. Potts, *Contraceptive Practice*, Cambridge, 1969, 255. See also Guillebaud, *The Pill*, 6, 165–7.

32 Peel and Potts, *Textbook of Contraceptive Practice*, 255. See also Guillebaud, *The Pill*, 6, 165–7.

33 Dr Gabriel V. Jaffe, *British Medical Journal*, vol. 1, 1961, 1043. WHO also promoted oral contraceptives for this reason. See letter from G. G. Robertson to G. J. W. Hunter, 25 March 1966, Searle's archives, High Wycombe.

34 Inman and Vessey, "Investigation of deaths, 193–9; M. P. Vessey and R. Doll, "Investigation of Relations between Use of Oral Contraceptives and Thromboembolic Disease. A Further Report", *British Medical Journal*, 14 June 1969, 651–7; M. P. Vessey, and R. Doll, "Investigation of Relation between Use of Oral Contraceptives and Thromboembolic Disease, A Further Report", *British Medical Journal*, vol. 2, 1969, 651–7; W. H. W. Inman *et al.*, "Thromboembolic Disease and the Steroidal Content of Oral Contraceptives", *British Medical Journal*, 25 April 1970, 203–9; M. P. Vessey *et al.*, "Postoperative Thromboembolism and the Use of Oral Contraceptives", *British Medical Journal*, 3, 1970, 123–6.

35 Inman *et al.*, "Thromboembolic Disease and the Steroidal Content of Oral Contraceptives"; P. D. Stolley *et al.*, "Cardiovascular Effects of Oral Contraceptives", *Southern Medical Journal*, vol. 71. No. 7, July 1978, 821–4, table 3, 824; M. P. Vessey and J. I. Mann, "Female Sex Hormones and Thrombosis: Epidemiological Aspects", *British Medical Bulletin*, vol. 34, No. 2, 1978, 157–62; and R. C. Bennett, "The Safety and Utility of Oral Contraceptives Containing 50 Micrograms of Estrogen", unpublished paper prepared for FDA Fertility and Maternal Health Drugs Advisory Committee Meetings, 28 Oct 1993; "Oral Contraceptives and Myocardial Infarction – The Search for the Smoking Gun", *New England Journal of Medicine*, vol. 345, No. 25, 20 Dec 2001, 1841–2; M. P. Vessey *et al.*, "Mortality in Relation to Oral Contraceptive Use and Cigarette Smoking", *British Medical Journal*, 2003, 362: 185–91. *Lancet*, vol. 362, 2003, 185–91.

36 G. M. Bonser to E. Mears, April 1960, SA/FPA/A5/161/1, Box 251; CIFC Minutes, April 21 1960, p. 110, SA/FPA/A5/154.

37 *British Medical Journal*, 31 Jan 1970, 252. See also *The Pharmaceutical Journal*, 13 Dec 1975, 597; P. Vaughan, "The Pill Turns Twenty", *New York Times Magazine*, 13 June 1976. See also G. R. Huggins and R. L. Giuntoli, "Oral Contraceptives and Neoplasia", *Fertility and Sterility*, vol. 32, No. 1, July 1979, 1–23.

38 *Pharmaceutical Journal*, 18 Sept 1976, 257.

39 B. Seaman and G. Seaman, *Women and the Crisis of Sex Hormones*, New York: Rawson Associates, 1977, 13–24, 40–2; A. Direcks and E. Hoen, "DES: The Crime Continues", in K.Donnell (ed.), *Adverse Effects: Women and the Pharmaceutical Industry*, Toronto, 1986, 41–50; and D. B. Dutton, *Worse than the disease: Pitfalls of medical progress*, Cambridge, 1988, chapter 3.

40 E. R. Greenblatt *et al.*, "Breast Cancer in Mothers Given Diethylstilbestrol in Pregnancy", *New England Journal of Medicine*, vol. 311, 1984, 1393–7.

41 Seaman and Seaman, *Women and the Crisis of Sex Hormones*, 116.

42 G. Pincus to D. Norman, 7 June 1960, GP-LC, Box 45. See also G. Pincus and C. R. Garcia, "Studies in Vaginal, Cervical and Uterine Histology", *Metabolism*, 3, 1965, 344–7; "How Safe are the Birth Control Pills?", *Vogue*, 8 Jan 1961, 90–1, 128.

43 FDA, *Report on the Oral Contraceptives*, 1 Aug 1966, Appendix 5, 51. See also Watkins, *On the Pill*, 87.

44 M. P. Vessey, R. Doll and P. M. Sutton, "Investigations of the Possible Relationship Between Oral Contraceptives and Benign and Malignant Breast Disease", *Cancer*, vol. 28, 1971, 1395; M. Vessey, R. Doll and P. M. Sutton, "Oral Contraceptives and Breast Neoplasia: a Retrospective Study", *British Medical Journal*, vol. 3, 1972, 719–24; P. E Sartwell, F. G. Arthes and J. A. Tonascia, "Epidemiology of Benign Breast Lesions; Lack of Association with Oral Contraceptive Use", *New England Journal of Medicine*, vol. 288, 1973, 551; Boston Collaborative Drug Surveillance Program, "Oral Contraceptives and Venous Thromboembolic Disease, Surgically Confirmed Gallbladder Disease, and Breast Tumors", *Lancet*, 23 June 1973, 1399–404; L.A. Brinton *et al.*, "Risk Factors for Benign Breast Disease", *American Journal of Epidemiology*, vol. 113, No. 3, March 1981, 203–14.

45 M. C. Pike *et al.*, "Breast Cancer in Young Women and Use of Oral Contraceptives; Possible Modifying Effect of Formulation and Age at Use", *Lancet*, vol. 2, 1983, 926–30; and K. McPherson *et al.*, "Oral Contraceptives and Breast Cancer", *Lancet*, vol. 2, 1983, 1414–15. That same month, the pill was also linked with liver cancer in a new study: *Medical News*, 27 Oct 1983. For a medical discussion on the results in 1983 see *Lancet*, 22 Oct 1983, 947–8.

46 M. Thorogood and M. Vessey, "Trends in Use of Oral Contraceptives in Britain", *British Journal of Family Planning*, vol. 16, 1990, 41–53, table 4, p. 46. By 1987 over 80 per cent of all British general practitioners' prescriptions of the pill were for women under the age of 30. M. Thorogood and L. Villard-Mackintosh, "Combined Oral Contraceptives: Risks and Benefits", *British Medical Bulletin*, vol. 49, No. 1, 1993, 124–39, p. 125; R. Russel-Briefel, T. Ezzarati and J. Pelman, "Prevalence and Trends in Oral Contraceptive

use in Pre-menopausal Females – Ages 12–54, United States, 1971–1980", *American Journal of Public Health*, vol. 75, 1985, 1173–6.

47 *Sunday Telegraph*, 23 Oct 1983; *Guardian*, 25 Oct 1983; "More Worries About the Pill", *Nature*, vol. 305, 27 Oct 1983, 749–50.

48 G. C. Buehring, "Oral Contraceptives and Breast Cancer: What has 20 Years of Research Shown?", *Biomedicine and Pharmacotherapy*, vol. 42, 1988, 525–30; 526.

49 CASH, "Breast Cancer and Hormonal Contraceptives", *Lancet*, vol. 347, 22 June 1996, 1713–27; CASH, "Breast Cancer and Hormonal Contraceptives: Further Results", *Contraception*, 53/3s (1996), 1s–106s. See also *Lancet*, vol. 348, 7 Sept 1996, p. 683. The data collected together not only came from studies conducted in Britain, the United States, Australia, New Zealand, but also Chile, China, Colombia, Kenya, Mexico, Nigeria, Philippines and Thailand.

50 V. Beral *et al.*, "Mortality Associated with Oral Contraceptive Use: 25 Year Follow Up of Cohort of 46,000 Women from Royal College of General Practitioners' Oral Contraception Study", *British Medical Journal*, 9 Jan 1999, 96–100.

51 Skegg, "Risks and Benefits of Oral Contraceptives", p. 166.

52 Interview with Mrs J. A. S. by Ros O'Brien on behalf of present author, Autumn 1997, transcript, p. 7.

53 Betty Vincent, interview on *Timewatch* TV programme, "The Pill: Prescription for Revolution", National Sound Archives.

54 Mrs T, cited in B. Seaman, *The Doctors' Case Against the Pill*, 1969, Almeda, CA, reprint 1995, p. 19.

55 Seaman, *The Doctors' Case Against the Pill*, p. 46.

56 A. Cartwright, *Parents and Family Planning Services*, London, 1970, pp. 232–4.

57 For more information on this issue see Marks, *Sexual Chemistry*, chapter 8.

58 Seaman, *The Doctors' Case Against the Pill*, p. 218.

59 F. B. McCrea and G. E. Markle, "The Estrogen Replacement Controversy in the USA and UK: Different Answers to the Same Question", *Social Studies of Science*, vol. 14, 1984, 1–26.

60 E. F. Jones, J. R. Beninger and C. F. Westoff, "Pill and IUD Discontinuation in the United States, 1970–1975: The Influence of the Media", *Family Planning Perspectives*, 12, 6 (1980), 293–300; p. 294.

61 D. Grimes, "The Safety of Oral Contraceptives: Epidemiological Insights From the First 30 Years", *American Journal on Obstetrics and Gynecology*, vol. 166, No. 6, June 1992, part 2, 1950–4; p. 1951.

62 J. W. Goldzieher, "Are Low-dose Oral Contraceptives Safer and Better?", *American Journal of Obstetrics and Gynecology*, vol. 171, No. 3, Sept 1994, 587–90, p. 590.

63 Eleanor B., cited in Seaman, *The Doctors' Case Against the Pill*, p. 60.

12 Addressing uncertainties

The conceptualization of brain death in Switzerland 1960–2000[1]

Silke Bellanger and Aline Steinbrecher

Introduction

In 1968 the Swiss Academy of Medical Sciences (SAMW) set up a committee to define the criteria for diagnosing death and brain death. At one of this committee's last meetings a general debate ensued about the potential recovery of dying patients and the difficulties involved in grasping the different aspects of the process of dying. Those members, who had at one time vehemently argued in favour of the evidence and certainty of brain death, stressing their professional competency to confirm death properly, suddenly began to highlight the doubts and uncertainties associated with diagnosing death in general. Every one of them came up with a story about a patient who, after having been pronounced dead, had returned to life. The transplant surgeon who had initiated the SAMW committee and who later performed the first Swiss heart transplant, emphasized: "We can't demand that every single physician always makes the correct diagnosis. ... As sad as it is, we will always have and always have to have doubts."[2]

Even today, stories about living patients who appeared at one time to be brain-dead still circulate, both inside and outside the medical culture. They suggest that brain death is neither easy to observe nor easy to determine and is not a natural and self-evident phenomenon. Brain death only becomes real by definition, diagnosis and decisive action. However, the practice of determining and deciding upon the reality of brain death entails uncertainty. The risk associated with the possibility of misjudging a patient's condition has always existed and will always exist. We would like to describe how Swiss physicians have dealt with this permanent condition of potential uncertainty since the late 1960s and how they tried to anticipate and minimize the implicit risk of making the wrong decision, when pronouncing someone dead.

Decision-making is a crucial moment in risk production, risk perception and risk management.[3] Risk is thereby understood to be strongly related to the production, distribution and function of knowledge. Technological innovations, shifts in scientific research and new epistemic objects, such as the introduction of the new medical concept of death, bring about uncertainty.

Innovations generate an increasing differentiation of received knowledge, and changes in practice produce uncertainties about what might be considered an appropriate decision and action in a particular situation. Thus, the act of decision-making takes on a special role in this context of innovation and changes. When no shared body of knowledge exists to serve as a framework, the very act of conceiving something as certain and accurate or uncertain and false depends upon making a decision.

To deal with this kind of uncertainty, physicians have developed their own techniques and procedures. Renée Fox has shown that uncertainty in medicine has been a topic in medical education at least since the 1950s.[4] In the social sciences of medicine, studies have looked at the tools developed to aid in decision-making as well as their changing objectives, functionality and significance in relation to medical knowledge and practice. One central issue dealt with in these studies has been the relationship between contingency and the standardization of medical practice.[5] The concept of brain death has been analysed by historians and social scientists, chiefly in relation to transplant surgery,[6] and recent sociological and anthropological studies on the subject have focused on the question of how different professional actors cope with brain death and brain-dead patients.[7]

So far, however, the aspects of uncertainty, risk and decision-making have not been considered with respect to brain death in a historical dimension. This interrelation leads the historian to questions about medical knowledge and practice: how is brain death shaped as an object of knowledge and practice? How do knowledge and practice come to be recognized and formalized? Issues of risk and safety in relation to the concept of brain death point to substantial elements of the medical culture itself, as they are embedded in the daily medical procedures of clinical interaction with patients who are between life and death.

Ever since the introduction of the concept of brain death, physicians have emphasized the necessity of avoiding any kind of risk. All those involved have repeatedly stressed the need to be able to diagnose brain death accurately and with certainty, and instruments have been created or adapted to achieve these ends. The history of brain death is thus also a history of the construction of the means for dealing with the changing contemporary perceptions of uncertainty. During this very process, however, the criteria defining certainty have changed as well.

When we analyse the history of brain death in Switzerland from 1960 until 2000 we see that three tendencies influence these altering configurations: scientific objectification of the phenomenon of brain death, standardization of the management of brain death, and regulation of subjective dispositions.[8] These tendencies reflect a certain chronology in the history of brain death but never completely displace one another over time, and they can, to some extent, always be observed simultaneously. These strategies for obtaining certainty imply that the figure[9] of the individual professional generates uncertainty in the whole context of addressing, managing and deciding on brain death. The figure of the individual, with all the subjectivity this implies, functions in opposition to the concept of safe and certain medical knowledge and practice.

The historical setting

In the 1950s and 1960s innovations in intensive care medicine made it not only possible but also necessary to revise the definition and diagnosis of death. Intensive care technology and resuscitation, in particular artificial respiration, had created a condition in some patients that was described as the irreversible termination of all brain activity with circulatory and respiratory functions being maintained artificially. Physicians working in intensive care medicine were aware of the need to reformulate the concept behind what was considered in medical culture to be the line between life and death.[10] But the eventual redefinitions and regulations of this hitherto unknown state were imposed internationally according to the needs of transplantation medicine. During the 1950s, thanks to developments in immunology, kidney transplants in humans were re-started initially using organs from living donors, mostly family members, and later from cadavers.[11] With the first human heart transplant, performed by Christiaan Barnard in Capetown in 1967, it immediately became clear that if transplants were to be a part of routine clinical care, organs would have to be made available on a regular basis and, in the case of hearts, could not come from cadavers of patients who had died of cardiopulmonary arrest.[12]

Medical literature on transplantation surgery proposed comatose patients and patients with serious brain injuries as ideal organ donors without, however, specifying the particular condition of these patients. The general subject of brain death was not explicitly addressed in Swiss medical journals before the late 1960s, nor were there any discussions in the mass media about new or different ways of diagnosing death. Debates about brain death as a distinct topic arose with the first heart transplants or, to put it more precisely, with the media's interest in and the public's increased awareness of this kind of medical activity. It was precisely the interrelation between brain death and transplantation surgery that made the act of decision-making in diagnosing brain death such a risk-laden topic. As the treatment of patients who were deemed brain dead might prove crucial for the management of transplantation, the fear was repeatedly expressed that the concept of brain death might only serve the purpose of organ transplantation. Hence, the link between brain death and transplantation demanded that a non-medical party – such as the relatives of the patient or the media – should understand the procedure as legitimate.

This new demand for legitimation led to the introduction of a number of committees concerned with the definition of death, particularly brain death, such as the ones at the Harvard Medical School and the German Society of Surgery.[13] In 1969 the SAMW committee, consisting of intensive care physicians, transplant surgeons and neurologists, worked out criteria and guidelines for diagnosing brain death and cardiopulmonary arrest in Switzerland. The results were published as the Guidelines in Swiss medical journals shortly after the first heart transplant had been performed at the university hospital of Zurich in April of that year.[14]

Objectifying brain death

Neither the minutes of the discussions of the SAMW committee, nor the Guidelines themselves, nor any medical articles mentioned explicit doubts about the objective existence of brain death. But there were nevertheless a number of crucial questions concerning the issue: at what moment in the process of dying could one speak of brain death, and which criteria were to be considered relevant for diagnosing this state with certainty? Even for medically trained professionals, it was a difficult task to convert the signs provided by the patient's body and registered by various technological devices into a single, homogeneous concept of death. In the light of such a heterogeneous and inconsistent phenomenon, decision-making, and thus medical practice in general, were considered to be uncertain.

The committee reacted by trying to define the phenomenon in the Guidelines. Matters of recurrent debate concerned the extent to which brain death should be regulated by criteria delineated in the Guidelines, and if so, which elements of knowledge and practice were essential to this definition and which could be disregarded. The solution to the problem of striking an appropriate balance between regulation and flexibility was reached by transferring the dilemma from the Guidelines' quasi-normative context to the practical context of diagnosis. To some extent, the published version of the Guidelines left the concrete decision about brain death to local management in local medical settings. Although it had been their intention to remain vague about the degree of professional knowledge and skill necessary for appropriate diagnosis, the committee's members expressed concern that any heterogeneity might render brain death a doubtful subject in general, despite their attempts to regulate its specific features by means of the Guidelines. Several members therefore strongly recommended a survey of current knowledge and medical practices in the diagnosis of death.[15]

"Have we committed two crimes?":[16] Surveying brain death in Switzerland

In the course of these recommended surveys two neurologists from the university hospital in Lausanne studied 90 local cases of brain death diagnosis in 1970 and discovered that, in two cases, the data conflicted with the SAMW's definition.[17] Two patients had been declared brain dead even though they had still shown reflexes of the extremities, whereas according to the Guidelines, such automatic responses should no longer have been possible. With a hint of irony, the authors asked if they had killed the two patients by accident. They compared their diagnosis with the international literature and ultimately ruled out the possibility of murder. Instead they remarked that – in contrast to the Guidelines – reflexes of the extremities were compatible with brain death if all of the other criteria were fulfilled.

Physicians at other Swiss university hospitals also started analysing their case material systematically.[18] The explicit aim of providing a systematic overview of knowledge and practice concerning brain death was to support the implementation of the Guidelines. On the one hand, the overviews were intended to confirm the appropriateness of the criteria and procedures determined by the SAMW and to show that the international medical standards, which were incorporated into the Guidelines, did not differ from the understanding based on experiences made locally in Switzerland. On the other hand, the overview illustrated in the eyes of contemporary medical actors that the previously existing framework of decision-making had been already adequate and had not led to any wrong decisions, or any accidental harm, let alone the death of patients. By comparing contemporary knowledge and current practice from various Swiss hospitals, the overviews thus functioned as a retrospective explication of brain death. The surveys produced numerical results confirming that no cases had been observed which differed in general from the SAMW assumptions about brain death, but revealed that the Guidelines had to be slightly adjusted with respect to the reflexes of the extremities.[19]

The statistical analysis and quantified correlation of the diagnostic criteria, procedures and data concerning patients declared brain-dead in Swiss hospitals was expected, furthermore, to serve as the foundation for a wider or even universal knowledge base for decision-making. Theodore Porter has argued that this notion of objectivity, as characterized by quantification and statistics, is closely related to the construction of accountability and legitimacy in wider contexts than that of an isolated group like the physicians who were concerned with defining and diagnosing brain death.[20] Such a concept is associated with public, explicit and impersonal rationality. In this case, quantification functioned as an instrument to address uncertainties that existed within the medical culture and were understood to be the result of the heterogeneity of ideas about the diagnosis of brain death.

As mentioned above, the physicians who proposed the surveys about death had also explicitly articulated their concern that any kind of diagnostic variation might lead to the risk of diagnosing death prematurely. Indeed, it was the figure of the individual physician, believing himself capable of judging both a situation and a patient's condition on his own, that embodied the contemporary perception of uncertainty in regard to the concept of brain death. The traditional ideal of medical expertise, according to which knowledge is constituted through individual experience, did not correspond with the emerging idea of and need for an objective, uniform and controllable object of knowledge and practice. In this context, the possibility of alternative definitions of brain death and a variety of different procedures invited suspicion concerning a lack of medical expertise and competence. This suspicion, it was feared, could ultimately lead to a general feeling of mistrust concerning medical knowledge itself.

Therefore, a framework for uniform decision-making was required. Accordingly, the first step was to create a unified body of knowledge and practices, which, with the help of a quantified survey of accepted characteristics and effects, was expected to transform difference and heterogeneity into a homogeneous object of knowledge and practice. Alternative approaches or variation in defining and diagnosing brain death were to be excluded in order to eliminate the dimension of subjectivity. The transformation of the individual physician's knowledge into a statistically quantified body of knowledge opened up the concept of brain death to scrutiny and control. Decision-making and medical practice came to be considered certain and legitimate when they occurred within the limits of this generalized body of knowledge and were guided by its rules.

Visualizing brain death

Other medical discussions that took place in the 1960s and 1970s illustrate that certainty about brain death was not only a matter of having a coherent set of diagnostic criteria and a corresponding justified framework for decision-making. The possibility of optical illusion also seemed to create uncertainty, and physicians were recurrently suspected of not being able to properly observe the criteria of brain death or of not being able to interpret the signals revealed by the body of the potentially brain-dead patient.

Articles used the topoi of apparently dead as well as apparently living patients in order to illustrate the illusive nature of brain death.[21] The outward appearance of the brain-dead patient's body did not correspond to the general suppositions about what a dead person would look like. Since the process of dying took place beneath the surface of the body and remained invisible to the observer, the physician's naked eye was considered to be an unreliable instrument for observing and diagnosing brain death. Thus, confiding the diagnosis to the capacities of perception of an individual human seemed a potential source of uncertainty.

At the same time, several medical articles were published on visualization techniques for the diagnosis of brain death.[22] They did not explicitly refer to possibly misleading appearances of life and death, as did the range of articles mentioned before, but they stressed instead the diagnostic significance of visualization techniques. Various technologies were discussed, the two most prominent being electroencephalography (EEG), a graphic recording of brain waves, and cerebral angiography, a radiographic image of the blood vessels after injection with a contrast medium. Although many physicians favored angiography, EEG was the more popular technique. One possible reason was that angiography was thought to be potentially harmful to the patient,[23] while EEG was widely perceived as a technique without any associated dangers. Above all, it was the electroencephalogram's graphic persuasiveness, the zero-line, that made it so popular.

The use of visualization techniques in medicine and science has been studied in depth in recent years.[24] Particular attention has been drawn to the technologically mediated visualization of otherwise invisible phenomena and to the correlation of visualization, evidence and objectivity. Crucial to these historical and sociological analyses is the question of how such normative ideals of modern science as objectivity, non-intervention and self-restraint were conceptualized in opposition to the idea of researchers as being humans with restricted perceptual capacities. Having studied the configurations of nineteenth-century science, Lorraine Daston and Peter Galison have argued that individuality was viewed by scientific actors as being in opposition to the normative values to which science referred in order to stabilize scientific knowledge production.[25] The limits of human perception, the associated link between sensory perception, subjectivity and emotions, or even the presence of individuals at the site of scientific research, threatened to subvert the reliability of knowledge production. Technological devices promised a solution to this dilemma by offering a way of enhancing or replacing individual human perception and participation in research. Daston and Galison characterized this understanding of objectivity, which equated scientific and medical reliability with the exclusion of subjectivity and which attributed supportive and reassuring functions to technological devices as mechanical objectivity.

Though EEG is a twentieth-century technological and scientific device, the hopes associated with its use as a supportive framework for medical knowledge and action with respect to brain death still function according to the concept of mechanical objectivity. With the introduction of EEG it became possible to objectify the unseen dimension of brain death by visualizing it with the help of mechanical devices. Brain death seemed to gain visual evidence through the graphic representation of brain activity or its absence. In particular, the visual evidence made it possible to understand brain death as a coherent phenomenon. As it was depicted as a zero-line, it could be addressed as a given fact. This way of obtaining evidence provided a stable and acceptable frame for managing brain death and promised to be purely objective, excluding any subjective dispositions or interests that may have otherwise come into play. Thus, the neutral visualizing device ideally guaranteed that any human weaknesses would be counterbalanced – if not excluded altogether. It was the machine-aided production of knowledge that was considered safe and certain and that allowed appropriate decision-making.[26] The EEG served as an additional monitor of the physicians' diagnosis.

Up to this point, we have argued only that EEG had been accepted for its reassuring quality with respect to diagnosis and decision-making. At the same time, however, it was considered by some to be less appropriate because the scientific evidence it produced was questionable. The employment of EEG did not put an end to concerns about the uncertainty of the brain death diagnosis. What was to be considered accepted medical knowledge and practice remained an ongoing process of negotiation. Back in the late 1960s, the SAMW committee had questioned whether EEG was scientifically necessary for diagnosis and recommended its use only for the purpose of documenting and illustrating brain death. Other medical actors outside of the SAMW voiced their doubts more strongly by insisting that EEG should never be used as the sole criterion for brain death. One of their concerns was that as a recording technique EEG was quite susceptible to outside influences that could alter the results of the recording.[27] Others feared the technique's incorrect use by unskilled staff, in which case, while the device itself was judged safe, the individual using it constituted a potential source of uncertainty. Still other critics dismissed the idealistic reception of EEG as an objectification technique free of any individual human interference, because they considered it to be strongly linked to individual operations. In order to avoid any ambiguity or misjudgment resulting from the use of electroencephalographic equipment or from its operator, they recommended that the EEG be conducted and the electroencephalogram interpreted exclusively by experts.

In addition to this practical skepticism concerning the use of EEG, some physicians articulated more general concerns about the medical use of machines. As one physician commented during an SAMW committee meeting: "[C]ontemporaries live with the idea that the machine can decide for them, which isn't actually the case."[28] Or, as Werthemann, then president of the SAMW, was reported to have stated on television, "the 'so called electroencephalogram' ... is not the only decisive criterion for the physician. He dispelled the doubts that a machine is deciding between life and death."[29]

The same device that served in one medical context to guarantee the scientific objectivity of medical knowledge and action was considered in another medical context to constitute a troubling and uncertain element. One reason was probably that different notions of medicine existed alongside each other during the 1960s and 1970s,[30] implying different concepts of certainty, safety and risk with respect to medical knowledge and practice: on the one hand, medicine was understood to be based upon scientific principles and ideas. The use of EEG and its visual evidence stood for the practice of rational medicine, in keeping with modern scientific principles. On the other hand, medical practice and decision-making were understood to be based upon personal experience and knowledge. In this latter context, the reliance on technological devices was perceived as rather disturbing.

Despite the aforementioned objections to the use of EEG, the SAMW Guidelines included it as a criterion for establishing brain death until the late 1980s.[31] But by the 1990s its status had changed, as other modes of diagnosing brain death such as clinical criteria were considered to be more meaningful. Other ways of documenting the physician's intervention had also been institutionalized, in particular standardized diagnostic protocols.

None the less, many physicians interviewed for our study still adhered to the EEG for diagnosing brain death, although they were aware of its uncertainty and its potential superfluity in comparison with other devices, as well as purely clinical criteria. The zero-line was just "comforting", as one retired nephrologist put it.[32] Many medical actors emphasized that the electro-encephalogram made particular sense and was helpful when talking to non-medical actors. Physicians highlighted the power of visual evidence and assumed that the image of a zero-line would more easily convince the relatives of the deceased that brain death was a real phenomenon. In doing so, the physicians attributed to non-medical and non-scientific actors a willingness to accept a logical connection between visual evidence, objectivity and truth.

Medical and non-medical actors alike have learned to understand the significance of a fever curve or the electrocardiogram's output as a representation of the presence or absence of physiological activity. Although the curve and the zero-line are not figurative representations, they have nevertheless made brain death accessible and plausible. The electroencephalogram is readable and understandable to some degree because of its similarity to these medical images that are already integrated into culture.[33] The zero-line of the electroencephalogram became a culturally shared symbol of death in the second half of the twentieth century.

The visual evidence thus not only served as a means for constructing scientific objectivity but also permitted the objectification and construction of brain death more generally as an existing, real and manageable phenomenon. For both medical and non-medical actors, then, the EEG remained a crucial guarantee of certainty and an important supportive device in the context of deciding on matters of brain death.

"A check list for brain death":[34]– the standardization of management

In the 1960s and 1970s proof of brain death was generally documented by visualization techniques. Subsequently, however, the idea of evidence providing certainty and the means to determine such certainty changed. The younger generation of physicians who had to deal with brain death conceived clinical criteria such as fixed pupils as a symbolic representation of brain death, in much the same way as the older generation had thought that EEG represented brain death. The increasing formalization and standardization of the diagnostic procedures for brain death was crucial for this development. Starting in the late 1970s and early 1980s, the routines of clinical practice coupled with experience in the treatment of brain-dead and comatose patients have stabilized medical knowledge. Furthermore, in the course of an increasing institutionalization of brain death in medical practice, there was no longer only a single physician in charge of the diagnosis; instead it became the task of teams to organize and take responsibility for medical work in the context of brain death. Hence, uncertainties and risks as well as their management were no longer simply a problem of medical knowledge, but rather a problem of practical procedures and coordination of the various actors and work routines involved.

It is possible to distinguish three ways of dealing with the uncertainties in relation to medical procedures and the organization of medical staff since the 1970s: the SAMW Guidelines; local hospital guidelines, which were set up only for internal needs; and the brain death protocol. The SAMW Guidelines aimed at providing a knowledge-based overview and a structure for handling brain death. They served not only as a normative and legal framework for diagnosis but also as a kind of instruction manual stipulating diagnostic parameters – though they were not specifically intended to be used as work manuals. Explicit rules of practice and action were also framed by guidelines established by local physicians. These local guidelines were intended to regulate any kind of interaction with the brain-dead patient. Finally, the protocol prescribed the individual steps of procedure taken in diagnosing and declaring brain death, since it also functioned as a record and proof of death.

The physicians interviewed repeatedly stated how glad they were to have the SAMW Guidelines as an orientation and a form of legal backing, and many of them emphasized that their hospitals had their own additional testing procedures and guidelines for diagnosing brain death.[35] The objective of introducing diagnostic procedures by means of internal or local guidelines was not identical with the objective of documenting brain death using protocols, although these two were, at least until the 1990s, interconnected in the way they were implemented. This meant that most of the intensive care units were using more tests than the Swiss Academy required.[36] For the physicians, the additional tests and their local guidelines were essential to proper diagnosis. As one intensive care physician expressed it: "It's the multitude of tests that gives me, rationally speaking, the assurance that he [the patient] is brain dead."[37]

The intensive care physicians were eager to standardize medical practice by using these local hospital guidelines. Diagnosis of brain death, they thought, should always be conducted according to the same rules, regardless of the time, place and identity of the physician. This was especially important for the doctors in charge of clinical units, who were interested in establishing an instrument of control so that in their absence any staff member would follow the same rules.[38]

Besides the in-house checklists, brain death was also regulated by additional records such as the protocols. Not only did the protocols teach the diagnostic procedure, but they also functioned as long-term written evidence for brain death that the actors of our study welcomed as a good means of documentation. It satisfied their need for a document proving brain death to others, since the doctors were wary of officially pronouncing someone dead based solely on their personal judgment. As one intensive care physician put it:

> I've always said, I will never just say someone is dead. If I leave later on and someone looks at the hospital record of Mr. Meier, who donated his organs, then they can only read, xy has found he's dead, and there is no document that proves that I did the right thing. ... It was always a desideratum to have a document. Normally you always have documents for everything in medicine. Just my observation of the patient was not enough for me.[39]

As this quotation shows, the protocol could be used when addressing colleagues, legal authorities and relatives of the brain-dead patient. It was considered essential to have a clearly structured procedure for contact with a patient's relatives. Only then did physicians feel capable of communicating freely, and show a willingness to let the relatives take part in every step of the procedure. This observation corresponds with sociological and historical analyses of medical protocols: the protocols served not only to make the medical procedure visible and comprehensible for the entire medical team, but also to structure social conflicts extending beyond mere operational needs. As already stated, they gave family members the opportunity to come to terms with the patient's death.[40] But the prior purpose of the protocols was, like the one of the local guidelines, to regulate and standardize medical action in general, as is illustrated in an article by two physicians at the Chur Hospital who wrote:

> The practical realization [of the diagnosis of brain death] repeatedly gives rise to debate. Therefore, we have stipulated the exact procedure and created a corresponding, printed protocol in order to carry out the diagnosis, to document it and to report on potential organ donors. Such a pre-established and documented procedure regulates competences, allows an objective judgment, avoids useless discussions and convinces relatives and team members.[41]

In the 1980s, nurses and physicians no longer viewed brain death as an uncontested and objective fact but, rather, as an issue that required repeated discussion, and as a source of conflict and difficulty in organizing everyday work in clinical units. Ethical concerns were thus mingled with organizational issues.

The implementation of standardized protocols was intended to prevent the potential uncertainty arising from heterogeneous diagnostic procedures and conflicting individual attitudes. Questions were expected to be resolved by the strict and regulated schedule of steps involved in the procedures prescribed by the protocols. For this reason, a brain death protocol was published in the third edition of the SAMW Guidelines in 1996 to serve as a model at the national level. Subsequently, local guidelines and protocols lost their importance and brain death became nationally standardized. Uncertainties concerning knowledge disappeared behind procedural standardization. The rules were supposed to provide uniformity, reproducibility and comparability of diagnosis as well as guaranteeing equivalent working patterns.[42] Risks were no longer perceived as caused by uncertain medical knowledge but by varying medical procedures in social settings that involved many different actors. Accordingly, the efforts to manage risk focused on brain death in its social and practical context.

"We've been abandoned emotionally": regulating subjectivity

From the 1960s up until the 1980s the heterogeneity of the phenomenon of brain death and the potential heterogeneity of situated knowledge and practices were perceived as being the factors that needed to be controlled in order to minimize the risk of the harmful effects of decision-making. And the previous passages on scientification, visualization and standardization of brain death have shown that this uncertainty in decision-making, being caused by heterogeneity, was tackled using strategies that aimed at rendering brain death a clear-cut object of medical knowledge and practice. At the same time the problem was addressed using strategies to avoid and exclude any individual intervention by delegating human activity to technical devices and integrating the individual range of action, as far as possible, into a body of generalized medical professional procedures.

Nevertheless, although this notion of objectivity, which referred to the absence of subjectivity, was the overriding contemporary professional ideal, subjectivity, emotions and personal attitudes had been always an integral part of the clinical everyday management of brain death.

In the 1980s and early 1990s the ways in which medical culture addressed individuality changed. In contrast to former tendencies to negate or exclude subjectivity altogether, now subjectivity, which had always been present as an implicit though significant element of medical practice and knowledge, became an explicit topic of medical discourse. Furthermore, the figure of the individual physician was recognized as being not only a trained professional but also a private individual, with his own individual cognitive and practical approach to medicine, and in particular an individual emotional approach to patients.

In the context of brain death, the explicit acknowledgement of subjectivity as part of medical knowledge and practice initially occurred in areas where the intensive care management of brain death intersected with transplant surgery.

Nurses were the first to address the subjective dimension of the management of brain death and organ transplantation publicly in the late 1980s. In professional journals of medical care and in general media forums, they voiced their anxieties and talked about the emotional burden of caring for potentially brain-dead patients or those actually declared brain-dead. They described their situation in the intensive care units as extraordinarily stressful. The conditions required to remove transplantable organs confronted them with the paradox of a dead person who was still warm and breathing. Expressing their unease, they stated: "We've been abandoned emotionally. It can be explained rationally, but the fact still exists: we are caring for a dead body."[43]

At first, emotional stress was only attributed to the nursing staff. Accordingly, the doctors welcomed new instruments for the emotional training of nurses.[44] Among physicians themselves, the acknowledgment of the emotional dimension took place only hesitantly. Initially, they held on to the ideal that the professional was not involved in the emotional, private aspects of his or her job and considered it to be an important source of problems when the emotions and attitudes of the various actors became manifest at the site of medical work. Emotions and attitudes threatened to subvert and destabilize the assured order of knowing, practicing and deciding on brain death, for the reason that they rendered possible once again a variety of ways of managing brain death. The interviews with physicians of different generations illustrate that different moral attitudes and understandings of death and dying and the linkage between brain death and transplantation surgery had resulted in different ways of diagnosing death and brain death. Physicians had thus interpreted and performed stabilized bodies of scientific medical knowledge and practices differently, and were able to produce different ways of dying, according to their opinions and attitudes.[45] Even if this were not the case, the physicians assumed and feared that their colleagues had done so. Several surveys in the 1980s and 1990s, conducted with the aim of supporting transplantation surgery, also exemplified that the personal attitudes and subjective dispositions of the medical staff significantly influenced which therapeutic measures were taken.[46] The differing attitudes conditioned whether patients died of brain death or cardio-pulmonary arrest, and whether or not they were reported as potential organ donors. These surveys were meant to identify the reasons why there were not more organ donations in Switzerland and which factors could be changed in order to raise this number. Beyond these intentions, the studies revealed that the strategy of excluding or negating subjective and individual dimensions of medical work had not produced uniformity of medical decision-making. Moreover, the problem seemed to be that subjectivity had not been explicitly addressed before and that no mechanism existed for dealing with this element of medical work and for ensuring transparency and legitimacy in decision-making.

In addition, the surveys had highlighted that the kind of communication between the medical staff and the patients' relatives was another factor that had predetermined organ donation. Having to communicate with brain-dead patients' relatives put considerable strain on medical staff, and having to ask them to think about the possibility of an organ donation was even worse. The survey brought to light established tactics for avoiding such situations.

But beyond the context of transplantation surgery, the communication of brain death to non-medical actors always implied the difficulty of making brain death plausible as an object of medical knowledge as well as a comprehensible phenomenon in a non-medical context. Brain death had always been a matter that was relevant and important to non-medical actors who were present at the site where brain death was managed. Nevertheless, up until the late 1980s the medical actors tried to establish brain death as exclusively an object of medical culture. This exclusion of non-medical conceptualizations and meanings of brain death became more difficult in the 1980s, when the spectrum of social groups demanding a voice in the debate broadened and medical culture itself was increasingly seen as being more heterogeneous than was previously assumed. It became a "wave of questioning",[47] as one physician told us in an interview, and the different demands in terms of legitimating medical knowledge and practice now required new ways of communicating brain death. An alternative way of posing the problem is to say that the failure of successful communication threatened the legitimacy of the decisions taken by the medical actors. The non-acceptance and even rejection of the medical concept of brain death by non-medical actors pointed once again to the general uncertainty concerning which framework was appropriate for making decisions about the status of patients without taking the risk of harming them. From the 1980s onwards, the medical profession not only attempted to minimize uncertainty within medical culture but also tried increasingly to communicate their position to a wider audience. The message was supposed to be that brain death was a safe and certain object of knowledge and practice, and it was intended to dispel any doubts about brain death and about medical expertise in general, which had become common in public debate.

From the mid-1980s on, and particularly once Swisstransplant, the Swiss foundation for organ donation and transplantation, had been founded in 1985, the Swiss media gave increasing coverage to the topic of organ transplantation and the lack of donors. The style of the articles stressed the human interest of the situation. Even though the main topic was still organ donation, brain death came under scrutiny in articles and interviews, which publicized the doubts expressed by some medical actors. Brain death received further public attention in the 1990s when a bill on transplantation medicine was submitted to a referendum.[48] With the increasing involvement of diverse groups in the discussion, various difficulties and ambiguities concerning brain death became noticeable.

But communication of medical topics in the mass media was only one way of addressing the changed notions of uncertainty and risk in the area of medical decision-making. To cope with personal uneasiness about brain death, something referred to by one nurse as "psycho-hygiene" started to be introduced into the education and advanced training of intensive care staff.[49] Special proposals for supervision and further training were initiated in order to counter individual uneasiness and uncertainty concerning the management of brain-dead patients.

Once more the initiatives emerged in close connection with programs for enhancing rates of organ donation. In 1991 the European Donor Hospital Education Programme (EDHEP) was devised and created by the Eurotransplant Foundation in Leiden, the Netherlands, working in close collaboration with professional communication skills coaches. EDHEP was created to meet the widely perceived need for helping health professionals feel capable of dealing with bereaved relatives while making donation requests. The Swiss program was under the patronage of Swisstransplant. The program offered – and still offers – a one-day skills awareness workshop, conducted outside the hospital setting and moderated by qualified trainers. One of the program's explicit aims, as stated above, was and still is to increase confidence and skills in dealing with death and organ donation. Furthermore, the interactive training program is based on the premise that a request for organ donation, if made with sensitivity, yields better results in the rate of donation and can, in the meantime, offer solace to those who have lost a loved one. The workshop not only teaches communication skills and appropriate behaviour in dealing with mourning relatives, but also encourages participants to reflect on their own opinions and attitudes towards death.[50]

The individual person with his or her subjective, moral and emotional concerns was no longer to be excluded from the medical and scientific domain, but was rather to be included and play a more prominent role. Now, acknowledging one's own individuality was not just seen as an integral part of medical knowledge and practice but as a necessity. In the field of medicine, handling personal cognition and levels of emotion in decision-making became part of professional training, as illustrated by the workshops and seminars offered by the EDHEP.

The uneasiness of the medical staff in relation to brain death has remained at the focus of these ongoing workshops. Surveys have shown a close interrelation between the decision of relatives to consent to an organ donation upon request and the attitude towards brain death and organ donation on the part of the medical actor who makes the request. The EDHEP workshops conceptualize the individual practitioner simultaneously as an object for self-improvement and as a key element in the problem of communicating about brain death and the possibility of organ transplantation. On the one hand, the workshops provide a forum for rehearsing procedures and behaviours that will be useful for the individual in a difficult situation, while on the other it is expected that a self-assured and self-reflexive individual will be able to contribute to the general acceptance of the concept by communicating a convincing image of brain death.

The preamble of the Guidelines of 1996 responds to this new kind of uncertainty and to doubts formulated both within and outside the medical culture. For the first time, the psychological and emotional components of diagnosing brain death, which until then had only been debated internally, were picked up as a central theme. The 1996 preamble described the dilemma confronting physicians who could not avoid considering the potential of organ donation while caring for a dying patient. Such situations were difficult for all parties involved, which is why the Guidelines called for "ethically as well as psychologically adequate behaviour on the part of all physicians involved in excising organs".[51] An additional requirement was the nomination of a competent contact person to accompany the relatives through the entire procedural process. With these regulations, the Guidelines tried to minimize the risk that brain death was seen in the wrong light. The images the medical individual communicated outside the profession were expected to contribute to the acceptance of the concept of brain death by a wider public. Thus the risk that was associated with explaining the concept in the context of organ transplantation was perceived as being inherent both to the perception of the concept by non-medical actors and to the communication process between medical and non-medical actors.

Medical culture had started to acknowledge the attitudes and emotions of the individual professionals involved and developed instruments to regulate them, rather than just trying to suppress them. This acceptance of subjectivity can be interpreted as the objectified ascertainment of subjectivity. The subjective dimension was partially standardized: processes of reflection were regulated in order to obtain a degree of homogenization and to render subjectivity a manageable and predictable factor.

This development shows a tendency towards individualization of risk. Social researchers, who refer to the later works of Michel Foucault and who have established a field of research called "governmentality studies", have stressed this new notion of risk perception and risk management with regard to the exposure to disease in relation to genetic predisposition, as in the case of breast cancer or psychic illness.[52] They argue that institutionalized mechanisms of risk control and regulation have been replaced by individual strategies of coping with uncertainty and risk, which imply a high degree of self-regulation. So far, governmentality studies have primarily analysed how social and political institutions shift the responsibilities of dealing with uncertainty and risk associated with medical knowledge onto the individuals who are the potential victims of a given disease. Less attention has been paid to the ways in which actors within the medical professional are instructed to face structural uncertainties in a self-regulative mode, too.

Conclusion

Since the late 1960s, brain death has generated various kinds of uncertainty in medical culture. The phenomenon destabilized institutionalized bodies of medical knowledge as well as routines of medical practice by virtue of being both a product of technological and therapeutic innovations and inherently an innovation concerning common concepts of death.

Brain death was not a well-defined object of knowledge and action but a heterogeneous phenomenon that blurred the familiar boundaries between life and death. The link between brain death and transplantation surgery in particular provoked considerable confusion and uncertainty. There was always the risk that a patient's condition could be misjudged, thereby leading to particular therapeutic measures that might in retrospect prove to have been wrong, inadequate, harmful, or even "murderous", fears articulated by the physicians we quoted at the beginning of this chapter. Dealing with such uncertainties and, moreover, conceptualizing brain death in a reassuring manner were important issues both within and outside medical culture.

Swiss medical culture generated three means of addressing these uncertainties: objectification of knowledge about brain death; standardization of medical practice; and regulation of subjectivity in dealing with brain death. In the 1960s and 1970s physicians tried to convert brain death into a homogeneous and consistent object of knowledge in two ways: first through a retrospective and quantified construction of a definite object of knowledge characterized by a set of criteria; and second through the creation of an idea of visual evidence, provided by the electroencephalogram. With the help of quantification and visualization techniques, brain death was transformed into an observable, identifiable and reliable object.

Starting in the 1980s, physicians also focused on questions raised by the stress of daily medical work and by the moral attitudes of the medical actors involved. With the fields of intensive care and transplantation medicine becoming more and more routine, these issues were assumed to hinder the efficient operational procedures on which intensive care medicine and transplantation medicine were ideally based. To cope with the morally charged concept of brain death in everyday intensive care, physicians established standardized protocols that prescribed the sequence of steps in the diagnostic procedure and the appropriate documentation. Individual responsibility was objectified through a unified and standardized protocol and the individual physician had to defer to the rules of the procedure. Several hospital guidelines were set up, designed to adapt to local circumstances in order to eliminate uncertainty and discussions among the staff members.

The strategies of both objectification and standardization led to the perception that the individual professional and the dimension of subjectivity were risky elements in the context of brain death. The means to minimize uncertainty were also the means to minimize the range of individual actions and decisions regarding life and death.

Since the late 1980s individuality and subjectivity have explicitly been taken into consideration. The discrepancy between professional demands and daily routine on the one hand, and individual attitudes and ideas on the other, had become visible and was perceived as a disruptive element. The articulation of personal problems in relation to brain death was recognized as an integral part of medical culture, resulting in attempts to introduce a highly self-conscious, regulated and managed notion of subjectivity. The implications of regulation and control, which were inherent in the objectification and standardization of brain death, were thus transferred to the individual.

The change of instruments for managing brain death and the risks inherent in its diagnosis indicate an expansion of regulative measures: at first medical knowledge was objectified, then medical action and medical staff became standardized, and finally the subjective disposition of the individuals working in medical contexts was regulated. This tendency might be interpreted as an increasing objectification of social life – which would suggest in turn that objectification has become a dominant ideal of society that now reaches beyond medical and scientific cultures.

But the change in instruments should also be seen in the light of shifting boundaries between medical culture and other segments of society. Different actors and social groups outside the clinical context have been involved with brain death since the concept first arose in the late 1960s. Despite this, however, the medical culture regarded brain death as an exclusive object of medical knowledge and practice for a long period of time. This exclusion of non-medical conceptualizations and meanings of brain death began to become difficult in the 1980s when several social and political groups started to discuss and question the concept of brain death. In this context, medical culture itself was increasingly seen as being more heterogeneous than had previously been assumed and the boundaries between medical culture and other segments of society became increasingly permeable. The regulation of subjective dispositions is, then, the contemporary strategy for conceptualizing the knowledge and practical management of brain death in different contexts as being something safe and legitimate.

Thus the perception of and responses to the uncertainties and potential risks involved in brain death can be seen to have shifted between the late 1960s and 2000. In the 1970s and mid-1980s the focus of interest was the conceptualization of the phenomenon and its management, while in the 1990s the principal preoccupations became the subjectivities and individualities of the healthcare personnel involved, and how to deal with them.

Notes

1 We would like to thank the editors for suggestions on former drafts of this paper. We also have to thank Margaret Andergassen and Alexis Heede for reading and correcting this paper so carefully. Finally, we would like to thank the Swiss National Science Foundation, the Jaques Brodbeck-Sandreuter-Foundation and the Swiss Academy of Medical Sciences for financing this research project.

2 Minutes of the Working committee of the Swiss Academy of Medical Sciences (SAMW), 6th meeting, 25.1.1969.

3 U. Beck, *Risk Society: Towards a New Modernity*, London: Sage, 1998; and K. P Japp, *Risiko*, Bielefeld: Transcript-Verlag, 2000.

4 R. Fox, "The Evolution of Medical Uncertainty", *Milbank Memorial Fund Quarterly*, 58 (1), 1980, 1–49; D. R. Gordon, "Clinical Science and Clinical Expertise: Changing

222   *Silke Bellanger and Aline Steinbrecher*

Boundaries Between Art and Science in Medicine", in M. Lock and D. Gordon (eds) *Biomedicine Examined*, Dordrecht, Boston, London: Kluwer, 1988, 257–95.

5 M. Berg, "Turning Practice into a Science: Reconceptualizing Postwar Medical Practice", *Social Studies of Science*, 25, 1995, 437–76; M. Berg, "Problems and Promises of the Protocol", *Social Sciences of Medicine*, 44, 1997, 1081–8; S. Timmermans and M. Berg, "Standardization in Action: Achieving Local Universality through Medical Protocols", *Social Studies of Science*, 27, 1997, 273–305; G. C. Bowker and S. L. Star, *Sorting Things Out: Classifications and its Consequences*, Cambridge MA: MIT Press, 2000.

6 M. S. Pernick, "Brain Death in Cultural Context: The Reconstruction of Death 1967–1981", in S. Youngner *et al.* (eds) *The Definition of Death: Contemporary Controversies*, Baltimore and London: The Johns Hopkins University Press, 1999, 71–82; W. Schneider,"*So tot wie nötig – so lebendig wie möglich!*": *Sterben und Tod in der fortgeschrittenen Moderne*, Münster, Hamburg, London: Lit-Verlag, 1999; Th. Schlich, "Tod, Geschichte und Kultur", in Th. Schlich and C. Wiesemann (eds) *Hirntod: Zur Kulturgeschichte der Todesfeststellung*, Frankfurt a. M.: Suhrkamp, 2001, 9–42; C. Wiesemann, "Notwendigkeit und Kontingenz: Ist der Hirntod ein Kind der Transplantationsmedizin?: Zur Geschichte der ersten Hirntod-Definition der Deutschen Gesellschaft für Chirurgie von 1968", in Th. Schlich and C. Wiesemann (eds) *Hirntod*, 209–35.

7 M. Lock, *Twice dead: Organ Transplants and the Reinvention of Death*, Berkeley: University of California Press, 2002; G. Lindemann, *Die Grenze des Sozialen: Zur sozio-technischen Konstruktion von Leben und Tod in der Intensivmedizin*, München: Wilhelm Fink Verlag, 2002; A. Manzei, *Körper, Technik, Grenzen: Kritische Anthropologie am Beispiel der Transplantationsmedizin*, Münster: Lit-Verlag, 2002.

8 Articles from Swiss medical journals dating from 1960 to 2000, unpublished minutes of the Swiss Academy of Medical Sciences (SAMW) and interviews with Swiss physicians from the disciplines of transplant surgery, surgery, intensive care medicine and neurology have been our source material.

9 We use the term "figure" in this article with reference to traditions in the social studies of science. See e.g. D. Haraway, "Syntactics. The Grammar of Feminism and Technoscience", in D. Haraway: *Modest_witness@second_millenium.Femaleman_meets oncomouse: Feminism and Technoscience*, New York: Routledge 1997, 1–22. According to Haraway and others, scientific cultures are analysed as cultures that use and produce rhetorical narrations. "Figure" should therefore be understood in its rhetorical dimension; the formulation "figure of the individual professional" intends to highlight the individual as real as well as fictional and rhetorical.

10 S. Schellong, "Die künstliche Beatmung und die Entstehung des Hirntodkonzepts", in Th. Schlich and C. Wiesemann (eds), *Hirntod*, 187–208.

11 Th. Schlich, *Die Erfindung der Organtransplantation. Erfolg und Scheitern des chirurgischen Organersatzes (1880–1930)*, Frankfurt a. M.: Campus, 1998.

12 Lock, *Twice dead*, pp. 64–5.

13 G. S. Belkin, "Brain Death and the Historical Understanding of Bioethics", *Journal of the History of Medicine*, 58, 2003, 325–61; Wiesemann, " Notwendigkeit und Kontingenz".

14 Schweizerische Akademie der Medizinischen Wissenschaften, Richtlinien für die Definition und die Diagnose des Todes, Basel, 25.1.1969. The SAMW Guidelines have been adapted several times. After the first guidelines were published in 1969, a second version was produced in 1983, a third in 1996 and a fourth edition is currently in preparation.

15 Minutes of the Working Committee of the Swiss Academy of Medical Sciences (SAMW), 1st meeting, 7.5.1968.

16 E. Zander and O. Cornu, "Les critères de la mort cérébrale: Revue critique de 90 cas", *Schweizerische Medizinische Wochenschrift*, 100 (9), 1970, p. 408–14; 412.

17 E. Zander and O. Cornu, "Les critères de la mort cérébrale", p. 412.

18 E. Ketz, "Beitrag zum Problem des Hirntodes (Beobachtungen an 100 Fällen von totalem Hirnfunktionsausfall)", *Schweizer Archiv für Neurologie, Neurochirurgie und*

Psychiatrie, 110 (2), 1972, 205–21; F. Robert and M. Mumenthaler, "Kriterien des Hirntodes: Die spinalen Reflexe bei 45 eigenen Beobachtungen", *Schweizerische medizinische Wochenschrift*, 107, 1977, 335–41.

19 F. Robert and M. Mumenthaler, "Kriterien des Hirntodes", pp. 335–41.

20 T. M. Porter, "Statistics, Social Sciences, and the Culture of Objectivity", *Österreichische Zeitschrift für Geschichtswissenschaft*, 7 (2), 1996, 177–91.

21 F. Schwarz, "Rechtliche Fragen bei der Transplantation", *Schweizerische Ärztezeitung*, 48, 1976, 331–3.

22 J. M. Mantz *et al.*, "A Propos des critères de la mort cérébrale: la fluoroscopie rétinographique", *Revue Medicale de la Suisse Romand*, 91 (10), 757–66.

23 F. Robert and M. Mumenthaler, "Kriterien des Hirntodes"; N. De Tribolet *et al.*, "Diagnostic radio-isotopique de la mort cérébrale", *Schweizerisch medizinische Wochenschrift*, 107, 1976, 464–7.

24 L. Daston and P. Galison, "The Image of Objectivity", *Representations*, Special Issue: *Seeing Science*, 40, 1992, 81–128; D. Gugerli, "Soziotechnische Evidenzen: Der 'Pictorial Turn' als Chance für die Geschichtswissenschaft", *Traverse*, 3, 1999, 131–58.

25 L. Daston and P. Galison, "The Image of Objectivity".

26 Daston and Galison name the similarly characterized notion of objectivity of nineteenth-century "mechanical objectivity", L. Daston and P. Galison, "The Image of Objectivity".

27 Minutes of the Working committee SAMW, 1970.

28 Minutes of the Working committee SAMW, 7.5.1968.

29 "Fernsehen – nachbetrachtet: Grundsätzliches zur Herzverpflanzung", *Schaffhauser Nachrichten*, 23 April 1969.

30 D. R. Gordon, "Clinical Science and Clinical Expertise".

31 Schweizerische Akademie der medizinischen Wissenschaften, Richtlinien für die Definition und Diagnose des Todes, Basel 6.5.1983.

32 Interview, carried out on 5.2.2002.

33 V. Hess, "Die Bildtechnik der Fieberkurve: Klinische Thermometrie im 19. Jahrhundert", in D. Gugerli and B. Orland (eds) *Ganz normale Bilder: Historische Beiträge zur visuellen Herstellung von Selbstverständlichkeit*, Zürich: Chronos, 2002, 159–80; W. Schneider, "So tot wie nötig – so lebendig wie möglich!", 279–317; C. Wiesemann, "Notwendigkeit und Kontingenz", 209–35.

34 Interview, carried out on 24.1.2002.

35 Interview, carried out on 24.1.2002.

36 G. Lindemann, *Die Grenze des Sozialen*, 116.

37 Interview, carried out on 7.2002.

38 Berg discusses in his works the general attempts in standardization of medical practices in order to regulate medical action and to prevent any alternatives since the mid-20th century. M. Berg, "Problems and Promises of the Protocol", 447–51.

39 Interview, carried out on 7.2002.

40 S. Timmermans and M. Berg, "Standardization in Action", 273–305; p. 291.

41 A. Leutenegger, S.-Y. Oh and A. Frutiger, "Hirntoddiagnose und Organspende", *Schweizerische medizinische Wochenschrift*, 112 (24), 1982, 864–6; 865.

42 S. Timmermans and M. Berg, "Standardization in Action", 273–305; p. 292.

43 "'Wir bleiben emotional auf der Strecke'. Interview mit der I-P Schwester Gisela Zumsteg. Geführt v. Fred Arm, Francoise Taillens", *Krankenpflege*, 9, 1990, 20–4.

44 K. Appert, "Organspende in der Schweiz. FMH unterstützt Aufklärungs-Aktion von SWISSTRANSPLANT", *Schweizerische Ärztezeitung*, 71 (24), 1990, 1006–8.

45 Interviews, carried out on 20.11.2001 and 5.2.2002.

46 D. Candidas, "Aktuelles zur Transplantationsmedizin und Organspende", *Schweizer Ärztezeitung*, 78 (34), 1997, 1223–6; K. Laeceracher-Hofmann and B. Isenschmid Gerster, "Einstellungen und Bedenken von Studierenden der Medizin gegenüber der Organtransplantation: Resultate einer Fragebogenerhebung im ersten Studienjahr", *Schweizerische Medizinische Wochenschrift*, 128, 1998, 1840–9.

47 Interview, carried out on 28.2.2002.
48 The referendum is the most widespread form of direct democracy. By means of the referendum the sovereign people in Switzerland approve or reject the bills and resolutions agreed upon by the legislative authority.
49 *Ibid.*, 23.
50 The passage about EDEHP is based on the courseware of EDEHP Switzerland and on our own observations when attending two seminars in 2001.
51 SAMW, "Richtlinien zur Definition und Feststellung des Todes im Hinblick auf die Organtransplantation", *Schweizerische Ärztezeitung*, 77 (44), 1996, 1773–80; p. 1774.
52 U. Bröcklin, S. Krasmann and T. Lemke (eds), *Gouvernementalität der Gegenwart: Studien zur Ökonomisierung des Sozialen*, Frankfurt a. M.: Suhrkamp, 2000.

13 Risk on trial

The interaction of innovation and risk in cancer clinical trials

Peter Keating and Alberto Cambrosio

These are difficult times for the nation's system of protection for human subjects in research.[1]

On June 2, 2001 a 24-year-old healthy volunteer, enrolled in a clinical trial at Johns Hopkins University School of Medicine, died following administration of a compound designed to mimic asthma as part of an investigation of the patho-physiology of the disease.[2] Her death quickly resulted in the suspension (lifted just as quickly)[3] of federally supported research projects at Johns Hopkins. Subsequent investigations highlighted the inadequacies and shortcomings of the safeguards for protecting human subjects. The Johns Hopkins case was not an isolated incident. Prompted in part by the creation of a new Office for Human Research Protection by the Secretary of Health and Human Services in 1998,[4] between 1999 and 2001 federal regulators suspended eight different clinical research projects because of safety problems.[5]

The debates surrounding these recent cases confirm a trend that dates back at least to the 1960s (see below), namely that the ethical dilemmas concerning risk to patients in clinical trials have become an integral part of the clinical trials process. Although generally deemed amenable to rational and ethical calculation and assessment within successive medical conceptions and definitions of cancer, the trade-offs between risk and innovation that emerge within clinical trials are, we would argue, more a moving target than a stable object. By that, we mean that just as the institutions for clinical research have evolved, so, too, have the risks and benefits to patients and the ways in which these risks and benefits are framed and calculated. We suggest, in other words, that there is a historical and institutional dimension to issues that are often presented as exclusively methodological or ethical.

The rise of clinical trials since World War Two has reorganized what, at first sight, appears to be a rather clear-cut distinction between therapy and research.[6] Within the field of cancer, therapy and research, rather than autonomous activities, now constitute two poles of a spectrum of clinical inquiry within which the distinction between the two first emerges and is then constantly reshaped. As a consequence, and as acknowledged by practitioners, risks and their assessment are located in "the gray zone between safety and science".[7] It is through the clinical trial process that a treatment moves from experiment to accepted therapy and, in some cases, back to the status of unacceptable therapy. The logical or ethical distinctions that are presumed to manage this process are, under our description, the historically contingent products of the clinical research enterprise itself. To understand how this is so, we begin with a brief overview of the clinical cancer trial system. We then describe how a series of different risk–innovation issues have emerged over the years and have prompted a variety of solutions.

The cancer clinical trial system

Cancer clinical trials are a complex enterprise: as we enter a new century, approximately 50 years after the establishment of the first institutions devoted to this activity in the US, more than 10,000 investigators at approximately 3,000 sites are registered with the largest sponsor of clinical trials, the US National Cancer Institute (NCI). Each year approximately 160 Phase III trials (see below) are actively pursued, with an average of 100 sites participating in each trial.[8] Clinical cancer trials are thus not isolated events. They are, moreover, part and parcel of the larger framework of modern biomedicine and, as such, they are generally carried out within the context of a national research *system*. Such a complex, multi-layered configuration of material, socio-institutional and epistemic components was obviously not designed in a single stroke. Rather, it is the cumulative result of an evolutionary process beginning in the 1950s.

The NCI organized the first randomized clinical cancer trial (in acute lymphocytic leukemia) in 1954, drawing collaborators from five cancer research centers. The success of the trial led to the formation of the Children's Cancer Study Group and the Cancer and Leukemia Group B (CALGB), subsequently referred to as cooperative oncology groups. The NCI organized the first "solid" (as opposed to the "liquid" leukemias) cancer cooperative group shortly thereafter. The resultant Eastern Solid Tumor Group become the precursor of the largest cooperative group in the United States, the Eastern Cooperative Oncology Group (ECOG). By the 1960s, most Phase I and Phase II clinical cancer trials in North America were conducted by cooperative groups.

As the cooperative groups evolved, so too did clinical trial practices and the kinds of risks that confronted patients faced with therapeutic innovation. Initially devoted to testing drugs provided by the NCI's drug research program, the cooperative group system has changed considerably since the mid-1950s. First and foremost, from small networks the cooperative groups have grown into large, distributed research organizations. The largest, such as the aforementioned ECOG, presently have over 4,000 members and span the entire United States in addition to conducting collaborative studies in Canada, the UK, Israel and elsewhere. Initially centered in research organizations like the NCI or the Roswell Park Institute, in the 1970s the cooperative groups spread into the community through programs designed to increase accrual to clinical trials that brought clinical investigators and "trialists" into direct contact with community oncologists (most of whom had initially trained with the "trialists").

Therapeutic modalities have likewise evolved. Initially restricted to chemotherapy, in the 1970s the cooperative groups expanded to include other modalities such as surgery and radiotherapy. Subsequently, the 1980s saw the first wave of immunotherapies produce relatively disappointing results. In turn, the 1990s have seen the emergence of a entire panoply of biologicals often referred to as cytostatic agents, given their mechanism of action.

The trials themselves have been transformed in many respects. At first confined to the testing of chemical compounds across a spectrum of cancers, they have since become disease-oriented, testing therapies across the prognostic and pathological stages of specific tumors.[9] Moreover, following the initial successes in the mid-1960s and early 1970s with the leukemias and the lymphomas, clinical trials have moved from relatively short-term studies using single agents and patients in advanced-stage disease, to much longer-term, multi-modality studies implicating maintenance therapies and, in some case, cures (as conventionally defined).

Finally, as a result of the widespread application of chemotherapy protocols first developed through clinical trials, but also of debates concerning biological differences among trial subjects,[10] trial patients and their diseases have undergone important transformations.

These cumulative shifts of emphasis connect the evolution of clinical cancer trials with a recurring theme of the larger history of clinical trials in general. Clinical trials for both cancer and other diseases can be alternatively described as testing devices for new drugs and procedures (i.e., tools for the management of therapies) or as research devices. There is a tension between the two, an explicit statement of which can be found in the distinction between a *pragmatic* and an *explanatory* approach to clinical trials first introduced by Daniel Schwartz and Joseph Lellouch in the late 1960s.[11] Simply put, the pragmatic approach is designed to test the efficacy of a given therapy in real-world clinical conditions, while the explanatory approach aims at answering biological questions under experimental (ideal) conditions. In other words, one can conceive of clinical trials pragmatically as a technology for deciding whether drug X works (or works better than drug Y) for patients affected by disease Z, the disease itself being a given. The explanatory approach conceives of clinical trials as a sort of human experiment to find out more about the disease under study: its etiological mechanisms, its prognosis, its reaction to therapeutic intervention, or its nosological status (i.e., whether it is one or many diseases). In both cases, of course, trials resort to human subjects but, according to Schwartz and Lellouch, in so far as they aim at the solution of "two radically different kinds of problems ... the resulting ambiguity affects the definition of the treatments, the assessment of the results, the choice of subjects and the way in which the treatments are compared" and – we would add – the kind of risks they produce.[12] Rather than further exploring the foundations of Schwartz and Lellouch's argument, we will examine how the tension they identified is reflected in the evolution of the NCI's clinical cancer trial system.[13]

The beginnings of the cancer clinical trial system

Since the mid-1960s, members of the NCI's Cooperative Oncology Group Program have continued to debate whether cancer clinical trials are designed primarily to select the best drug or therapeutic regimen or whether they serve principally to improve therapy through a better understanding of the bio-pathological mechanisms implicated in the treatment process.[14] While they clearly do both, the question of where to put the emphasis has remained controversial.[15]

When the groups were first set up as units for testing drugs, they were confronted with terminally ill patients and a dearth of therapies. Clinical trials consequently targeted small groups of patients and did not initially compare therapies as there were none to be compared. A major tool for managing the trials and the risks they engendered was the trials' division into phases. By the late 1950s, clinical researchers within the NCI distinguished between "Phase I" and "Phase II" trials. The former sought "toxicological and pharmacological information" and the latter sought "data on therapeutic response, optimum route of administration and optimum dosage regime".[16] The methodological division between Phase I and Phase II trials was further reinforced in the early 1960s when Edmund Gehan of CALGB developed specific statistical methods for Phase II trials.[17]

Phase II trials were further divided in the late 1950s into two types, which should not be anachronistically confused with the present-day division between Phase II and Phase III trials.[18] As defined by the NCI, these two types of study primarily separated multi-disease from single-disease studies, i.e., "short term, preliminary trial of new agents in a broad spectrum of human malignancy" from "quantitative, comparative studies in human malignancies responsive in some degree to chemotherapeutic agents to establish a ranking of relative therapeutic ability of agents".[19] The exploratory nature of the comparisons carried out in clinical cancer trials becomes clear when we consider the relation between the second type of Phase II trial and animal models. This relation is explicitly set out in the 1960 definition of this type of trial: "If comparative rankings are found in animal tumor "rating systems", this will aid immeasurably in the selection of the agent of choice for trial in specific human malignancy."[20]

The relative risk for patients in Phase I and Phase II trials was and remains quite high. Unlike other classes of drugs that are tested in healthy volunteers, anti-cancer agents, because of their toxicity, are tested on patients. In Phase I trials, patients (chosen among the terminally ill) have to abandon other forms of therapy in order for the toxicity testing to be practicable. Thus, the first risk run by patients comes from relinquishing "their rights to established effective therapy".[21] In the 1950s and early 1960s, with the absence of established therapy, this kind of risk was obviously minimal. Even by the late 1950s, however, there was at least palliative therapy. From the research point of view, this raised a second problem – a risk for the research data – namely what had been the effect of prior therapy on the test subjects? Based on results obtained in animal models, investigators initially believed that late-stage patients would be unresponsive to even relatively effective drugs. As CALGB researchers pointed out in the early 1960s, however, this was not necessarily the case. In their well-known paper published in *Blood*, they argued:

A problem in clinical cancer chemotherapy studies is that new agents are for the most part studied in patients with late, i.e. advanced disease. In transplanted rodent tumors there is ample evidence that responsiveness to a given agent decreases with time. Were this true in man, studies of new agents in patients with late, refractory acute leukemia would be relatively ineffective in that drugs which might be active earlier in the disease would be missed. Our studies indicate strongly that this is not the case.[22]

Further studies confirmed this belief. As the researchers wrote several years later:

These findings support the concept that chemotherapeutic agents can be adequately tested at any phase of the disease and that patients are not characterized as "responders" or "non-responders" on the basis of response to other chemotherapy.[23]

The research component of clinical trials was reinforced, as the cooperative oncology groups progressively detached themselves from the NCI's chemotherapy program in the mid 1960s to become autonomous clinical research organizations. A decisive turning point in this respect came in 1968, when the Cancer Chemotherapy Collaborative Clinical Trials Review Committee established by Kenneth Endicott, Director of the NCI, held a "Cooperative Studies Workshop". Participants at that meeting saw themselves at a novel juncture: "Justification for the cooperative chemotherapy groups, formerly based on their role as a testing facility for the NCI's drug development program, now resides solely in the quality of the research they propose and conduct."[24] Accordingly, the cooperative groups now saw their mandate expanded "to the clinical investigation of cancer epidemiology, etiology, diagnosis and prevention as well as cancer therapy",[25] and in keeping with this expanded mandate the Committee's name changed to the more expansive "Clinical Cancer Investigation Review Committee".

Both terms of the therapy vs. research distinction were, in principle, covered by this mandate. At the time, however, research was clearly privileged over therapy. As the Committee went on to point out: "While it is recognised that good multi-institutional clinical studies will extend and improve patient care, and that education and training are important facets of the Program, it is emphasized that meritorious research must be the primary criterion for the evaluation of grant applications."[26] Indicative of the idea that the cooperative groups did more than test drugs was also the incorporation of pathologists into the groups. Rare prior to 1966, they become common thereafter.[27]

The definition of clinical treatment research and the expansion of Phase II trials

The research orientation of clinical cancer trials was further reinforced in the 1970s with the appointment of Vincent DeVita as director of the Division of Cancer Treatment. Espousing an expansive view of clinical research, DeVita argued that clinical trials should be justified in terms of the biological rationale behind them. The inability of rodent models to predict the relative value of two treatments known to work contributed to the idea that: "[t]he bedside is the laboratory; the patients are the ingredients of the experiment."[28] Despite their research orientation, the groups came under attack for the pedestrian nature of the research they conducted. Henry Kaplan, a well-known Stanford pathologist and member of the Division of Cancer Therapy's Board of Scientific Counselors, openly criticised the cooperative groups as useless, claiming that they had too often conducted "what I call me-too trials, that have added trivial data and accomplished essentially nothing".[29] None the less, during a subsequent review of the cooperative group program, DeVita sided with the groups, saying: "It is my personal view that clinical trials often test fundamental therapeutic hypotheses. At the very least, they represent the effector arm of a wide variety of pre-clinical research programs and they have clearly yielded important results."[30] This was a view echoed by the Board of Scientific Counselors who had conducted the review and who, in the process, redefined the kind of research carried out by the cooperative groups as clinical treatment research which they defined as follows:

> Clinical treatment research refers to research on human subjects encompassing any or all aspects of treatment involving individuals or groups of cancer patients, including validation of preclinical research findings in a clinical setting. Clinical treatment research is particularly concerned

with efforts to determine the best possible treatment of each type of human cancer based on knowledge of the natural history of the disease. Clinical treatment research includes all clinical trials, but not all clinical research involving human subjects and materials.[31]

The 1970s also saw an expansion of Phase II trials with an explicit curative intent. Once again, because of the nature of anti-cancer agents and the cancer process, Phase II cancer clinical trials created a specific blend of risks and rewards. To begin with, anti-cancer agents have a cumulative effect. Eligibility criteria for Phase II trials had therefore to exclude patients who had developed resistance to anti-cancer drugs in order to avoid generating too many false negative results. This was not always and everywhere the case. As knowledge of specific cancers, stages and types of resistance accumulated, criteria for eligibility became increasingly strict. Two consequences flowed from the selection. On the one hand, the greater the selection, the more the trial became associated with the research end of the clinical spectrum – a consequence, as we have seen, that was actively promoted within the NCI. On the other hand, the greater the selection, the longer the trial took to complete as accrual rates slowed, and thus the greater the risk that the answer to the question asked would no longer be relevant as the underlying science and alternative therapies moved on. When the answer was no longer relevant, the patient consequently ran the risk of participating in an irrelevant exercise.

Yet another risk created by the widespread adoption of chemotherapy in this period resulted from the disappearance of the untreated patient and thus from the emergence of a penury of uncompromised research subjects. One example will suffice: in 1970, when the NCI introduced doxorubicin for Phase II testing in breast cancer, 54 per cent of the patients in the trial had not received chemotherapy. In 1979, when they tested aclarubicin, not a single patient had not already had chemotherapy.[32] The full impact of the transformation was not felt until the mid-1980s when the Cancer Therapy Evaluation Program (CTEP), originally established in 1968 as a branch of the NCI Chemotherapy Division, realized that with fewer and fewer uncompromised patients, Phase II clinical trials were becoming more and more indeterminate because of decreased patient accrual. In an analysis of Phase II trials carried out between 1970 and 1985, Wittes and his colleagues noted that "Nearly one-third of the drugs tested in leukemia and lymphoma and nearly one-half of the drugs in head and neck cancer are indeterminate with respect to their activity ... which reflects insufficient numbers of patients accrued in a given disease to establish the lower confidence limit >10% or the upper confidence limit <15%."[33]

In addition to generating novel risks, the 1970s also ushered in the era of informed consent in the biomedical world in general. The milestones here are well known. Beginning with the Thalidomide scandal of the early 1960s, Henry Beecher's subsequent catalogue of "questionably ethical studies" published in the *New England Journal of Medicine* in 1966,[34] and the denunciation of the Tuskegee Syphilis Study in 1972,[35] reforms followed with the passage of the National Research Act of 1974 that established the National Commission for the Protection of Human Subjects of Biomedical and Behavioral Research. Less well known is the fact that the NCI had required written informed consent from the beginning of the 1960s[36] and that, by the mid-1960s, the NIH required independent review of research projects.[37] In particular, the NIH set out guidelines in 1966 covering all federally funded research involving human experimentation that mandated "reviews of the judgement of the investigator by a committee of institutional associates not directly associated with the project".[38] As Rothman has commented, the effects were mixed:

> The new rules were neither as intrusive as some investigators feared nor as protective as some advocates preferred. At their core was the superintendence of the peer-review committee, known as the institutional review board (IRB), through which fellow researchers approved the investigator's procedure. With the creation of the IRB, clinical investigators could no longer decide unilaterally on the ethics of their research, but had to answer formally to colleagues operating under federal guidelines.[39]

The clinical cancer trial system, however, had already been under the surveillance of de facto IRBs, namely the previously mentioned Cancer Therapy Evaluation Program (CTEP), long before the former had come into existence. Cooperative group protocols had routinely been reviewed by the CTEP and thus the emergence of the IRB system initially had little impact. As we will see in the next section, however, in the mid-1980s yet another monitoring instrument, the data monitoring committee, emerged to police the risks to research and patients. Here the impact would go directly to the heart of the clinical trial system.

The rise and (controversial) role of data monitoring committees

Much cooperative group activity in the 1980s and 1990s revolved around Phase III trials – large-scale trials that compared new with standard therapies – and the attempt to make them both more pragmatic and more exploratory and, at the same time, more expeditious. The need for a more efficient system was prompted in part by the fact that, with the improvement of therapy, cancer patients lived longer and so Phase III trials stretched into decade-long operations; hence the concern with speed and the emergent risk to patients that they would be left behind in a sort of research backwater as new fashionable approaches to cancer research and therapy, such as immunology and molecular biology, moved ahead. The increased length of trial contributed to the production of a new institution to deal with the research and patient risks produced by clinical cancer trials: the data monitoring committee. Although the committees themselves were not specific to cancer trials, we will see that many of the problems that they dealt with and continue to deal with, are once again, the interplay between research and therapy and the associated research and patient risks figure prominently in the trialists' concerns.

The first data monitoring committees emerged in the mid-1980s within the cooperative groups themselves, even though informal monitoring by group statisticians had long been the case beforehand.[40] In the 1980s, the CTEP set up guidelines requiring all cooperative groups to establish data monitoring committees. Although data monitoring committees do, in principle, protect patients from running unforeseen risks, they were originally set up for other purposes. As members of the Southwest Oncology Group (SWOG) explained, prior to the establishment of their data monitoring committees in 1984:

> [I]nterim results were presented periodically to the entire membership of the Group and were often published in the course of the study, either in abstract or in manuscript form. As a result, some trials could not be carried to completion because accrual declined after apparent trends became public, and other trials were published early as being positive, and published later as being negative.[41]

In other words, SWOG initially created data monitoring committees to protect the data, not the patients, even though the latter were not entirely absent from the scene.[42] Indeed, as SWOG monitors reported after a decade of monitoring:

> Nearly ten years of experience with Data Monitoring Committees that are composed of study investigators, with some outside representation, has demonstrated to the satisfaction of the SWOG leadership that this system is practical, has appropriate patient safeguards, and functions in the best interest of clinical science.[43]

Indeed, by the early 1980s, it had become evident that without some kind of formal procedure data monitoring could manipulate the trial process itself.[44] The paradigmatic case was the replacement of single-agent chemotherapy by combination chemotherapy in advanced breast cancer in the 1970s. The prior success with combination chemotherapy in the leukemias and the lymphomas had created expectations that were met in the interim analyzes of trials conducted by ECOG and the Western Cancer Study Group. The trials were thus closed and the conclusion drawn that combination chemotherapy was superior to single-agent chemotherapy. When, however, the long-term survival data became available towards the end of the 1970s, the opposite conclusions were drawn.[45] In response, the Western Cancer Group conducted an autopsy of the original interpretation in an attempt to discover why the erroneous conclusions had been drawn. Their analysis pointed to a number of factors, such as, for example, the fact that a subset of the patients with liver metastases did indeed benefit from the combination chemotherapy. None the less, the members of the group could not ignore that: "[a] final factor influencing the early interpretation of this study was the fact that this trial achieved the 'expected' result. The results of three [successful] combination chemotherapy trials involving 150 patients with breast cancer had been reported when the study was begun in 1971."[46]

By the early 1990s, a number of issues had emerged with regard to data monitoring committees, and they were sufficiently serious to prompt the NCI to organize a meeting devoted to the discussion of interim analysis and the various statistical techniques invented to deal with the evaluation of clinical trials. The presentations and much of the discussions surrounding them were quickly published in the journal *Statistics in Medicine*. The resulting special issue constitutes an important historical document, for behind this seemingly technical topic lay a lively and enlightening discussion of the problems encountered and the variety of qualitative and quantitative measures taken to balance research and patient risks in clinical cancer trials.

One of the first issues to emerge at the conference was the problem of incompatible stopping rules. By the time participants met in Bethesda, statisticians had invented a number of ways of establishing the statistical boundaries beyond which a trial would have to be stopped. Not all methods gave the same answer. As one trialist reported: "I was involved in a trial in which there were no boundaries in advance and the coordinating centre said that if we had used Pocock [stopping rules] we would have just barely crossed, if we used O'Brien-Fleming [stopping rules] we wouldn't have, if we had used stochastic curtailing ... and it became completely meaningless."[47] There were thus clear advantages to stipulating the stopping rules beforehand. According to ECOG representatives, if the rules (statistical and otherwise) were clearly stated prior to patient accrual, then future grief was largely avoided:

> [O]ur sense in the cancer co-operative group has been that the choice of statistical rules for interim monitoring will generate a fair bit of heat, some light, and lots of argument. We found it best to finish that discussion before the trial starts accruing patients, because if we delay the discussion into the midst of the trial very close to the actual presentation of data, then we find it very hard to be sure that the ultimate choice of a monitoring rule isn't to some extent data driven.[48]

None the less, participants admitted that the rules themselves should not necessarily be slavishly followed. As the previous speaker averred, "most of us who have worked in the methodology of interim stopping rules ... will often say that we acknowledge that the interim stopping boundaries are a guideline." Indeed, following the rules too closely could become counter-productive, as the previous speaker further explained:

> But in the clinical literature, it has become much more than a guide-line: it has become essentially a litmus test for whether something is published. I am also very nervous about specifications that statisticians understand how to balance and treat, but that for others with less experience in interpreting randomness become more than a guideline, almost a lab assay in measuring whether a trial was done properly.[49]

Similarly, pre-defined statistical endpoints did not foresee the unforesee-able. As a clinician sitting on a data monitoring committee reported:

> I believe my role on such [data monitoring] boards, in addition to the obvious, is to recognize unexpected problems that surface, trends that appear in subgroups that have not been previously defined or even known about, so that I provide a clinical alertness quite different from just arbitrarily accepting whether a line has been crossed.[50]

Unforeseen information could also emerge from concurrent clinical trials which, although perhaps not identical, were sufficiently similar to change beliefs about plausible outcomes. Trials, in other words, partook in a system of trials:

> When you have a large ongoing research programme with trials going on around the world, there are instances where the original intent of the trial can be contradicted by results that are appearing elsewhere. In fact, in a trial where we had a statistically significant result, which according to the design would dictate stopping, there were other trials that contradicted that result. I think that only highlights the fact that the monitoring committees have a very complicated business on their hands.[51]

Finally, patients seemingly ran different risks depending on whether it was the individual physician or the statisticians or the clinical investigators who decided whether or not to continue or discontinue a particular trial. In other words, it was not clear who would benefit in any given scenario given the emerging mix of public and private interests. Here, for example, is how Richard Simon, head of the Biometrics Research Branch of the NCI, summarized discussion of the issue during the aforementioned conference:

> It's interesting to me to hear the discussion of the issue of collective ethics in how it relates to independent monitoring committees. I thought

the critique of not having an independent monitoring committee was that the members of the committee would not necessarily be protecting the patients because of the investment they might have in terms of their career or seeing the study continue. But yet, as the discussion proceeded, it sounds like having an independent monitoring committee is used as an excuse to extend the accrual of the study beyond which you could ever extend it if you had a committee that included clinicians who were entering patients. I'm very concerned about continuing the studies to a size that is thought by some small group of people to be convincing. I feel that, at least in this country, doing that endangers public support for clinical trials.[52]

Decisions were further complicated by the fact that many trials had (and continue to have) multiple endpoints. For data monitors, problems arose when data on one endpoint contradicted data on another end-point or when a primary endpoint had not been specified so that the contradiction could not be characterized as real or trivial. According to a data monitor:

I am part of a [data-monitoring] board where a year and a half after we convened as a board, the study investigators still didn't know what the primary question was. I know it sounds silly, but it's absolutely true. We kept coming together and saying, what's the primary endpoint?[53]

Finally, there was the complex issue of the statistical price to be paid for looking at the data.[54] Consider the following exchange.

DR. JOSEPH PATER: I'd like to return to a question, which I don't think was answered, that is of practical interest to me: whether it's appropriate to show relative efficacy data to a monitoring committee more frequently than specified in terms of formal interim analysis, and if so, do you have to pay some form of statistical penalty for having done it?

DR. SIMON: First of all, in many cancer groups, it is common practice for the monitoring committee to see relative efficacy data at times other than the official interim analysis times. Is that common practice in other areas?

DR. BRISTOW: No, at least in the trials that I've dealt with it's a very serious matter to decide to do an additional analysis that is unplanned, and a plan is made to pay a penalty for it.[55]

Yet, when the cooperative group statistician looked in an informal manner at the data as it came in, he did so "for free", i.e., without incurring any statistical penalty. According to one such statistician:

Where I work, there is an interesting distinction between the monitoring committee and the study statistician. Even in the cancer groups ... one can say that we present interim formal analysis to a monitoring committee only at the times at which they were preplanned. However, the study statistician seeing an emerging difference, will look almost daily, and I think that's not always an exaggeration, because you are sitting on a time bomb. ... I know that we have discussions that sound rather silly: one of our working statisticians will come in to me and say "Do you remember the analysis of that melanoma study back in January?" I'll say yes. "Did that count?" And be very serious about wondering whether the subsequent P-values should be adjusted for that.[56]

Conclusion

In the course of this paper, we have examined the co-production of a new approach for generating biomedical knowledge in the cancer field – clinical trials – and of new forms of risk. Where do we stand today? Members of the Cancer Therapy Evaluation Program of the NCI, discussing in 1997 the issue of data monitoring committees, described three different kinds of risk that result from the development of clinical cancer trials.[57] The first, most obvious kind of risk follows from patients' participation in clinical trials and concerns the toxicity of the chemotherapeutic compounds being tested. Toxicity data, unlike efficacy data, are generally not blinded, a fact that creates a qualitative distinction between this first category of risk and the following ones. Researchers directly involved with the trial provide patient protection for this first kind of risk.

A second, more subtle kind of risk follows from the activities of data monitoring committees and refers to the possibility that patients who are in one of the two arms of the trial (say, the control arm not receiving the new drug) run the risk of being offered an inferior treatment if it should happen that the other arm (say, the experimental arm) is receiving a drug of demonstrably superior efficacy. This second kind of risk concerns an issue technically known as clinical equipoise. Defined as "the state of genuine uncertainty within the expert medical community about the preferred treatment", equipoise, according to bioethicists, should exist *before* staging the trial and last *throughout* the entire trial.[58] Its disappearance puts patients receiving the inferior regimen at a relative risk, by comparison to the other patients receiving the superior treatment. This risk category can be further subdivided into two different sub-categories: a) receiving an inferior treatment when there is a *confirmed* superior treatment compromises the safety of the person receiving the former; and b) receiving an *alleged* superior treatment (based on the analysis of interim data) puts one at risk in so far as the treatment can turn out not to be superior after all.

The third kind of risk puts the trial itself, not actual patients, at risk, but thus also, one could argue, puts at risk future patients who will suffer from the resulting lack of therapeutic knowledge. This is the "risk that the study will not obtain a reliable answer" and the risk of "compromising the moni-tored study".[59] If, for instance, on the basis of interim (but misleading) data a given trial is stopped, a promising chemotherapeutic agent could be over-looked or an unpromising one accepted. As others have noted: "the system has to be set up in this way [i.e., with no knowledge of interim trends] to have science move forward. Both the patients and the clinical investigators involved voluntarily accept temporary ignorance and rely on an independent body to make judgments on their behalf."[60] From this point of view – and as we have previously seen, data monitoring committees exist not only to protect the human subjects enrolled in a given trial but also to protect the data – these two goals can potentially conflict.

Yet, the stated overall goal of institutions such as data monitoring committees is to protect "patient-subjects from potential research risks asso-ciated with participation in clinical trials".[61] Such a formulation may lead one to believe that the risks "associated" with them have a timeless quality and little or no relation to their shifting methodology and the evolving kinds of bodies enrolled in the trial, and can thus be assessed independently of the trials' evolving design. Not all practitioners agree with such a stance: the statisticians for the seven major US cooperative oncology groups, for instance, have claimed that it is impossible to separate questions of risk from the scientific questions involved in the innovation process.[62] In this chapter we have argued that, because of the interpenetration of research and testing, risk issues are tied to knowledge issues and thus evolve in ways that make their management different from risk management in other fields of biomedical research. Trialists can easily maintain that the reduction of risk to zero would stifle the research process and thus reduce benefits to future patients. In such instances, "risk" is consequently not ultimately reduced; the burden is merely shifted from the present to the future. The historical–dynamic nature of risk and innovation within the field of clinical cancer research renders strictly ethical or logical analyzes partial and ulti-mately unsatisfactory: they are, in fact, epiphenomena of the historical development of trials and of the qualitatively different kinds of risk the latter have produced over time.

Notes

Research for this chapter was made possible by grants from the Social Science and Humanities Research Council of Canada (SSHRC), the Canadian Institutes of Health Research (CIHR), and Quebec's Fonds de Recherche sur la Société et la Culture (FQRSC). An initial version of this chapter was presented at the 2003 Cain Conference on "Risk and Safety in Medical Innovation", organized by Arthur Daemmrich, Thomas Schlich and Ulrich Tröhler at the Beckman Center for the History of Chemistry at the Chemical Heritage Foundation and the Wood Institute for the History of Medicine at the College of Physicians of Philadelphia. We would like to thank the organizers and the other participants for their comments and suggestions.

1 M. C. Christian *et al.*, "A central institutional review board for multi-institutional trials", *New England Journal of Medicine* 346, 2002, 1405–8.

2 R. Steinbrook, "Protecting research subjects: the crisis at Johns Hopkins", *New England Journal of Medicine* 346, 2002, 716–20 (correction: 1678). The compound, in other words, was not a drug to treat a condition but, rather, a substance designed to investigate a disease mechanism.

3 D. S. Greenberg, "Johns Hopkins research returns to normal", *Lancet* 359, 2001, 393.

4 On the events leading up to the creation of this Office, see Institute of Medicine, *Preserving Public Trust: Accreditation and Human Research Protection Programs*, Washington: National Academy of Sciences, 2001, pp. 29–32.

5 Steinbrook, "Protecting research subjects", pp. 716 and 1678. In 1998, Federal regulatory actions against Institutional Review Boards rose sharply from one in 1997 to fourteen in 1998; see W. J. Burman *et al.*, "Breaking the camel's back: multicenter clinical trials and local institutional review boards", *Annals of Internal Medicine* 134, 2001, 152–7.

6 F. Rolleston and J. R. Miller, "Therapy or research: a need for precision", *IRB* 3(7), August/September 1981, 1–3.

7 Christian *et al.*, "A central institutional review board", p. 1407.

8 Christian *et al.*, "A central institutional review board", p. 1405.

9 S. J. Pocock, *Clinical Trials: A Practical Approach*, New York: John Wiley, 1983, p. 22.

10 See, e.g., S. Epstein, "Bodily differences and collective identities: the politics of gender and race in biomedical research in the United States", *Body and Society*, 10, 2004, 183–203.

11 D. Schwartz and J. Lellouch, "Explanatory and pragmatic attitudes in therapeutic trials", *Journal of Chronic Diseases* 20, 1967, 637–48.

12 Schwartz and Lellouch, "Explanatory and pragmatic attitudes in therapeutic trials", p. 637.

13 Virtually ignored in the first years after its publication, the Schwartz and Lellouch paper, following major reforms in clinical cancer trials in the mid-1980s and the rise of the bioethics business, went on to become the widely-cited (321 citations) source for the distinction.

14 P. Keating and A. Cambrosio, "From screening to clinical research: the cure of leukemia and the early development of the cooperative oncology groups, 1955–1966", *Bulletin of the History of Medicine* 76, 2002, 299–334.

15 A survey of members of the American Society of Clinical Oncology showed that many American oncologists believe that therapy constitutes the principle purpose of clinical trials; see S. Joffe and J. C. Weeks, "Views of American oncologists about the purposes of clinical trials", *Journal of the National Cancer Institute* 94, 2002, 1847–53. The investigators that conducted the survey observed that this stance directly contradicted the principles of research ethics set out in the Belmont Report; see National Commission for the Protection of Human Subjects of Biomedical and Behavioral Research, "The Belmont Report: Ethical Principles and Guidelines for the Protection of Human Subjects of Research", in J. Sugarman, A. C. Mastroianni and J. P. Kahn (eds), *Ethics of Research with Human Subjects*, Frederick, MD: University Publishing Group, 1998, pp. 9–30.

16 G. Burroughs Mider, "Annual report of the scientific director", *National Cancer Institute* vol. 1, 1959, p. 73.

17 E. A. Gehan, "The determination of the number of patients required in a preliminary and follow-up trial of a new chemotherapeutic agent", *Journal of Chronic Diseases* 13, 1961, 346–53. See also E. A. Gehan and M. A. Schneiderman, "Historical and methodological developments in clinical trials at the National Cancer Institute", *Statistics in Medicine* 9, 1990, 871–80, and C. G. Zubrod, "Clinical trials in cancer patients: an introduction", *Controlled Clinical Trials* 3, 1982, 185–7. For a brief history of clinical cancer trial statistics in general, see E. A. Gehan and N. A. Lemak, *Statistics in Medical Research: Developments in Clinical Trials*, New York: Plenum, 1994.

18 The "phase" terminology itself is not cast in stone: the FDA, together with the International Committee on Harmonization, have proposed new definitions of clinical trials according to the different purposes they suit rather than the different phases into

which they fit; see Food and Drug Administration, "International conference on harmonization: guidance on general considerations for clinical trials", *Federal Register* 62(242), 1997, 66113–19.

19 National Institutes of Health, National Cancer Institute, *Annual Report of Program Activities*, vol. 1, 1960, p. 20.

20 National Institutes of Health, National Cancer Institute, *Annual Report of Program Activities*, vol. 1, 1960, p. 20.

21 S. K. Carter and P. S. Schein, "Clinical evaluation of new anticancer agents", in P. Calabresi, P. S. Schein and S. A. Rosenberg (eds) *Medical Oncology: Basic Principles and Clinical Management of Cancer*, New York: Macmillan, 1985, p. 393.

22 E. Frei III *et al.*, "Studies of sequential and combination antimetabolite therapy in acute leukemia: 6-Mercaptopurine and Methotrexate", *Blood* 18, 1961, p. 451.

23 E. J. Freireich *et al.* (Acute Leukemia Group B), "The effect of 6-Mercaptopurine on the duration of steroid induced remissions in acute leukemia: a model for evaluation of other potentially useful therapies", *Blood* 21, 1963, 699–716; p. 711.

24 Report of the Cancer Clinical Investigation Review Committee on the "Cooperative Studies Workshop" held in Williamsburg Virginia, 20–23 October 1968. NCI Archives, p. 1.

25 Report of the Cancer Clinical Investigation Review Committee on the "Cooperative Studies Workshop" held in Williamsburg Virginia, 20–23 October 1968. NCI Archives, p. 1. This "new and broader charge" to the Committee had been made in February of 1968 by the National Advisory Cancer Council (NACC) Subcommittee on Diagnosis and Treatment and adopted by the NACC. Report of the Cancer Clinical Investigation Review Committee on the "Cooperative Studies Workshop" held in Williamsburg Virginia, 20–23 October 1968. NCI Archives, p. 2.

26 Report of the Cancer Clinical Investigation Review Committee on the "Cooperative Studies Workshop" held in Williamsburg Virginia, 20–23 October 1968. NCI Archives, p. 4.

27 Regarding single disease or organ groups, seven of the eight groups with pathology sections all added pathology to their Group in the period 1967–73. By 1977, within the groups as a whole, there was one pathologist (total: 400) for every four medical oncologists (total: 1,600), a not insignificant number. See V. Loeb, G. C. Lewis and J. Newall, "Cancer education", in B. Hoogstraten (ed.), *Cancer Research: Impact of the Cooperative Groups*, New York: Masson, 1980, 365–9; p. 368.

28 V. T. DeVita, "Human models of human diseases: breast cancer and the lymphomas", *International Journal of Radiation Oncology, Biology, Physics* 5, 1979, 1855–67.

29 "Cooperative group reorganization to be offered by DeVita at clinical trials review next March", *The Cancer Letter* 4(42), 1978, p. 2. Similar charges were laid against the groups five years later by the former head of NCI's cancer centers program, John Yarbro; see "Feds short on money long on regs: Yarbro", *The Cancer Letter* 9(12), 1983, 2.

30 "New funding mechanisms – cooperative agreement consortium grant – proposed for clinical groups", *The Cancer Letter* 5(14), 1979, p. 4.

31 "New funding mechanisms – cooperative agreement consortium grant – proposed for clinical groups", *The Cancer Letter* 5(14), 1979, p. 3. In the "Minutes" of the Board of Counselors Meeting, these remarks were attributed to Vincent DeVita. See V. DeVita, "Opening remarks", *Minutes, Board of Scientific Counselors, Clinical Trials Review*, 26–27 March 1979, NCI Archives.

32 S. Marsoni *et al.*, "Clinical drug development: an analysis of phase II trials, 1970–1985", *Cancer Treatment Reports* 71, 1987, 71–80.

33 S. Marsoni *et al.*, "Clinical drug development", p. 79.

34 H. Beecher, "Ethics and clinical research", *New England Journal of Medicine* 274, 1966, 1354–60.

35 J. Heller, "Syphillis victims in US study went untreated for 40 years", *New York Times* 26 July 1972, Sec. A-1.

36 *Ethics Oral History Project – Preliminary Findings*, January 13, 1995, p.12.

37 Institute of Medicine, *Preserving Public Trust*, p. 25.
38 D. J. Rothman, *Strangers at the Bedside: A History of How Law and Bioethics Transformed Medical Decision Making*, New York: Basic Books, 1991, p. 89.
39 Rothman, *Strangers at the Bedside*, p. 90.
40 See the retrospective remarks by one of the statistical innovators in this area, P. Armitage, "Theory and practice in medical statistics", *Statistics in Medicine* 20, 2001, 2537–48.
41 J. Crowley *et al.*, "Data monitoring committees and early stopping guidelines: the Southwest Oncology Group experience", *Statistics in Medicine* 13, 1994, 1391–9; p. 1391.
42 For other groups and the NCI, see S. Green, T. Fleming and J. O'Fallon, "Policies for study monitoring and interim reporting of results", *Journal of Clinical Oncology* 7, 1987, 1477–84.
43 Crowley *et al.*, "Data monitoring committees and early stopping guidelines", p. 1398.
44 S. K. Carter, "The potential lack of comparability between interim and final results of cancer clinical trials", *Cancer Chemotherapy and Pharmacology* 8, 1982, 1–2.
45 For the re-analysis of the Western Cancer Group trial data, see R. T. Chlebowski *et al.*, "Survival of patients with metastatic breast cancer treated with either combination or sequential chemotherapy", *Cancer Research* 39, 1979, 4305–6; for the ECOG data, see P. P. Carbone *et al.*, "Chemotherapy of disseminated breast cancer: current status and prospects", *Cancer* 39 (Suppl.), 1977, 2916–22.
46 R. T. Chlebowski *et al.*, "Factors influencing the interim interpretation of a breast cancer trial: danger of achieving the 'expected' result", *Controlled Clinical Trials* 2, 1980, 123–32; p.128.
47 M. Proschan, in "Panel discussion: scientific issues in data monitoring", *Statistics in Medicine* 12, 1993, 583–600; p. 586.
48 D. P. Harrington, in "Panel discussion: scientific issues in data monitoring", *Statistics in Medicine* 12, 1993, 583–600; p. 584.
49 Harrington, in "Panel discussion"; p. 584.
50 D. Bristow, in "Panel discussion; p. 584.
51 Harrington, in "Panel discussion"; p. 587.
52 R. Simon, in "Panel discussion", 521–5; p. 525.
53 W. Friedewald, in "Panel discussion", 583–600; p. 588.
54 This issue is popularly known as the Monty Hall problem and is too complex to be discussed in detail here: basically, it relates to the fact that any "peek" at interim (statistical) results modifies the statistical end results.
55 "Panel discussion"; p. 594.
56 Harrington, in "Panel discussion"; p. 594.
57 M. A. Smith *et al.*, "Role of independent data-monitoring committees in randomized clinical trials sponsored by the National Cancer Institute", *Journal of Clinical Oncology* 15, 1997, 2736–43; p. 2736. For an angry reply to their argument, followed by the authors' rebuttal, see R. J. Wells, "Secrecy for data monitoring committees: inferior ethics, bad policy", *Journal of Clinical Oncology* 16, 1998, 390–1.
58 For a bioethical discussion of clinical equipoise, see B. Freedman, "Equipoise and the ethics of clinical research," *New England Journal of Medicine* 317, 1987, 141–5.
59 Smith *et al.*, "Role of independent data-monitoring committees", p. 2740.
60 L. Walters, "Data monitoring committees, the moral case for maximum feasible independence", *Statistics in Medicine* 12, 1993, 575–80, discussion 580–1. For a criticism of this kind of statement, see R. J. Wells, P. S. Gartside and C. L. McHenry, "Ethical issues arising when interim data in clinical trials is restricted to independent data monitoring committees", *IRB* 22(1), January–February 2000, 7–11.
61 Smith *et al.*, "Role of independent data-monitoring committees".
62 D. Harrington *et al.*, "The case against independent monitoring committees", *Statistics in Medicine* 13, 1994, 1411–14; p. 1413.

14 BioRisk: interleukin-2 from laboratory to market in the United States and Germany

Arthur Daemmrich

Risk and the political economy of biotechnology

In a remarkable congruence, three events in 1980 stimulated the emergence of a new industrial sector in the United States and around the world. First, in a pivotal Supreme Court decision, the chief justices decided that genetically manipulated organisms could be patented. Second, the US Congress passed the Bayh-Dole Act, allowing recipients of federal research funding to secure patents. Third, Genentech – the first publicly traded "biotechnology company" – set a record in its initial public offering, as its stock price soared from $35 to $89 per share in 20 minutes. Within a few years, several thousand biotech companies were founded in the United States, raised funds from venture capitalists, and in many cases went public at early stages. Investors accepted "surrogate markers" for sales and income, including prominent scientists on boards of directors, patents on untested medicinal compounds, and ambitions to cure major diseases, including cancer, diabetes, and AIDS.[1]

The sequence from university spin-off to venture capital funded firm to publicly traded company was not followed universally. For example, by the early 1980s European countries and the United States shared advanced capital markets, well-educated scientists and physicians, and had high-tech-based medical treatment. Yet a biotechnology sector did not immediately arise across Europe. In Germany, large chemical and pharmaceutical firms set up new in-house research labs and invested in partnerships with biotech ventures and academic research centers in North America.[2] However, without investors eager to take the risk of supporting new ventures, and in the face of strict federal and state laws on effluents from production facilities, few small biotech companies were created until the mid-1990s.

In effect, the stakes for corporations and risks for investors were very different on the two sides of the Atlantic. In the United States, small biotech companies lived and died based on the outcomes of laboratory research, clinical testing, and regulatory decisions on one or two medicines. Large German corporations, by contrast, spread risks among a variety of technologies and could hedge bets on the success of any one new drug. More recently, new firms have been created in Germany through the joint infusion of venture funding and government support. Nevertheless, the risk context for investors, patients, and biotech firms remains different in important ways.

This chapter examines the risk context of the biotechnology industry in the United States and Germany through a focus on the anti-cancer treatment interleukin-2 (IL-2). Its testing, regulatory review, and market introduction in the two countries illustrate the enduring nature of cultural differences in risk perception and the importance for medical innovation of national styles for regulating risk. As in other cases described throughout this book, questions about the competence of medical experts were intertwined with debates over the safety of the therapy. At the same time, this chapter's chronological jump to events in the 1980s and 1990s documents some key changes in medical and regulatory conceptions of risk and their impact on innovation. IL2's clinical testing and regulation in the United States took place under intense public scrutiny, and a focus on quantitative risk measures produced a specific treatment regimen for a single type of cancer. In Germany, the company faced less publicity of interim results and IL-2 was integrated into regular clinical practice, giving physicians greater flexibility to employ alternative treatment regimens. Public concerns with the human health and environmental risks posed by biotechnology also differed in the two countries, prompting American physicians to use the therapy as an aggressive treatment in hospitals, whereas German physicians more cautiously integrated it into regular medical practice. More generally, the IL-2 case suggests that, despite recent convergences in government policies regarding medicinal biotechnology, significant national differences remain when physicians and regulators define medical risks and decide on the market status of new therapies.

Biorisk

From its inception, the biotech industry has held out the promise of major therapeutic breakthroughs in order to attract funding for research and clinical testing. Entrepreneurs launching new companies in the 1980s looked at the formal requirements for pre-market testing and expected a smooth path from laboratory to market. After all, regulatory authorities in Europe and North America based approval decisions on nearly identical statutes for "safety and efficacy".[3] Entrepreneurs likewise anticipated that biotech medicines, unlike traditional pharmaceuticals, would beat the typical ten- to twelve-year development timeline, estimated in the mid-1980s to cost $231 million per new drug.[4]

For physicians running clinical trials and regulators assessing the safety and efficacy of new therapies, biotech came of age simultaneous with changes in patients' roles and increased public scrutiny of regulatory decisions.[5] From a comparatively simple calculus of gauging whether a new medication would benefit more patients than it might harm from side effects, regulators at the US Food and Drug Administration (FDA) increasingly had to accommodate patients with fatal diseases clamoring for medicines, as well as greater publicity of even interim testing results. When clinical trials went well, government officials were criticized for preventing apparently safe and effective medicines from reaching patients. When clinical trials went poorly, critics wondered why regulators were failing to protect patients from dangerous drugs.

In Germany, developments in biotech stimulated broader political debates about genetic testing and the safety of interventions into "normal" life processes, not just in humans, but also in plants and bacteria. The specter of Nazi-era human experimentation and discrimination loomed large in public policy.[6] With a significantly less visible and powerful regulatory apparatus, the Federal Health Office (*Bundesgesundheitsamt*, or BGA) played almost no role in these discussions.[7]

A new form of "BioRisk" thus emerged in each country, driven by different trajectories in medical risk assessment, clinical testing approaches, financial investment, and public responses to visions for the future of biotechnology. American companies tightly coupled publicity and fundraising to research and testing, while German firms kept these categories more distinct. The promise of therapeutic breakthroughs and safety guarantees issued by a well-respected government agency ameliorated concerns about side effects and contamination from genetically modified organisms in the United States. In Germany, on the other hand, the potential for environmental contamination from biotech-based production methods raised concerns – even about potentially life-saving medicines – that neither industry nor government officials could easily resolve. As a result, the medical profession played a significant role in defining and balancing risks for patients.

Interleukin-2 and the biotechnology revolution

In the mid-1970s, scientists at the US National Cancer Institute (NCI) identified a set of compounds in the human body that appeared to control the immune system. Further research demonstrated that these "interleukins" regulate the production of T-cells, a class of white blood cells. Key to the immune system's ability to recognize and destroy bacteria and viruses, T-cells can also control and even eliminate cancers. Interleukin-2 (IL-2) was first isolated in the early 1980s, and NCI scientists were excited to learn that it encouraged white blood cell reproduction. The ability to generate white blood cells in the laboratory, it was hoped, would revolutionize cancer therapy.

Efforts to produce billions of white blood cells and then inject them into patients, however, were plagued by a variety of technical difficulties. Early treatments contained impurities, including remnants of T-cell cultures and other compounds. Patients responded poorly to the lab-generated cells and had allergic responses to the impurities. Small doses appeared to have little impact, while larger doses led the immune system to attack diseased and healthy cells indiscriminately.[8]

Concurrent with the NCI work, scientists at the biotech firm Cetus began exploring therapeutic uses for interleukins. Founded in 1971 by three scientists from the University of California at Berkeley, Cetus achieved fame when its initial sale of five million shares in 1981 netted the company $115 million and set its market value at $600 million.[9] Cetus soon began working on a therapeutic dosage of IL-2 as a means to bypass the problems created by laboratory-produced white blood cells. Company researchers expected direct injection of IL-2 to stimulate internal white blood cell growth with minimal adverse reactions. They also hoped that internally produced T-cells would better differentiate between cancerous and normal cells.

Whereas NCI scientists extracted IL-2 from mice spleens, using huge numbers of expensive rodents in the process, Cetus turned to recombinant DNA techniques for mass production. The company designed a strain of *E. coli*, a bacterium found in the human digestive tract, to carry the IL-2 gene. In order to distinguish their product from the IL-2 found in the human body, Cetus began using the name "Proleukin" for the recombinant version. Once greater amounts of IL-2 were available, Cetus carried out *in vitro* and animal tests. The company quickly moved on to human tests, in collaboration with Steven Rosenberg at the NCI.[10] In 1984, Cetus launched a clinical trial, started on 75 terminally ill patients. Likewise, the NCI administered a "high-dose therapy" of IL-2 to ten patients.

Reports of success in 1985 produced glowing cover stories in *Fortune* and *Newsweek*. Warning that "cautious clinical investigators fear the familiar phrase 'cancer breakthrough' almost as much as laymen dread the word cancer itself", *Fortune* nevertheless stated that IL-2 could control a wide spectrum of cancers, and would perhaps cure all cancers. The article concluded:

> Even if lymphokines live up to only half of their promise, there will be a lot of joyful faces − not only in the research clinics and in the boardrooms of companies well placed to profit from the breakthrough, but also ... in countless households that the disease will touch.[11]

Newsweek began its article similarly warning of the potential for a "wreckage of false hopes", but then claimed that a major breakthrough was imminent. The *Newsweek* article also suggested that techniques of "adoptive immunotherapy" would treat cancer bodywide, unlike more narrowly targeted surgery or radiation.[12] Coupled to the media exposure, Cetus's stock climbed from $14 to $40 per share. By the middle of 1986, the company had a market capitalization of over $1 billion, despite annual sales of only $50 million from diagnostics and no pharmaceuticals ready for FDA review.[13]

When NCI scientists published the results of their initial tests in *JAMA* later the same year, the journal included an editorial critical of IL-2's side effects and its likely price tag.[14] Two of the ten patients in the NCI study had partial tumor regression, five were listed as "dead of disease", and the remaining three showed no change, or experienced slight additional growth of their cancers. According to Charles Moertel, a physician at the Mayo Clinic, the treatment was "an awesome experience" of long hospitalization and multiple visits to intensive care units. Furthermore, "the price in dollars for treatment and management of toxicity may reach six figures. Such high human and financial costs demand commensurate therapeutic benefit."[15] According to Moertel, patients had few benefits, leaving the majority to suffer debilitating side effects. These included serious infections and capillary leak syndrome, a potentially life-threatening condition where plasma and proteins leak into the extravascular space. Capillary leak can produce a variety of ailments, including heart attacks, respiratory problems, gastro-intestinal bleeding, and kidney damage. Nevertheless, Moertel's criticism of IL-2 therapy as too expensive and too toxic had little immediate impact on its further development by Cetus. The company proceeded to larger clinical trials in collaboration with the NCI, and by the late 1980s was ready to seek regulatory approval for Proleukin in the United States and Europe.

Although clinical studies reported by *JAMA* in 1986 offered a far more sobering assessment of IL-2's efficacy than was found in popular magazines, it would take another two years for business journals to warn investors that the compound was not a "one-stop cancer breakthrough".[16] In the stock market crash of October 1987, biotech companies were criticized for relentless media hype and few marketable products. Entering what Robert Teitelman has characterized as an "iron age", only cooperative research agreements, the sale of successful testing technologies, and licensing agreements with large pharmaceutical firms kept small biotech companies fiscally solvent.[17] IL-2's revenue potential was assessed down to $275 million annually from as high as $400 million two years earlier. Nevertheless, Cetus, the NCI, and competing firms sponsored over 80 clinical trials with recombinant IL-2 during the late 1980s. Even analysts critical of the hype regarding most anti-cancer agents anticipated a healthy revenue stream for the compound.

Proleukin in the United States

Before Cetus could begin earning money from Proleukin, it needed FDA marketing approval. By the time the company submitted a new drug application (NDA) for Proleukin to the agency in 1988, physicians had narrowed its proposed use to treatment of metastatic renal cell carcinoma, a disease affecting some 25,000 Americans per year. Cetus expected Proleukin to gain rapid approval for this indication, since on average only 10 per cent of patients survive beyond five years from diagnosis. When the FDA's Biological

Response Modifiers Advisory Committee met to review the application, however, company hopes were dashed. Committee members requested additional studies and demanded that the company clearly specify which patients would benefit from the therapy. Cetus had included results from studies on "metastatic cancer" in the NDA, but did not differentiate the source or type of cancers. As a result, FDA advisory committee members were not convinced of Proleukin's specific efficacy to treat kidney cancer.

Two years later, the advisory committee met again to review a revised Proleukin application. Like their predecessors, advisory committee members requested that Cetus perform further research and carry out more specific data analysis. In particular, they challenged the selection of control groups, methods for compiling data, and, most importantly, the narrow selection of clinical trials for the NDA. Cetus attracted extensive publicity in the late 1980s with claims that it would soon cure a broad spectrum of cancers. Each of the many trials carried out on Proleukin, successful or not, drew media coverage. While integral to the sequence of stock offerings that kept the company afloat financially, this media attention ultimately made it difficult for the company to justify its selection of studies to include in the NDA.

Widespread testing ultimately hurt the company, since reviewers felt unclear about the dosage and precise treatment regimen advanced by Cetus. The advisory committee demanded specifics on which patients benefited from Proleukin treatment. Furthermore, some members expressed concerns that the therapy required too much expertise on the part of physicians. One committee member noted:

> It may be fine in Steve Rosenberg's hands [at NCI] where he has a good staff to treat the side effects, or here at [Johns] Hopkins or other big places. But what about little hospitals? If this drug were widely used, we could see drug-related mortality go way up.[18]

In effect, the advisory committee wanted a clearly specified treatment regimen that relied less on physician skill and institutional experience with the treatment. They were concerned that these prerequisites would translate poorly to other clinical settings.

After this advisory committee meeting in 1990, Cetus's stock went into a slide, eventually bottoming out at $8.75 per share. Failure to gain FDA approval cut the company's market value by 75 per cent to $276 million. Analysts speculated that parts of the company would be sold. Instead Chiron, a competitor located across the street from Cetus, purchased the entire company for $660 million in 1991. As part of the deal, Cetus sold several patents including the DNA replication system known as the polymerase chain reaction.

In order to prepare a revised FDA application, Chiron focused on a smaller group of patients during an additional two years of clinical testing. Consequently, its 1992 application described just seven clinical studies with

255 patients, each of whom had metastatic or unresectable (not removable through surgery) renal cell carcinoma. Four of the seven studies were carried out at a single clinic, while the others were multi-clinic trials. Three of the trials were of Proleukin alone, while the other four involved comparisons with treatments such as Interferon or injections of lymphokine-activated killer cells.

In the revised application, Chiron claimed that the duration of patient responses and stabilization of their ECOG Performance Status proved Proleukin's efficacy. The ECOG scale (Table 14.1), devised by the Eastern Cooperative Oncology Group, consists of five levels that gauge the influence of cancer on the "daily living abilities of the patient". For the Proleukin trials, Performance Status (PS) served as a surrogate for more precise quantitative measures of patient response.

Of the 255 patients used for the revised application, 28 (11 per cent) were classified as "partial responders", meaning that their tumors had shrunk by half or more, and existing lesions had not expanded in size. Between the ECOG status and uncertainties in how to define "partial" and "complete" responses, proof of efficacy required patient assessment and communication between physicians and patients in the clinical trial. Furthermore, the company and FDA officials had to negotiate appropriate measures of efficacy and how to scale data from various tests.

Proleukin's side effects continued to plague the application. Just as Moertel noted years earlier, the therapy was an "awesome experience" for patients who suffered damage to nearly every internal organ. Of the 255 patients, 11 died during the clinical trials, nearly half as many as experienced "partial" improvement. Once the drug was approved, the FDA published a two-page list of side effects, with detailed tables showing that patients suffered damage to their cardiovascular, pulmonary, gastrointestinal, neurological, renal, hepatic, hematological, dermatological, musculoskeletal, and endocrine systems. Even a full week after therapy ended, some 14 per cent of patients remained hospitalized. To help assuage concerns about adverse reactions, the company announced that it would monitor patients indefinitely following IL-2 therapy.

Table 14.1 ECOG performance status

ECOG	
0	Fully active, able to carry on all pre-disease performance without restriction.
1	Restricted to physically strenuous activity but ambulatory and able to carry out work of a light or sedentary nature, e.g., light housework, office work.
2	Ambulatory and capable of all self-care but unable to carry out any work activities. Up and about more than 50% of waking hours.
3	Capable of only limited self-care, confined to bed or chair more than 50% of waking hours.
4	Completely disabled. Cannot carry on any self-care. Totally confined to bed or chair.
5	Dead.

Source: Eastern Cooperative Oncology Group

Following the 1992 meeting, the advisory committee recommended FDA approval only under specific conditions. Committee members endorsed a drug regimen under which patients receive Proleukin over the course of two five-day treatment cycles, separated by a rest period. Fourteen injections are given in each cycle involving a fifteen-minute intravenous infusion, followed by an eight-hour rest period. After 9 days of rest, the schedule is repeated for another 14 doses, resulting in a total of 28 doses per course of therapy.[19]

From a therapy intended to treat all cancers, Proleukin evolved in the course of clinical trials and FDA review to a treatment for largely asymptomatic kidney cancer patients. Patients with an ECOG status greater than PS–1, those most eager for treatment, were denied the drug outside of clinical trials. Though the advisory committee's minutes hardly read like a ringing endorsement, the application soon earned FDA approval. Reporting on the decision, *Business Week* suggested that revenue would start slowly and climb to $100 million yearly, a sharp reduction from earlier estimates of a $500 million blockbuster drug.[20] By early 1993, over 1,000 patients had been treated with Proleukin, and Chiron announced sales of $12.5 million, still far short of previous estimates.[21]

Interestingly, Chiron's efforts to monitor patients closely following treatment were supported by the National Kidney Cancer Association (NKCA), an organization founded in 1989 to help patients secure reimbursement for experimental therapies. Like other disease-based organizations, NKCA expanded its mission by early 1990s to play a role in clinical trials and patient care. Its publications promoted a shift in decision-making authority from the physician to the patient by reminding cancer patients that "your doctor works for you ... you are his boss".[22] The organization also distributed a "Patient Symptom Record" to promote record-keeping and draw attention to adverse reactions among patients undergoing IL-2 therapy.

One clear benefit to the company from sponsoring ongoing patient treatment and observation was demonstrated in 1997, when the FDA approved Proleukin for the treatment of metastatic melanoma. Based on a "retrospective analysis of patients" carried out to meet FDA requests for additional data, the company identified a cohort of 270 skin cancer patients helped by the treatment.[23] Advisory committee members were receptive to the therapy, noting that "metastatic melanoma is a disease that gives cancer a bad name", since it strikes young patients, progresses rapidly, and has extremely low long-term survival rates (only two to three per cent of patients survive five years once the disease is identified). Out of 270 patients with melanoma treated between 1985 and 1993, 17 experienced a complete return to health and an additional 26 had a partial recovery.

FDA representatives at the advisory committee meeting raised some concerns by noting that the response rate was offset by the large number of patients who suffered severe adverse reactions without discernible benefits. Advisory committee members nevertheless decided that the therapy merited

Patient Symptom Record (Photocopy as needed)

Using the rating scales below, please record the symptoms you may be experiencing while receiving IL-2 therapy. If you feel hot or have chills during the day, record your temperature and the time this occurred.

Rate each symptom for severity using the following scale:

0=No symptoms
1=Mild (aware of symptoms but does not interfere with normal activity)
2=Moderate (symptoms interfere with normal activity)
3=Severe (unable to continue normal activities because of symptoms)

Record the duration of each symptom using the following:

C=Continuous symptom present most of the time
I=Intermittent symptom which comes and goes

Cycle_____   Week _____

Treatment Day	1	2	3	4	5	6	7
DATE:							
IL-2 injection time							
IL-2 injection site*							
Temperature/time							
Weight							
Chills							
Headache							
Bone/muscle pain							
Fatigue							
Nausea							
Vomiting (number)							
Loss of appetite							
Diarrhea (number)							
Nightmares/vivid dreams							
Confusion/clouded thinking							
Dizziness							
Shortness of breath							
Chest pain/tightness							
Injection site pain*							
Hand/feet swelling							
Skin: Dryness, swelling, redness, pain							

*Site: RA = right arm; LA = left arm; RH = right hip; LH = left hip; RT = right thigh; LT = left thigh.

Figure 14.1 Patient-recorded assessment

Source: National Kidney Cancer Association, *Interleukin-2 and Biologic Therapy: A Booklet for Patients and Their Families*, Evanston, IL: NKCA, 1999.

approval, so long as it was accompanied by ongoing clinical studies. Reflecting a shift in risk perception, committee members, like many of the patients they treated, were primarily concerned with reasonable access to the treatment. The agency, on the other hand, still faced political pressures to approve "risk-free" medicines that produced few or no adverse reactions.

During debates on how best to shape future Proleukin studies, concerns about adverse reactions mingled with consideration of the therapy's cost, even though drug prices are supposedly not a factor in approval decisions. Echoing the FDA reviewers, one advisory committee member commented: "We are talking about a very, very small number of patients that will receive a very, very toxic and extremely expensive therapy."[24]

Despite concerns about its side effects and cost, the FDA ultimately approved Proleukin for metastatic melanoma, recommending a treatment regimen identical to that for kidney cancer. The agency again requested Chiron to monitor patients for at least five years after therapy. By the time of this decision in 1998, the FDA had developed greater flexibility about allowing therapies on the market despite evidence of serious side effects and limited statistical proof of efficacy. Historically strict boundaries separating clinical trials from market approval had given way to a more flexible regime that allowed market access conditional upon long-term patient monitoring.

German biotechnology policy and politics

In contrast to the United States, Germany historically has had a relatively fluid approach to determining a new drug's marketing status.[25] The sharp boundary between clinical trials and post-market surveillance implemented in the United States after the 1938 Food, Drug, and Cosmetic Act and strictly enforced after the 1962 Kefauver-Harris Act was not a major feature of the 1961, 1964, or 1976 German Drug Laws. As a result, whereas IL-2's testing and regulatory review in the United States was dragged out over a lengthy period, in Germany it proceeded comparatively quickly. At the same time, public concern with the human health and environmental risks posed by biotech prompted very cautious integration of the treatment into medical care. Published reports of clinical trials and documentation prepared in the company's application to the BGA consequently illustrate more attention to risks to the healthcare system writ large, and greater concern about individual patient autonomy than in the United States.

Unlike the case-by-case review of biotech drugs and foodstuffs in the United States, Germany in the 1980s and 1990s employed a process-based regulatory approach marked by cautious assessment of risks to public health from recombinant DNA research and its industrial-scale applications.[26] Responding to public protests, federal and state regulations required firms to document not just the safety of their products, but also the physical containment of biological materials used in research labs and factories. Changes in the "Federal Nuisance Act" during the late 1980s required that effluent from industrial production facilities be completely free of micro-organisms. Citizen groups concerned with biotech-based drug production agitated for additional government regulation and directly monitored company compliance with existing laws. They reported violators to government authorities and even sued manufacturers. As a result, production facilities, including BASF's Tumor-Necrosis-Factor plant, Behringwerke's Erythropoietin factory, and a Hoechst facility for insulin production were all prevented from operating at various points in the 1980s.[27]

A variety of local disputes concerning biotech-based medicine production prompted federal hearings on the "Risks and Opportunities of Biotechnology" in 1985 and 1986. Organized by newly-elected Green Party parliament members, hearings were led by a Commission of Inquiry (*Enquete-Kommission*).[28] In the course of the hearings, witnesses repeatedly challenged the necessity of promoting biotech in Germany. Their opposition ranged across a spectrum, from moral and ethical concerns to fears of medical and environmental risks. Seeking to balance these criticisms with the desire to promote economic development, the parliament approved a Genetic Engineering Law that permitted biotech research and production contingent upon the use of containment facilities. The law also regulated the marketing of products that contained genetically modified organisms.[29]

During and after these hearings, Germany's drug approval process also came under critical scrutiny. Specifically, Green Party member Erika Hickel criticized German regulations for not requiring manufacturers to demonstrate a pressing "need" for their medicines prior to market approval.[30] Hickel used IL-2's production by means of genetically modified *E. coli* to argue that biopharmaceuticals should be assessed differently from other medicines. Along with other critics, she claimed that existing regulatory approaches failed to address the new hazards posed by biotech.

Public opposition to biotech in Germany, however, did not completely stymie cancer research and testing using interleukins. Concerns about biotech became highly differentiated; German citizens worried about environmental impacts of modified micro-organisms and feared harm to humans from DNA manipulation, but simultaneously hoped for new therapeutics to treat life-threatening diseases. Reports in German press and medical journals about IL-2 and other biotech therapies in the mid-1980s described the outcomes of animal tests and early clinical trials, but also discussed the influence of private commercial interests on medicine in the United States.

Proleukin in Germany

Cetus's newly formed European branch, Eurocetus, began clinical tests of IL-2 in 1986. Eurocetus trials eventually drew together data on 3,000 patients from Western and Central Europe, Russia, Hungary, and Israel. Unlike studies carried out in the United States, these tests sought to develop a dosage regimen that would not require intensive care. European physicians soon hit upon subcutaneous application as an alternative to the intravenous infusion used in the United States.[31] This approach reduced Proleukin's toxicity since the compound was absorbed into the body more slowly than after intravenous injection. Significantly, it also eliminated capillary-leak syndrome, one of the main side effects of intravenous infusions. Furthermore, since this mode of administration was less invasive, patients could be treated in an ambulatory (outpatient) setting.

German and other European physicians also latched on to combination therapy of Proleukin with interferon-alpha as helpful to outpatient or home care. A series of reports in German medical journals suggested that subcutaneous infusion and combination therapy would result in fewer side effects, less strain on patients, and more successful cancer treatment.[32] The approach drew sufficient interest from physicians to encourage the company to sponsor tests to document its efficacy and Cetus eventually presented data to the BGA to support this treatment method. Cetus used a database of 425 patients to compare 225 patients who received Proleukin as an intravenous drip infusion with 200 patients who injected themselves with Proleukin combined with Interferon-alpha. The two approaches did not result in statistically different outcomes in terms of cancer remission, but were strikingly different in their toxicity. Intravenous application had a remission rate of 15 per cent, while 30 per cent of the patients suffered from severe adverse reactions. In contrast, the subcutaneous application had a 20 per cent remission rate while only 5 per cent of the patients experienced side effects.[33]

In the BGA application and in reports sent to German physicians, Eurocetus (absorbed into Chiron after the 1991 Cetus purchase) explicitly criticized American treatment methods. In particular, side effects were seen as an outcome of the treatment *method*, not the treatment itself:

> The treatment regimen developed by the NCI in Bethesda, Maryland, USA, is an intensive high-dose therapy protocol, which results in serious adverse reactions and in many cases, requires treatment in an intensive care unit ... patient compliance can be greatly improved through the development of a less aggressive treatment regimen and better management of adverse reactions.[34]

Employing a scale similar to ECOG, physicians divided patients with metastatic kidney cancer into four risk groups and oriented their treatment efforts to patients in lower risk categories.[35] The miracle drug status first accorded to IL-2 in the United States had by this time given way to a much more nuanced approach. German physicians accordingly were less concerned with saving terminal patients than with treating patients in early stages of cancer.

Despite the success with Proleukin in ambulatory settings, BGA officials who approved the therapy in 1989 still recommended treating metastatic kidney carcinoma only in hospital oncology departments or clinics with

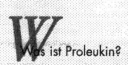
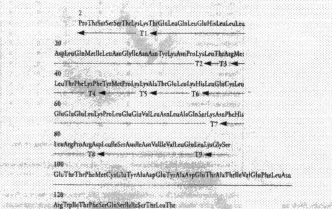

Figure 14.2 German Proleukin monograph
Source: Chiron, *Proleukin Produktmonographie*, Ratingen: Chiron GmbH, 1995.

intensive medical supervision. Government reviewers were concerned that its impact on patients varied so widely. Physicians who reviewed clinical studies for the BGA noted that the therapy only helped 25 per cent of kidney cancer patients, while even fewer – 10 per cent – had complete remission of their cancers.[36] The BGA therefore required Eurocetus to file regular reports of patient "experiences" after Proleukin's marketing. Physicians also were to measure white blood cell counts and platelets to further weed out patients who should not be on the therapy. These restrictions helped BGA officials justify Proleukin's rapid approval in Germany. They also helped physicians select a controlled and homogenous patient population for therapy. Just as advisory committee members in the United States wanted the company to supply the FDA with reports of ongoing studies, the German BGA wanted more laboratory data and clinical reports than were found in the initial marketing application.

In Germany, the interleukins generally, and IL-2 specifically, were often cited as prime examples of biotech's promise and failings. Critics claimed the treatment was inadequately tested and that, even with BGA approval, recombinant Proleukin needed greater study and broader "societal consensus" before admission to widespread use.[37] As a result, when Eurocetus began marketing Proleukin in Germany, the company went to great lengths to document both the "natural" presence of IL-2 in the human body and the environmental safety of its production methods.

The German product monograph reveals the company's desire to convince government officials, physicians, and patients that Proleukin posed no special risks. A bold sidebar states: "the biological activity corresponds to that of natural IL-2", while the main text provides a detailed explanation of the manufacturing process. The monograph even reproduced the recombinant Proleukin amino acid sequence. More generally, the company emphasized that "natural and recombinant IL-2 induce comparable biological effects ... both forms possess the same spectrum of biological activity and effects."[38]

Public concerns about the equivalence of "natural" and "recombinant" ultimately had little direct impact on Proleukin's regulatory approval. They did, however, influence physicians to exercise great caution with the treatment. German physicians thus employed strict criteria to select patients, advanced a treatment method that could bypass the life-threatening capillary leak syndrome, and observed patients very closely for adverse reactions. In this manner, they helped assuage some of the concerns about the risks of biotechnology-based therapies that were articulated in Germany.

The ebb and flow of bio-enthusiasm

The United States

Just as IL-2 eventually gained FDA approval, other biopharmaceuticals increasingly came on the US market in the mid-1990s. By the end of 2003, over 155 biotechnology-based drugs and vaccines were approved for disease treatment. Advances in gene sequencing provided the basis for a new wave of firm growth. The number of biotech stock offerings thus skyrocketed from 15 in 1999 to 68 in 2000.[39] At the same time, other companies went out of business or were acquired by larger firms. Thus, in the last decade, the total number of biotech firms has held relatively constant; the range was from 1,272 in 1993 to 1,466 in 2002.[40] In the United States, the industry appears to be caught in a cycle of venture capital influx and hyped stock offerings, followed by the bankruptcy or purchase of companies unable to generate marketable testing technologies or therapies. Three years ago, the sequencing of the human genome and expectations for a new generation of therapies helped underwrite some $32 billion in new support. Within a short time, a much harsher operating environment meant that biotech companies raised only $10 billion in new capital in 2002, primarily through debt offerings. Only six biotech companies had initial public offerings (IPOs) that year. By mid-2004, the market had improved and a new genera-tion of firms queued up for IPOs.[41] Contrary to predictions that a major shake-out would inevitably leave large pharmaceutical firms in control of the market, repeated influxes of new capital, cooperative research and cross-licensing agreements, and the introduction of new technologies have preserved an economic and social space for small biotech ventures.

While cures for diseases such as cancer or AIDS have been proven more elusive than thought during biotech's early years, one-third of all new drugs now reaching the market are based on recombinant proteins (interferons, growth hormones, blood clotting factors) or monoclonal antibodies.[42] Coupled to the FDA's tight vigilance, the potential for these areas of research to produce significant breakthroughs has generally reduced public concerns regarding biotech in the United States.

Germany

As a result of public opposition to bioengineering, more conservative invest-ment trends, and strict controls on research and production, comparatively few new biotech firms were founded in Germany during the 1980s and early 1990s. Companies had to dedicate personnel to meet regulatory demands and found it difficult to move into new research areas. Some analysts blamed Germany's anti-business culture for inhibiting innovation, stifling market growth, and inducing large firms to shift their research personnel overseas. For example, *Forbes* reported in 1989 that uncertainties about federal and local approval for experiments and mass production had "virtually paralysed Germany's fledgling biotech industry".[43] Employing the term "risk" for lost potential benefits rather than physical or social hazards, promoters of biotech in the early 1990s frequently lamented the absence of *Risikokapital* due to a skeptical German public.[44]

Within a few years, however, the tide turned for medical biotech in Germany. Life-science firms lobbied to reduce regulatory controls. They drew on Germany's high unemployment in the mid-1990s and reports of declining patent filings to claim economic hazards from the absence of a biotech sector.[45] Responding to these concerns, the Federal Parliament (the *Bundestag*) revised the Genetic Engineering Law in 1994 to reduce government oversight of research protocols and abandoned regulations on experiments that posed no risk of releasing viable organisms, including tests using genetically modified *E. coli*. Whereas researchers previously had to submit nearly 100 forms for every set of experiments, they now could carry out laboratory studies with less oversight and needed only the approval of an ethics board to launch clinical tests.[46]

In addition to lessening regulatory burdens, the German government began supporting start-up companies. In one successful program, the government provided direct financial assistance through *BioRegio* competitions. Even regions that did not get a large influx of federal support promoted greater cooperation between industry and government officials at a local level and campaigned for greater public acceptance of biotech.[47] Their efforts had some impact: a widely cited poll conducted in 1996 indicated that 59 per cent of the respondents believed Germany should gain a leading position in biotech.[48]

Many of the same critics who disparaged excessive caution regarding biotech in the 1980s and early 1990s, now lauded a "boom" in German biotech sector. By the end of the 1990s, Germany led Europe in small-firm growth. Listing 279 firms in 2000 (360 by 2002), analysts stated: "Germany can now claim to be Europe's most densely populated biotech kindergarten."[49] Newly established firms received upwards of $4 million each from the federal government, which disbursed over $900 million annually for biotech research. A "German model" comprised of regional research parks and no-interest loans from federal and state governments thus contributed to the rapid emergence of a biotech industry.

The success of this medical biotech industry relies to some degree on its differentiation from the still hotly contested agricultural biotech business. On the one hand, Germans vigorously oppose genetically modified foods; on the other, medical research and drug production through biotech now has a greater degree of acceptance than in the 1980s. Nevertheless, the opposition to biotech was overridden less by institutionalized mechanisms for guaranteeing safety or clinical effectiveness than by concerns of industrial competitiveness and the apparent necessity to mimic developments in the United States. A hybrid set of social, political, and economic motives thus proved more important than establishing new regulatory mechanisms for ensuring the validity of medical evidence.

Conclusion: clinical trials, patient care, and biorisk

The clinical testing, regulatory review, and marketing of IL-2 illustrate significant differences in the healthcare systems and BioRisk portfolios of the United States and Germany. First, responsibility for patient monitoring and treatment – especially after Proleukin had gained provisional approval in both countries – lay with the manufacturer in the United States and with the medical profession in Germany. Clinical trials in the United States were strongly oriented to the collection of data for FDA approval. In Germany, the medical profession had greater authority to shape the treatment regimen, and individual physicians served as crucial nodes in the flow of information between patients and the company and even between the company and the government. Physicians thus not only recorded and responded to side effects, they also played a formal role in determining Proleukin's marketing status during meetings with government officials and company representatives.

Second, American physicians advocated a testing protocol and treatment method that required long hospitalization periods for intravenous administration. German patients, considered by physicians to be reliable participants and subject to observation and control outside of hospitals, often received treatment on an ambulatory basis through subcutaneous application. These two methods of administering Proleukin and structuring the clinical trials and therapy are revealing of broader differences in patient autonomy and risk perception in Germany and the United States. German physicians shied away from the financial costs and loss of authority associated with treating patients in intensive care units. They instead configured their own clinics, or even outpatient settings, to meet the demands of Proleukin therapy. Patients had the appearance of greater autonomy and ability to lead "normal" day-to-day lives while on Proleukin. In the United States, on the other hand, treatment in intensive care units offered more controlled data collection, helped ensure insurance reimbursement, and reduced potential legal liability from adverse reactions. Patients had little control over either the treatment regimen or any other aspect of their daily lives while receiving Proleukin.

The interplay among investors, drug innovation, clinical testing, and government regulation that eventually saw IL-2 to the market has only increased in saliency since the mid-1990s.[50] For biotech ventures, the BioRisk identified here has a particular hazard; when products perform poorly in clinical trials, companies are pushed to cut testing short and drop potentially useful therapies. As IL-2 – and even the recent introduction of Thalidomide in the United States – illustrate, drugs sometimes find different end-uses than originally anticipated. In addition to its uses for renal carcinoma and metastatic melanoma, IL-2 has been tested as an adjunct therapy for patients with HIV. Facing uncertain results and a small potential market, Chiron recently found itself unable to support clinical trials estimated to cost $20 million per year. The company first transferred responsibility for the trial to an independent scientific committee, then terminated it nine months later.[51] For patients, an analogous hazard has emerged as insurers – including Medicare – are increasingly reluctant to cover a $40,000 treatment regimen (of which only some $14,000 goes for IL-2).[52] Only intensive lobbying by hospitals, physicians, and the company reversed a Medicare decision in 2003 to reimburse just $7,000 for the therapy.

Recent studies have analyzed the risk tradeoffs inherent in modern biomedicine, especially in light of government involvement by means of regulating market approvals and specifying treatment methods.[53] Approving a drug too quickly can lead to "countervailing risks" in the form of severe (and publicly visible) side effects. Withholding or approving it too slowly can be problematic as well, most obviously when dealing with a potentially life-saving therapy like IL-2 for cancer. Yet the interplay of market and economic risks with medical risk assessment procedures is less well understood.

From a historical calculus of risk measured in relation to the benefit and harm of a therapy, risk in biomedicine now also incorporates probabilities of financial gain or loss. If investors gauge the likelihood of achieving therapeutic success as low, companies fail. The converse, as IL-2 shows, is not always true. Even with great faith and hope, the interleukins have not emerged as a cure for all cancers. Only carefully structured risk management systems, ones that account for national differences and can provide patients with access to life-saving treatments while also offering the assurance that, if something goes wrong, their individual suffering will be addressed and systemic learning will take place, will help biomedicine achieve some of its utopian promises.

Notes

1 See: R. Teitelman, *Gene Dreams: Wall Street, Academia, and the Rise of Biotechnology*, New York: Basic Books, 1989, pp. 11–14; *Diamond v. Chakrabarty*, 447 US 303 (1980); L. Branscomb and J. Keller (eds), *Investing in Innovation: Creating a Research and Innovation Policy that Works*, Cambridge, MA: MIT Press, 1998, pp. 14–20.

2 S. Jasanoff, "Technological Innovation in a Corporatist State: The Case of Biotechnology in the Federal Republic of Germany", *Research Policy* 14, 1985, 23–38; M. Sharp, "The Science of Nations: European Multinationals and American Biotechnology", *International Journal of Biotechnology* 1, 1999, 132–62.

3 A. Daemmrich, *Pharmacopolitics: Drug Regulation in the United States and Germany*, Chapel Hill: UNC Press, 2004.

4 J. DiMasi *et al.*, "Cost of Innovation in the Pharmaceutical Industry", *Journal of Health Economics* 10, 1991, 107–42.

5 S. Epstein, *Impure Science: AIDS, Activism and the Politics of Knowledge*, Berkeley: University of California Press, 1996.

6 H. Gottweis, *Governing Molecules: The Discoursive Politics of Genetic Engineering in Europe and the United States*, Cambridge MA: MIT Press, 1998; P. Weingart, J. Kroll, and K. Bayertz, *Rasse, Blut und Gene: Geschichte der Eugenik und Rassenhygiene in Deutschland*, Frankfurt am Main: Suhrkamp Verlag, 1988, pp. 680–4.

7 The BGA was divided into several smaller ministries in 1994, with the Robert Koch Institut subsequently responsible for biological therapies and vaccines.

8 I. Löwy, *Between Bench and Bedside: Science, Healing, and Interleukin-2 in a Cancer Ward*, Cambridge, MA: Harvard University Press, 1996, pp. 124–34.

9   T. J. Lueck, "Cetus Charting a Broad Course: Plans to Use Biotechnology in Many Fields", *New York Times*, 5 June 1981, 25.

10 S. Rosenberg and J. Barry, *Transformed Cell: Unlocking the Mysteries of Cancer*, New York: Avon Books, 1992; P. Rabinow, *Making PCR: A Story of Biotechnology*, Chicago: University of Chicago Press, 1996.

11 G. Bylinsky, "Science Scores a Cancer Breakthrough", *Fortune*, 25 November 1985, 16–21.

12 M. Clark *et al.*, "Search for a Cure", *Newsweek*, 16 December 1985, 60–5.

13 G. Slutsker, "Look Before You Speak", *Forbes*, 142, 26 December 1988, 116–17.

14 M. Lote *et al.*, "High-Dose Recombinant Interleukin-2 in the Treatment of Patients with Disseminated Cancer", *JAMA* 256, 1986, 3117–24. The critical review was published in the same issue: C. Moertel, "On Lymphokines, Cytokines, and Breakthroughs", *JAMA* 256, 1986, 3141.

15 Moertel, "On Lymphokines", p. 3141.

16 F. Lunzer, "Trials of a Cancer Drug", *High Technology Business* August 1988, 33–5.

17 Teitelman, *Gene Dreams*, pp. 186–97.

18 B. Culliton, "Cetus's Costly Stumble on IL-2", *Science* 250, 1990, 20–1.

19 Food and Drug Administration, "Summary for Basis of Approval: Aldesleukin", 5 May 1992, p. 2.

20 J. Hamilton, "Heartbreak and Triumph in Biotech Land", *Business Week*, 3 February 1992, 33.

21 D. Jenish, "A Risky Treatment", *Maclean's* 106, 22 February 1993, 52–3.

22 National Kidney Cancer Association, "13 Steps to World Class Cancer Care".

23 Oncologic Drugs Advisory Committee, Meeting 55, 19 December 1997, p. 11.

24 Oncologic Drugs Advisory Committee, Meeting 55, 19 December 1997, pp. 121–2.

25 Daemmrich, *Pharmacopolitics*; A. Murswieck, *Die staatliche Kontrolle der Arzneimittelsicherheit in der Bundesrepublik und den USA*, Opladen: Westdeutscher Verlag, 1983.

26 S. Jasanoff, "Product, Process, or Programme: Three Cultures and the Regulation of Biotechnology", in M. Bauer (ed.), *Resistance to New Technology*, Cambridge: Cambridge University Press, 1995, pp. 311–31.

27 U. Dolata, *Internationales Innovationsmanagement: Die deutsche Pharmaindustrie und die Gentechnik*, Hamburg: Institut für Sozialforschung, 1994.

28 Deutscher Bundestag (ed.), *Chancen und Risiken der Gentechnologie: Der Bericht der Enquete-Kommission*, Bonn: Deutscher Bundestag, 1987.

29 "Gesetz zur Regelung von Fragen der Gentechnik", *Bundesgesetzblatt I* 20 June 1990, 1080.

30 E. Hickel, "Arzneimittel und Gentechnik", *Deutsche Apotheker Zeitung* 128, 1988, 297–303.

31 C. Franks *et al.*, "EuroCetus-Coordinated Clinical Trials", in M. Atkins and J. Mier (eds), *Therapeutic Applications of Interleukin-2*, New York: Marcel Dekker, 1993, pp. 311–25.

32 J. Atzpodien *et al.*, "Home Therapy with Recombinant Interleukin-2 and Interferon Alpha-2b in Advanced Human Malignancies", *Lancet* 335, 1990, 1509–12; H. Steinmetz, "Rekombinantes Interleukin-2", *Deutsche Apotheker Zeitung* 130, 1990, 2483–4.

33 Chiron, *Proleukin: Produktmonographie*, pp. 8–12.

34 Chiron, *Proleukin: Produktmonographie*, p. 18.

35 Bundesverband der Pharmazeutischen Industrie, "Chiron: Proleukin", *Fachinformation* Aulendorf: BPI, 1994, p. 3.

36 "Krebstherapie mit Interleukin-2 noch zu optimieren", *Pharmazeutische Zeitung* 135, 1990, 1116–17.

37 R. Kollek, "Neue Kriterien für die Abschätzung des Risikos", in M. Thurau (ed.), *Gentechnik – Wer kontrolliert die Industrie?* Frankfurt am Main: Fischer Verlag, 1989; Gottweis, *Governing Molecules*, pp. 237–61.

38 Chiron, "Proleukin: Produktmonographie" Chiron, 1995, pp. 6–7.
39 Biotechnology Industry Organization, "U.S. Biotech IPOs".
40 Ernst and Young, *Beyond Borders: The Global Biotechnology Report 2003*, New York: Ernst and Young, 2003.
41 "Biotech Uptick", *Chemical and Engineering News*, 8 March 2004, 11.
42 A. Thayer, "Great Expectations", *Chemical and Engineering News*, 10 August 1998, 19–31.
43 R. Bailey, "Brain Drain", *Forbes*, 27 November 1989, 262; see also H. Henzler, "Politics and Culture thwart German Innovation", *Wall Street Journal Europe*, 27 August 1996, 25.
44 Verband Forschender Arzneimittelhersteller, *Eine Erfolgsgeschichte mit Zukunft: Chancen Innovativer Arzneimittel für Deutschland* Bonn: VFA, 1995, p. 32.
45 K. L. Miller, "Biotech Blooms in Germany – Again", *Business Week*, 23 January 1995, 70–1.
46 M. Simm, "German Geneticists Get Some Relief", *Science* 263, 1994, 23–4.
47 H. Domdey, "Germany as a location for Biotechnological Entrepreneurship: Achievements and Challenges", in S. Silvia (ed.), *Reversal of Fortune? An Assessment of the German Biotechnology Sector in Comparative Perspective*, Washington, DC: American Institute for Contemporary German Studies, 1999, 1–11.
48 EMNID Survey, reported in: Verband Forschender Arzneimittelhersteller, *Gentechnik*, Bonn: VFA, 1996.
49 P. Short, "German Biotech", *Chemical and Engineering News*, 12 June 2000, 19–24; Ernst and Young, *Zeit der Bewährung: Deutsche Biotechnologie-Report 2003*, Mannheim: Ernst and Young, 2003.
50 D. Rasnick, "The Biotechnology Bubble Machine", *Nature Biotechnology*, 21 April 2003, 355–6.
51 "Chiron Corporation and SILCAAT Principal Investigators Agree on Transfer of Trial", *Chiron News*, 14 January 2002; B. Munk, "Activists Hold Conference Call with Chiron Re Termination of Interluekin-2 SILCAAT Study", *HIV and AIDS Top Stories*. URL: http://www.hivandhepatitis.com/recent/immunology/111302h.html (accessed 19.5.05).
52 C. Rowland, "Life-saving Therapies go under Budget Knife", *The Boston Globe*, 3 August 2003.
53 L. Kohn *et al.* (eds), *To Err Is Human: Building a Safer Health System*, Washington, DC: Institute of Medicine, 2000; J. Wiener, "Managing the Iatrogenic Risks of Risk Management", *Risk: Health, Safety & Environment* 9, 1998, 39–82.

15 The redemption of Thalidomide

Standardizing the risk of birth defects[1]

Stefan Timmermans and Valerie Leiter

How can risk be managed in a standardized drug distribution system, particularly when the risk is that babies might be born with severe congenital birth defects? The Food and Drug Administration (FDA) and the drug company Celgene faced this issue in the late 1990s when they intended to introduce the drug thalidomide to the US market. Currently, the drug is recognized as a promising treatment for a virtually endless list of conditions, including serious, life-threatening diseases such as AIDS wasting syndrome. But Thalidomide has a dark and dangerous past: it was promoted in the late 1950s as a sedative and treatment for morning sickness, before scientists and physicians discovered that it caused neurotoxicity among some patients, and devastating congenital malformations among babies born to women who took the drug. The problem with marketing thalidomide in the nineties is not just the drug's well-documented toxicity (many drugs on the market are as toxic, if not more so), but also its deep symbolic value. Thalidomide also played a key role in shaping US drug regulation. After thousands of babies were born with congenital malformations worldwide, and the disaster barely missed the US, a stringent drug regulation bill quickly became legislation. Thalidomide and the malformed babies symbolized the horror of unregulated drugs. With such a history, how could the FDA and Celgene introduce thalidomide to the North American market?

Much of the convincing case that Celgene built for Thalidomide rested upon a proposed *standardized* distribution system forging a unique collaboration between doctors, pharmacists, and patients. Attempts at standardization have been studied extensively by social scientists who have focused on what standardization means for achieving universality, rationality, factual knowledge, marginality, settling disputes, or advancing professional interests. Social scientists investigated how standards match with work routines and technological practices, until the standards become work practice and disappear in an invisible infrastructure only to reappear when violated. The Thalidomide drug distribution system adds a new variable to the analysis of standardization: risk. Thalidomide pits the risk of congenitally malformed babies against the promise of treating life-threatening conditions. How can one standardize the risk of fetal abnormality?

Standardization refers to the control of a diverse set of actors and actions conforming a standard to guarantee uniformity and predictability. Indeed, the hallmark of standardization is uniformity through control, at the expense of restricted or at least altered individual autonomy. But even with the most authoritative standards, control is never absolute. Inevitably, a certain margin of discretion is needed to lubricate a standardized system. Some personal or professional autonomy provides an incentive for actors to enroll in the standardization attempt, and is necessary to keep them enrolled. The possibility for standardization breakdown resides in the individual freedom of the actors, as well as in the system's controls. The actors' margin of freedom leads to a level of unpredictability: they might follow, bypass, or modify the prescriptions and procedures put in place by the designers of a standardized system. Control and safety checks lead to a similar increased risk. Controls that are too cumbersome or strict provide fertile ground for insubordination. Every standardization system is thus a precarious balancing act between control and flexibility, while keeping the system manageable.

What happens when serious risk enters a standardization attempt? When standardization is introduced after disaster has already struck and the consequences of insufficient regulation are well known, standardization system developers will need to carefully consider where they allow flexibility and where they require control. Ideally, Thalidomide pills should travel along short and narrow paths from the factory to the designated patients' mouths. Unfortunately, Thalidomide's path is long and treacherous, requiring the collaboration of patients, physicians, regulators, manufacturers, and pharmacists, each of whom may take shortcuts and detours leading to different destinations. In order to minimize the risk of fetal exposure, the distribution system will need to reconfigure the responsibilities and roles of the actors within the system. Too much flexibility in the distribution system might lead to unmonitored off-label use, pill sharing, noncompliance, and eventually to Thalidomide babies. Strict control of the drug might prevent fetal exposure within the system, but might lead to wider illegal use, and thus inadvertently lead to more fetal exposure. Even with the best distribution system possible, participants discussing Thalidomide at the regulatory meetings stated repeatedly that it was inevitable that Thalidomide babies would be born because of failure to use contraception, failure of contraception, or off-label prescription, or pill sharing.

The main argument of the paper is that the standardization attempt helped achieve a normalization of the risk of fetal abnormalities.[2] The architects of the distribution system successfully reframed a previously unacceptable risk as a permissible, residual risk. The distribution system's designers were able to enroll healthcare providers by preserving or expanding their professional autonomy, instead pointing to female reproductive behavior as the main source of risk. Patients were expected to tolerate this level of surveillance in order to get access to the drug. Furthermore, although this is the most stringent drug distribution system ever used in the US, the FDA's and Celgene's involvement is minimized – their role is to monitor the system. The risk of birth defects was rendered manageable and acceptable within this arrangement of autonomy and responsibility.

We explore the normalization of risk of teratogenic birth defects via this standardized distribution system through an abbreviated history of Thalidomide, an outline of the proposed distribution system, and an analysis of the major actors' reactions to the proposal at a public FDA advisory board meeting early in September 1997 and a public National Institutes of Health (NIH) meeting a week later.[3]

Short history of Thalidomide

Thalidomide was first synthesized in 1954 by Kunz in Germany as an anti-histamine, and was introduced as a sedative in 1956 by the German company Chemie Grunenthal. The drug was marketed as a sedative and mild hypnotic with 51 brand names in 46 countries. It quickly became the third-largest-selling drug in Europe, because of its prompt action, lack of hangover effect, and apparent safety. In many European countries, Thalidomide was available over the counter and physicians prescribed it to pregnant women to combat morning sickness.

In September of 1960, the FDA received a new drug application for Thalidomide. The application was assigned to a new medical officer, Frances Kelsey, who uncovered serious safety problems with the drug. Despite repeated pressures from the company and agency superiors, Kelsey delayed approval of the drug, and requested additional information from the company. In 1961, while the application was still pending, serious side effects of the drug were reported in Australia, Germany, and Japan. As a result of those reports, Thalidomide was not approved for marketing in the US.

Worldwide, more than 10,000 babies were born with serious birth defects due to exposure to Thalidomide. Most visibly, infants had stunted flipper-like extremities with missing fingers, and an absence of the proximal portion of the limb, or absence of entire limbs (phocomelia). Many infants also had affected internal organs. These birth defects were not reproduced in the few early animal models used to evaluate Thalidomide (but neither were the sedative properties of the drug). After the Thalidomide disaster, studies in which pregnant rabbits were given Thalidomide produced the birth defects.[4] Ten Thalidomide babies were born in the US: they were exposed to the drug sent to 1,200 US doctors for testing, or were exposed to Thalidomide that was obtained abroad.

Critics and supporters of the FDA agree that the averted Thalidomide disaster brought the agency under renewed public scrutiny. Since 1906, the FDA's role was largely limited to checking whether drug labels accurately reflected descriptions of the drug's effects. In 1938, a wave of sulfanilamide deaths had empowered the agency to impose stricter labeling and safety requirements but it was still the FDA's burden to demonstrate that a drug was not safe in order to keep it off the market. If the agency did not formulate its objections within a fixed time period, a drug became automatically marketable. Once approved, a drug was virtually immune to FDA challenge.

The Thalidomide disaster generated momentum for drug regulation among the general public, the Kennedy administration, and legislators, turning the FDA from a modest agency into one of the world's strongest and strictest regulatory bodies.[5] The Thalidomide episode was the catalyst of Congress passing the 1962 Kefauver-Harris amendments to the Food, Drug, and Cosmetic Act.[6] These amendments, which had been lingering in congressional committees for years as antitrust legislation, required that drug manufacturers not only had to prove the safety but also the efficacy of the drugs they intended to distribute on the US market. All new drug applications were required to show the drug's safety for use under conditions prescribed in the proposed drug label and were required to show evidence of effectiveness through adequate, well-controlled studies. Finally, the identity, strength, quality, and purity of the drug had to be established through information on the manufacture, quality control, and chemical process used by the manufacturer. Also, the FDA had to take positive action to approve a new drug application before it could be marketed, in contrast with default approval if the FDA did not disapprove the application within six months. Observers agree that the amendments installed important major public health protections, while at the same time lengthening the drug development process and skyrocketing the economic cost of drug approval.[7]

The Thalidomide compound did not disappear after its exposure as a dangerous teratogen.[8] Scientists conducted animal research to map the drug's toxicology and pharmacology. In 1965, an Israeli physician used Thalidomide as a sedative for patients with leprosy (Hansen's disease) and noted that patients who had a tissue inflammatory syndrome called Erythema Nodosum Leprosum (ENL) responded positively to the drug. Since then, the World Health Organization has recommended Thalidomide as the treatment of choice for ENL. In 1975, the FDA approved Thalidomide for leprosy treatment under an investigational new drug permission held by the country's major leprosy treatment center in Carville, Louisiana. Thalidomide has been available in Mexico for ENL since 1988, and for AIDS wasting syndrome since 1996. It has also been available in eight South American countries through leprosy treatment centers. In Brazil, which has the highest prevalence of leprosy, Thalidomide is available in some ordinary pharmacies. At least 33 Thalidomide babies have been born there since 1965.[9]

By the 1990s, laboratory research indicated that Thalidomide's anti-inflammatory and immunemodulary agency had potential as a treatment with relative few side effects for a virtually endless list of immunological, rheumatologic, hematologic, and oncologic disorders, including AIDS wasting syndrome. The FDA called a meeting of pharmaceutical companies in 1995 asking them to consider applying for approval to market Thalidomide in the US. The FDA provided two rationales for this strong action. First, the leprosy center in Carville had trouble securing a reliable supplier of Thalidomide because no US firm produced the drug. Foreign drug suppliers did not reliably provide the drug, leading to rationing at times and a pharmacologically inconsistent product. The second reason was more pressing. Biomedical researchers intended to test Thalidomide's effectiveness on conditions such as AIDS wasting syndrome in clinical trials. But the AIDS community did not wait for the trial results: once AIDS activists found out that Thalidomide could be used as a treatment for throat and mouth ulcers and to counteract the enormous loss of body mass and weight, drug buyer clubs imported the drug from Mexico and Brazil and made it available in the US via mail-order, sometimes unlabeled. Concerned with the illegal distribution of this potentially dangerous drug, the FDA's goal was to make Thalidomide legally available, while regulating its use.

A small New Jersey company, Celgene, took up the FDA's challenge and submitted a new drug application for the use of Thalidomide to treat ENL. Because there are only 100 to 200 new cases of ENL diagnosed in the US each year, Celgene was able to make the application under the Orphan Drug Act of 1983, which encourages companies to develop drugs for conditions with a low number of patients. As part of the approval system, the company proposed the most stringent drug distribution system in US history, the System for Thalidomide Education and Prescribing Safety (S.T.E.P.S.) program. In July of 1998, the FDA approved Celgene's application to market THALOMID™ in the US for use in treating ENL.

The S.T.E.P.S. program

Celgene presented scientific data about the safety, efficacy, and indications for Thalidomide to the FDA's Dermatologic and Ophthalmic Drugs Advisory Committee meeting in September of 1997. The FDA asked the members of that committee to answer eight questions about Celgene's application based on scientific and clinical data, and offer their recommendations to the FDA, which has the final decision and approval power. The committee consisted of nine dermatologists, four ophthalmologists, one biostatistician, and one consumer representative. Because it was a public meeting, any organization could present an opinion about the drug under consideration. At the time of the meeting, FDA scientists had already issued primary and secondary reviews of the company's clinical and toxicological data and a division director had issued a memo disapproving the application for Thalidomide. Yet the director of the FDA's office of drug evaluation explained at the beginning of the public advisory meeting that the decision was not set in stone. Working within a system of supervisory oversight, other directors could write overriding memoranda. Because of the important symbolic value of Thalidomide, the FDA staff repeatedly emphasized that the advisory committee's recommendations would carry a heavy weight in their decision-making. The pivotal question at the meeting was whether Thalidomide's benefits outweighed its risks. Among the committee members present at the meeting, only one member voted no, and another abstained from the vote.

Based on input from the Thalidomide Victims Association of Canada,[10] neuroscientists, physicians, teratologists, potential patients, academic public health officials, patient advocacy groups, women's health activists, staff from the Centers for Disease Control and Prevention (CDC), FDA, and NIH, and researchers who implemented a system for a teratogenic acne medication and an anti-schizophrenic drug, Celgene proposed the following "state of the art" system:[11]

- **education** of physicians, pharmacists, and patients;
- **contraceptive counseling** by the prescribing physician, or by a referring physician if the prescribing physician does not feel capable, competent or willing to provide adequate contraceptive counseling;
- **regimen of pregnancy testing** for women with child-bearing potential;
- **informed consent** of patients (copies of the forms go to the patient, physician, registry, and pharmacy);
- **managed distribution;** and a
- **mandatory outcomes registry survey.**

At the time of the meetings, Celgene envisioned the following scenario: when a patient and physician agree that Thalidomide would be the most appropriate therapy, the physician counsels the patient, using material from Celgene. If the patient understands the risks and responsibilities involved with taking the drug, the patient signs the informed consent form and agrees to participate in a registry survey. The physician then files a copy of the informed consent form, and may write a prescription for no more than four weeks' worth of Thalidomide. At that time, male patients receive extra counseling about dangers of pill sharing and are told to use a condom when engaging in sexual activity with a woman of childbearing age. Female patients receive contraceptive counseling, either by the prescribing physician, or through referral to a gynecologist. Before women begin taking the drug, they are required to provide a negative pregnancy test (or proof of missed periods for 24 months, indicating menopause),[12] and delay therapy until simultaneously initiating two forms of effective contraception after their next menstrual period. The patient then goes to a pharmacist who is registered and certified in the S.T.E.P.S. program. Pharmacies can only dispense Thalidomide for four weeks at a time. The drug will be packaged in a blister pack in a carded system with clear warnings, including the photograph of an affected infant. Dispensing can only occur if an informed consent form is presented, and subsequent refills require a new prescription. Each patient will be registered into a tracking system. The survey registry will track compliance with the program on a monthly basis for female patients and on a three-monthly basis for male patients. Both the FDA and Celgene will monitor the data from the registry, although no specifics were given regarding the frequency of the monitoring or any punitive actions.

Celgene's proposal for the S.T.E.P.S. program was discussed at the FDA advisory committee meeting, and interest groups offered their opinions about exactly where the risks and responsibilities lie, how they should be addressed, and which aspects of the proposal should be elaborated or changed. As a link between the drug manufacturer and the patient, the distribution system will confirm or alter power relationships, professional boundaries, agency, and responsibilities of a number of intermediaries. The system does not only standardize the distribution of Thalidomide, but also the risk of birth defects with their legal and financial accountability. In the process, the distribution system maps out a legal strategy and takes a positive stance on reproductive rights and abortion. In the next sections, we address how the major players – physicians, patients, Thalidomide victims, the FDA, and the drug itself – influenced and redefined this system, how in turn the players' jurisdictions and identities were redefined by the system, and how this process made the risk of fetal exposure acceptable.

Risk of fetal exposure in the S.T.E.P.S. program

Physicians

Physicians are the first point of access in the proposed distribution system. They will receive information about the drug and its risks from Celgene, and will be asked to inform their patients about the dangers associated with taking Thalidomide. They will also be asked to counsel patients about the use of birth control, in effect "playing the role of the social worker"[13] in ensuring that women understand the need for contraception, and then ensuring that they are able to get access to it. If a prescribing physician does not feel qualified or comfortable counseling female patients about contraception, Celgene will provide referrals to gynecologists who will do so. After informing their patients about the risks and responsibilities associated with taking Thalidomide, physicians have the patients' complete informed consent forms, which are filed at the physician's office. The physicians then enter the patients into the registry system.

But the physician's role is not over once the prescription for Thalidomide is written: patients must return for a new prescription every four weeks, and it is important that the physician monitors all patients carefully for neurotoxicity, and female patients for pregnancy. It was unclear, however, to what extent physicians would be willing or able to perform this unusually high level of monitoring. A woman's health advocate stated that some physicians do not adequately counsel their patients about the risks and benefits of treatment and suggested that educational information about off-label use be included in the packet.[14] The Canadian Thalidomide Victims Association representative, Randolph Warren, also noted that "we are not convinced that doctors will give consistent warnings and that doctors are necessarily aware of all aspects of their patients."[15] In turn, physicians questioned the degree to which the current health system would support such a time-intensive counseling system.[16] If the patient is covered by managed care, the physician could run into a number of barriers that may reduce the likelihood of being able to monitor patients according to the S.T.E.P.S. program rules. Managed care companies may set time limits on patient visits,[17] limit drug availability (particularly contraceptives), set caps on treatment costs, or limit second opinions.[18]

Physicians' discretion also poses a challenge to the viability of the distribution system. Although the physician's role is spelled out strongly in the S.T.E.P.S. program, physicians still have considerable flexibility and autonomy when making treatment decisions. Most importantly, physicians have a professional prerogative to prescribe drugs for indications other than those for which the drug was approved ("off -label" prescribing). A physician's ability to prescribe off-label erodes the control mechanisms build into the distribution system, because it allows physicians to experiment with the drug. The FDA's consumer advocate, Thalidomiders (Thalidomide victims), discussion participants, a lawyer, and some medical researchers were very concerned about off-label use and pressed repeatedly for a restriction of Thalidomide. According to one of the lawyers who spoke at the meetings, physicians may have the legal prerogative to prescribe off-label, but they do it at their own peril, risking greater legal liability.[19] FDA officials, the company, and practicing physicians resisted any off-label restriction on the grounds that physician's legal professional rights should not be undermined. One physician defended this autonomy, stating that: "The responsibility for using [Thalidomide] wisely falls I think with the medical profession."[20] But as an audience participant noted, precedents for restricting off-label use do exist. Methadone, for example, may only be prescribed for well-defined indications.

At several points during the discussion, participants suggested that physicians should be accredited or tested to verify their understanding of the information provided in the S.T.E.P.S. program. But when the Celgene representatives pointed out that it would not only be awkward but possibly illegal for a drug company to accredit physicians, this suggestion was quickly dropped. In the final version of the S.T.E.P.S. program, physicians only need to register their participation in the drug program. If they feel unqualified to conduct contraceptive counseling, they may refer the patient to a different physician. And if a patient becomes pregnant while using THALOMID™, the prescribing physician should refer the patient to an obstetrician-gynecologist experienced in reproductive toxicity.

Although physicians' full compliance with the S.T.E.P.S. program seemed questionable and their prescribing practice constituted a risk for congenital malformations, the only check on physicians' behavior is the administrative paper trail created by the informed consent procedure. Instead, the distribution system gives great latitude to physicians: they make the initial decision about the appropriateness of Thalidomide therapy, decide whether the patient is sufficiently informed, follow up with patients if more prescriptions are needed, and maintain the right to prescribe off-label. The system thus preserves and validates physicians' professional autonomy and does not locate the risk of fetal exposure in the medical profession.

Patients

While consumer and health advocates rather cautiously questioned the willingness of doctors to follow the drug distribution requirements, many of the physicians involved in the advising process – academics, clinicians, public health officials, laboratory researchers – suggested numerous potential complications regarding the patient's part in the distribution system. Patients' opportunities for non-compliance varied, depending on whether the discussion was about patients in general, female patients, or specific patient subpopulations (such as people with AIDS). In the end, however, the drug distribution system relied upon reproductive surveillance, resulting in an erosion of patient autonomy.

A great many factors enter into patients' willingness and ability to follow a drug protocol within the context of their everyday lives. During the meetings, physicians who had been involved with prior efforts to change patients' behavior described them as complex actors, with varying degrees of skill and reliability. The physicians pointed out that the potential population of Thalidomide patients is very heterogeneous: this fact calls into question the feasibility of truly standardizing behavior across patients in the distribution system. Potential patients would have varying levels of literacy (with 20 per cent of the US population considered illiterate and another 20 per cent functionally illiterate);[21] existing knowledge about the drug;[22] formal education, income, and insurance;[23] knowledge of English due to recent immigration status;[24] sickness;[25] and contraceptive skill.[26] They would also come with varying beliefs about sexual intercourse, contraception, and abortion.[27] Also, some patients could be expected to do their own research on available treatments and then actively seek them out; these patients might want a greater voice in deciding which treatment they will receive.

Perception of risk may vary tremendously among the potential patient population. Over 50 per cent of people over the age of 45 have very vivid associations with the word "Thalidomide", but only about one third of people under the age of 45 (largely, the reproductive age) know of the drug's history.[28] But it is not enough for patients to know that there is a risk. They must also understand how to prevent that risk from becoming a reality in their own lives. This kind of behavioral change requires that patients believe that the risk is real, intend to perform the change, and have the skills and environmental resources to make the change effectively. According to a discussion during the meetings, the most important environmental resource is the availability of contraceptives. If patients are not easily able to get access to contraceptives, because of lack of insurance, money or other barriers, the entire system may be compromised.

Three patient populations received special attention during the FDA and NIH meetings: leprosy patients, HIV and AIDS patients, and female patients. Leprosy patients had been receiving Thalidomide for decades and were, at least on paper, the intended drug recipients. At the time of the FDA meeting, only five patients were being treated with Thalidomide for ENL at Carville, four of whom were male.[29] Fueled by Biblical associations with impurity, the leprosy population in the US has had a long and sad history of civil rights violations as a consequence of mandatory institutionalization.[30] It therefore is not surprising that Carville required surgical sterilization or proof of menopause for female out-patients, and required that female in-patients receive two forms of contraception and weekly pregnancy tests.[31] In the public meetings, the Carville experience with leprosy patients was interpreted to mean that the risk of Thalidomide could be minimized with proper monitoring. No leprosy patients were present to corroborate or challenge this portrayal at the meetings.

HIV and AIDS patients, the second patient population discussed at length, offered a bigger challenge for the designers of the distribution system. In contrast with the assumed docility of the leprosy population, people living with HIV symbolized demanding, assertive, well-organized, activist-patients' bodies. Patient activists from the AIDS epidemic[32] have been aggressive about pressuring doctors for new treatments, or seeking drugs from buyer's clubs if physicians will not dispense them. HIV and AIDS patients, and their activists, therefore represented the real possibility of future Thalidomide patients bypassing the regulated distribution system if its requirements were too stringent.

Expected to be the largest consumers of Thalidomide, HIV patients may already be participating in demanding therapies, involving as many as 28 pills each day. And some people with AIDS may be living on the socio-economic fringe, with a significant amount of chaos involved in their lives.[33] Thalidomide may add to that chaos for some patients, on top of figuring out where their next meal will come from, where their next ride to and from the doctor will come from, whether they will still live in their house, and, for parents, how they will take care of their children. Poor populations may need extra support. Adding to these challenges, some patients may be illicit drug users, and such users do not have a good track record of contraceptive use.[34] The effects of Thalidomide also pose an additional problem: it is a sedative, and may impair the judgment of patients who take it,[35] reducing compliance with a contraceptive program.

Female patients were the third key patient population that was discussed during the meetings. Ultimately, the S.T.E.P.S. program aimed to influence their reproductive behavior. During the FDA meetings, women had a limited voice, but their possible future behavior within the distribution system was the subject of heated debate on several occasions. According to the discussion, much of the credit for the success or failure of the S.T.E.P.S. program will fall on female patients' shoulders. Throughout the meetings, women were alternately described as intelligent decision-makers, unsuitable patients, actors with varying degrees of ability and reliability, and unruly physical bodies.

Cynthia Pearson, director of the National Women's Health Network (NWHN), described women patients as intelligent decision-makers, who would make good choices if they understood the risks associated with their behavior. Hers was the one voice that specifically spoke on behalf of future women patients during the FDA and NIH meetings. Pearson advocated that women make their own choices about contraception, rather than having physicians or the FDA make those decisions, and challenged a stereotypical view that "all women who ovulate and have open fallopian tubes are at risk of pregnancy".[36] She emphasized that most women would not want to have babies with birth defects, and would take decisions accordingly after they are informed about the risks associated with taking Thalidomide.

The most conservative view of women, that they were unsuitable patients, was held by some of the research scientists who had been working with Thalidomide at the Carville leprosy center. They were accustomed to a clinical situation where zero risk was tolerated and institutionalization was a routine intervention. Leo Yoder, one of the physicians at Carville, advocated that women be required to use two methods of contraception, and stated that, ideally, women would use a method "that does not apply to compliance".[37] Others suggested that women should not receive the drug at all, or that it should only be made available to infertile women in clinical trials.

Female patients' bodies were also characterized as varying in ways that the distribution system, and the women themselves, cannot control. By instituting monthly pregnancy tests, the system hoped to guarantee that a pregnant woman will not receive Thalidomide. But women often do not have twenty-eight-day cycles,[38] making it unclear at what point in her cycle a woman is being tested if she is being tested every 28 days. Technological issues compound this problem: it takes nine to ten days for a serum pregnancy test to become positive, so a negative test only shows that the woman is not ten days or more pregnant. But the sensitive period is 21 to 36 days.[39] To be absolutely sure that a pregnant woman does not take the drug, women would have to be tested every ten days. The FDA did not require this frequency of testing, because it feared that the requirement would be too stringent and drive people to the buyer's clubs.[40]

In the end, a discursive construction of women as unreliable and unpredictable overwhelmingly shaped the S.T.E.P.S. program. In contrast to the relatively few controlling provisions for physicians, women's knowledge and behavior is counseled, questioned, verified, checked, tested, re-checked, and then continuously monitored via a compliance survey. Largely based upon the accumulated knowledge of AIDS prevention research,[41] the final version of the S.T.E.P.S. program is aimed at modifying female sexual behavior. If a woman has not undergone a hysterectomy or been sterilized, or has menstruated in the 24 months preceding Thalidomide treatment, she must agree to two forms of contraception. One of those methods must be highly effective (e.g., IUD, hormonal, tubal ligation, or partner's vasectomy), and be used in combination with one effective method (e.g., condom, diaphragm, or cervical cap). Women must also produce a written negative pregnancy test that was conducted no more than 24 hours prior to beginning treatment with THALOMID™. After receiving the drug, women of childbearing potential must receive a pregnancy test every week for the first four weeks, then every four weeks thereafter if their menstrual cycles are regular. If her cycle is irregular, a woman must receive a pregnancy test every two weeks thereafter. If all else fails, emergency contraception will be made available to female patients.

All patients, regardless of their sex, are monitored to some extent within the proposed S.T.E.P.S. program. Patients are instructed that they should not donate blood. Female patients cannot breastfeed while on THALOMID™, and male patients are instructed to use a condom every time that they have sexual intercourse with a woman (even if they have undergone a vasectomy) and are not allowed to donate sperm.[42] Each patient must fill out informed consent forms, take a quiz, register via a survey enrollment form, and participate in the registry survey (monthly for female patients and quarterly for male patients). This confidential survey asks questions about sexual behavior, pill sharing, and use of contraception, and requests the results of pregnancy tests. Every patient is assumed to be able and willing to freely discuss his or her sexual behavior with physicians and survey researchers.

These invasive and elaborate measures to assure patient compliance show that the system designers saw the real risk of fetal exposure as residing with patients, particularly female patients, rather than with the professional actors within the system. Although an ethicist at the NIH meeting quoted an attorney stating that "a woman has no legal or moral duty to be a procreative saint,"[43] the system singles out female patients. It is also clear that the system focuses on sexual activity and pregnancy as the locus of risk, not fetal exposure, even though a Celgene representative claimed that the opposite was true.[44] The standardized distribution system assumes that a woman is in charge of contraception, reproductive decisions, and her sexual relationships. But at the same time, all women wishing THALOMID™ are also presumed to be heterosexually active unless they can prove hysterectomy or menopause. Women's sexual behavior and their bodies are ultimately untrustworthy. At every point where female patients' behavior was interpreted, the strictest control (short of institutionalization) was chosen. The system works from the assumption that women are willing to trade a close supervision and regulation of their sexuality and reproductive privacy for access to a potentially life-saving drug.[45] Women are not trusted to make decisions to protect their unborn children.[46]

Thalidomiders

Randolph Warren, the CEO of the Thalidomide Victims Association of Canada, played a crucial role in developing the S.T.E.P.S. program. Warren attended the FDA and NIH advisory committee meetings, speaking for the handful of US Thalidomide victims, the Thalidomide victims and mothers in Canada, and future Thalidomide babies. During those meetings, he consistently and vocally demanded that the program do its best to minimize the risk of Thalidomide babies being born in the US Prior to the FDA meetings, Warren worked closely with Celgene to develop the S.T.E.P.S. program. Although he was unhappy about Thalidomide being available in the US, he preferred FDA regulation of the drug to the current situation.

Warren saw his role as an educator. He and the other members of his organization understood the potential impact of the drug in a way that none of the other actors could, and they wanted to serve as a lighthouse, showing the danger that lay ahead. It was important to Warren that the dangers be stated clearly, using photographs of infants and videos of adult Thalidomide victims, to show the extent of the damage that Thalidomide could cause. He believed that education was the key to protecting future babies: if women could see the devastating damage that Thalidomide could cause, they would prevent it. Throughout the meetings, he asked: "What will you tell the Thalidomide baby that inevitably will be born?", and demanded that Celgene work to develop a non-teratogenic substitute for Thalidomide, eliminating the need for the drug in the future.

As the living embodiment of the drug's major risk, the Thalidomiders had some direct effects on the S.T.E.P.S. program. They critiqued the drug packaging, offered to participate in the creation of an informative video to educate future patients, and offered to make themselves available as counselors for future Thalidomide babies. The final educational package includes a letter from the Canadian Thalidomide Victims Association, which is addressed to prospective patients and physicians. A picture of a (smiling) Thalidomide baby is included in the information folder. In turn, the renewed attention to Thalidomide and the S.T.E.P.S. program gave the Thalidomiders a forum to validate their concerns and questions. Aware of their living symbolic value and their dwindling numbers, Thalidomiders presented themselves as the spokespeople of affected children of the future. The Thalidomiders advocated for zero tolerance of the risk of fetal exposure, wanting to prevent the birth of similarly affected babies in the future, even if that meant that a picture of a Thalidomider would be used as a deterrent. Their main goal was to prevent more babies from being affected. Warren sadly expressed the irony that Thalidomiders "cannot fight Thalidomide. It wins every time."[47]

The FDA

The social-political context in which the FDA makes decisions about drug approval applications has changed significantly in the almost 40 years since the Thalidomide tragedy. The FDA is working in a macro-political climate of less regulation, less bureaucracy, and more independent decision-making by consumers.[48] Currently, there are calls for expanded access to clinical trials (notably by women and minorities), pressure from the pharmaceutical industry to accelerate approval for drug distribution and marketing, a strengthened anti-abortion movement, treatment activism (especially by HIV/AIDS activists), and stronger consumer awareness. Often, patients are now more involved in their treatment than they were in the past, and look to the FDA to provide them with a statement of the risks associated with drugs, so that they can participate in managing that risk.[49] The FDA's role is still to monitor the safety of drugs, but the agency is strongly criticized if it is seen to be getting in the way of distributing promising new therapies to people with severe diseases.[50]

When it invited drug companies to rethink Thalidomide, the FDA created a more proactive role for itself as a federal consumer protection agency that regulates industry based on scientific data.[51] But the invitation to apply, the less rigorous application process under the orphan drug status, and the disregard for the agency's own safety experts who argued that the application did not meet scientific criteria, created the impression that the approval of Thalidomide was virtually guaranteed. Indeed the Thalidomider Warren noted: "To be critical, as far as I'm concerned, the first application should have been an honest application that was involving HIV/AIDS wasting."[52]

Although the FDA played a key role in paving the way for the distribution of Thalidomide, and in the development of the S.T.E.P.S. program, it will play a backstage role in the implementation of the system. In response to a question during the NIH meeting about who will be responsible for overseeing the distribution system when it is in action, one FDA representative stated: "I think it's the responsibility of all of us."[53]

From a consumer's point of view, the distribution system would have had extra teeth if the FDA had insisted on a clearly defined set of criteria to evaluate the adverse effects of THALOMID™. A lawyer who represents injured victims asked the haunting rhetorical question: "[J]ust how many children will need to be harmed by this drug before the risks of the drug are deemed to outweigh the benefits?"[54] He added that, in his home state of Michigan, once the FDA has approved a drug, the drug is deemed to be safe. No lawsuit can be brought unless it can be demonstrated that the FDA approval had been procured by fraud. Although the FDA has a voluntary postmarketing reporting system – a database consisting of adverse drug reactions – in place, it remained unclear at what point the agency might step in to further restrict access to the drug. Researchers estimate that only about 5–10 per cent of adverse reactions are reported and that causality is difficult to establish.[55]

Some observers have noted the FDA's deft political move in the Thalidomide case:[56] the FDA showed its sensitivity to the needs of patients, while taking responsibility for the outcomes of a minute number of leprosy cases and avoiding responsibility for the estimated thousands of off-label prescriptions. Although this is not such a watershed event, compared with first time the FDA came into contact with Thalidomide, its approval of Thalidomide reflects the course the FDA hopes to set in the future as a regulatory agency. The FDA sent the message to its critics that, within the current regulatory system, it is possible to approve even Thalidomide. Major reform, budget cuts, or loosening of restrictions are not warranted.

Thalidomide

Thalidomide has been re-evaluated and redeemed. Once, it was an over-the-counter remedy for insomnia and morning sickness which caused devastating birth defects among infants. Now, it is an "essential' drug for patients with painful and often life-threatening diseases who are otherwise untreatable, such as people with ENL and AIDS wasting syndrome. Thalidomide is allowed to act again in the United States. Because of its "pharmacotherapeutic rehabilitation",[57] several patient groups have a new outlook on life, physicians have a new tool, the FDA a new standard for drug distribution, and Celgene prospects for profit. The rehabilitated Thalidomide is the linchpin holding all those groups together in a new configuration.

To indicate the break with the past, Celgene proposed the name Synovir for the transformed Thalidomide. But the discussion participants agreed that Synovir sounded too much like the name of an ordinary antiviral drug, and, to play on the name recognition among people over 45, the name became *THALOMID™ (Thalidomide)*. Thalidomide's transformation affected even its visual presentation. Instead of distributing the drug in a bottle, the meeting participants preferred blister packaging with a stale date.

In constructing the drug distribution system, medical researchers compiled and evaluated the available knowledge about the drug's absorption time, biological equivalency, etiology, toxicity, drug interactions (particularly with oral contraceptives), teratogenicity, peripheral neuropathy, efficiency for ENL, and immunological agency. A comparison with other teratogenic drugs already on the market further drew out the characteristics of Thalidomide until a picture of its pharmological consistence appeared. Instead of a horror drug of the past, Thalidomide appeared through the scientific work as any other chemical compound with known toxicological parameters, and, as was stated repeatedly, this picture proved less alarming than that presented by some other drugs currently approved by the FDA and widely available by prescription (e.g., Accutane). The discussants chiseled further away at Thalidomide's symbolic value when they emphasized the limitless therapeutic applications of the drug. The result of these defining acts was a symbolic, functional, and therapeutic make-over of Thalidomide, and the establishment of a new identity: THALOMID™.

But the drug's identity picture was not complete. Some identity features remained unknown or controversial. One of the biggest gaps in the drug knowledge was Thalidomide's mechanism of action, both globally and in specific conditions. Several hypotheses were circulated of how Thalidomide might cause congenital birth defects and neuropathy, but no consensus existed. A number of audience members demanded an acknowledgment of the drug's unpredictability in the informed consent form. Other very basic pharmacological data (for example, about dosing) was missing as well, and several participants called for more animal models, clinical trials, and research applications. Some of those new applications might lead to discovering Thalidomide's therapeutic role for life-altering conditions instead of life-threatening conditions, raising issues about the standard of the drug's risks and benefits. Researchers generally considered the lack of knowledge a stimulus for more research and they expressed cautious excitement about the future of Thalidomide. In the final version of the S.T.E.P.S. informed consent form, no disclaimers or warnings about the drug's unknowns were mentioned. A lawyer noted that the lack of clear causal path might limit the legal accountability of people suffering from the adverse effects of the drug, because some congenital malformations occur "naturally" in the general population.

At the same time that the drug distribution system rehabilitated Thalidomide, it also put the drug under strict control and severely limited its access to human bodies. Thalidomide is the most regulated drug in US history.[58] The rehabilitation of Thalidomide might also carry the seeds of its demise. Because of the enormous therapeutic promise and profit margin, the race is on for an analog with Thalidomide's healing qualities but without its teratogenic effects. A Celgene representative referred to the analog as "the holy grail of drug development".[59]

Standardization and the normalization of risk

Haunted by the Thalidomide disaster, in 1962 Congress gave the FDA unprecedented powers to regulate drugs. In 1998, the same compound with the same teratogenic potential was approved for distribution in the US. Among the factors which helped to overcome the heavy symbolic legacy of Thalidomide, and made its distribution possible, were the proactive role of the FDA, an evaluation of scientific expertise, cooperation with Thalidomiders, a presentation of the limitless benefits for hard-hit patient populations, the threat of unregulated black-market Thalidomide, and the strategically positioned S.T.E.P.S. program. In this paper, we have high-lighted the role of the distribution program in normalizing the risk of congenital malformation.

One of the merits of the S.T.E.P.S. program is that it satisfies the most powerful social worlds whose collaboration was needed for the system to operate. The designers preserved and enhanced their professional autonomy. Physicians' off-label prescription prerogatives were left untouched, and pharmacists were given desired counseling responsibilities. The federal regulators were satisfied that the proposed drug system set a new standard for restricted distribution. The fact that Thalidomide was approved showed that the current drug regulation system worked and that the agency paid attention to the needs of the pharmaceutical industry and patient populations. The program simultaneously positioned Celgene at the beginning of the distribution chain and minimized the company's participation once the system was put into place. The reluctant Thalidomiders played an important role in educating Celgene and the other actors about Thalidomide's dangers. As for the most silent actors – the patients – the system assumes that access to a life-saving drug will be a sufficient incentive to make the program a success.[60]

The distribution system also clearly identifies women's sexual and reproductive behavior as the primary locus of risk of congenital malformations. The standardization effort provided a sense of security because it imposed an ideal situation in which fetal exposure should not occur if all actors played their roles. The formalized distribution chain minimized the risk of adverse effects by defining a number of loopholes and then suggesting means to close them off. The risk of a Thalidomide baby is defined as the risk of a woman patient taking Thalidomide. It bears repeating that controlling women's reproductive behavior is not necessarily the only or most obvious choice: physicians' off-label use or pill sharing among male and female patients could have been the target of control. Or, instead of increasing the surveillance of female sexuality, the different actors could have pointed to the availability of abortion as a legal healthcare choice. Or they could have argued for greater acceptance of and accommodation to people with disabilities. By marking women's reproductive behavior the most important safety valve, the designers perpetuate a distorted view of women as untrustworthy decision-makers and delegate control to physicians and pharmacists.

Standardization thus re-establishes and solidifies social inequalities and professional power relationships in one more medical domain, revealing assumptions about trust, responsibility, and risk. Even in the design phase, the actors recognized the potential to by-pass the system (for example, with Mexican Thalidomide). As we know from studies of standardization in action, a reshuffling of control and leeway – often unanticipated by system designers – is necessary for any system to function.[61] The careful balance between control, flexibility, and manageability will need to be achieved anew during drug prescription and dispensing. The participants in the debate were aware of the tension between designing and implementing a distribution system because they stated repeatedly that Thalidomide babies would inevitably be born in the US. One of the lawyers at the meetings worried more specifically that "[t]he impact of noncompliance by literally everyone in the distribution chain is a high likelihood, not an isolated instance".[62] The lawyer's deeply-felt concern stood out because most meeting participants considered the probability of noncompliance insufficient to stop the distribution of Thalidomide.

Participants at the meetings hinted at several medical and political subtexts, each of which have the potential to reduce the effectiveness of the distribution program. Abortion politics, the role of managed care in the healthcare system, disability activism, and the reimbursement of drug prescriptions in government programs (including Medicare) all have the potential to reduce the viability of the S.T.E.P.S. program. The most important "invisible" topic was legal liability in case a Thalidomide baby is born. Legal liability seemed to be in the back of everyone's mind, but few participants addressed the topic directly. An FDA official stated at the end of the meetings that enforcing the system "is the responsibility of all of us".[63] The standardization attempt seemed to have absorbed individual responsibilities and located an ambiguous collective and formalistic responsibility in the distribution system.[64] At the outset of Thalidomide distribution, it seems that the system itself, and not one of the social worlds, will be to blame, put to trial, and patched up or overhauled for any adverse effects. The responsibility for adverse effects rests with the distribution chain made up of interconnecting links.

Similar to Diane Vaughan's analysis of the Challenger launch decision, the end result of the public meetings and the FDA approval process was the collapse of deviation into a new standard of acceptable risk. The standardized S.T.E.P.S. program leads to a normalization of risk of birth defects.[65] The FDA and Celgene admitted at the outset that the S.T.E.P.S. program would not completely prevent congenital malformations due to Thalidomide, yet the standardized distribution system made the residual risk of congenital disability acceptable. It shifted the cost–benefit ratio in favor of the benefits, by promising to reduce and control the risk of fetal exposure and disability. While this normalization of risk might be acceptable for the current actors in the distribution chain, the question still remains whether this justification of risk will satisfy the Thalidomide babies who will be born.

Notes

1 This chapter is a much shortened version of S. Timmermans and V. Leiter, 'The Redemption of Thalidomide: Standardizing the Risk of Birth Defects', *Social Studies of Science*, 2000, 30, 41–72 © Sage Publications, 2000; by permission of Sage Publications

Ltd. The original paper includes the reaction of pharmacists and Celgene to the meetings, a more extensive discussion of abortion and disability, and more references.

2 D. Vaughan, *The Challenger Launch Decision: Risky Technology, Culture, and Deviance at NASA*, Chicago: The University of Chicago Press, 1996.

3 This paper uses the transcripts of an FDA meeting (4 and 5 September 1997) and an NIH meeting (9 and 10 September 1997) regarding Thalidomide. When quoting from the transcripts, we will refer to the meetings by the speaker, function, date of meeting, and page number of the transcript.

4 R. A. Fine, *The Great Drug Deception*, New York: Stern and Day, 1972.

5 T. Connors, "Anticancer Drug Development: The Way Forward", *Oncologist*, 1, 1996, 180–1.

6 J. Abraham, *Science, Politics and the Pharmaceutical Industry*, London, New York: St Martins Press, 1995.

7 See, for example, C. H. Asbury, *Orphan Drugs: Medical versus Market Value*, Lexington: Lexington Books, 1985; L. E. Hollister *et al.*, "The Kefauver-Harris Amendments of 1962: A Critical Appraisal of the First Five Years", *Journal of Clinical Pharmacology*, 8, 1968, 69–73.

8 A National Library of Medicine bibliography listed 1,495 citations out of more than 4,600 between January 1963 and July 1997. K. Patrias, R. L. Gordner and S. Groft, *Thalidomide: Potential Benefits and Risks*, Bethesda: National Library of Medicine, 1997.

9 These numbers were provided during the meetings; we could not find anything else about these new Thalidomide cases.

10 Because of the low numbers of Thalidomide babies born in the US, no victims association exists there. The Canadian association has reached out to the US Thalidomiders and presents itself as their spokesperson.

11 Williams, Vice President, Sales and Marketing, Celgene Corporation (4 September), 78; Bruce Williams, (10 September), 26–31.

12 The participants did not explain how one "proves" a missed period.

13 Pearson, *National Women's Health Network* (9 September), 52.

14 Pearson, *National Women's Health Network* (9 September), 51.

15 Warren, Thalidomide Victim's Association of Canada (5 September), 54.

16 Povar, George Washington University School of Medicine (10 September), 18.

17 Allen, American Medical Association (9 September), 49.

18 Senak, AIDS Project Los Angeles (10 September), 22.

19 Bleakley Bleakley and P.C. McKeen (10 September), 57.

20 Povar, George Washington University School of Medicine (10 September), 18, note 16, 20.

21 Lumpkin, Deputy Center Director for Review Management, FDA (4 September), 75.

22 Morris, Division of Drug Marketing, Advertising, and Communications, FDA (10 September), 8.

23 Senak, AIDS Project Los Angeles (10 September), 22, note 18, 24.

24 Rea, Celgene Corporation (5 September), 90.

25 Hill, Division of Dermotological and Dental Drug Products, FDA (9 September), 97.

26 Fishbein, University of Pennsylvania (10 September), 12.

27 The physicians in this debate constructed patients' "non-compliance" in terms of demographic factors and healthcare beliefs. It did not occur that non-compliance could be a deliberate strategy. See N. Fineman, "The Social Constructions of Compliance: A Study of Health Care and Social Service Providers in Everyday Practice", *Sociology of Health and Illness*, 13, 1991, 354–73.

28 Morris, Division of Drug Marketing, Advertising, and Communications, FDA (10 September), 8, note 22, 8.

29 Moore, Centers for Disease Control and Prevention (9 September), 106.

30 People diagnosed with leprosy were escorted by law officials to Carville, their possessions were burned, and, if they died, their graves would often be marked with assumed names. Z. Gussow, *Leprosy, Racism, and Public Health*, Boulder: Westview Press, 1989.

31 Yoder, American Leprosy Mission (4 September), 44.

32 Senak, AIDS Project Los Angeles (10 September), 22, note 18, 93.

33 AIDS Project Los Angeles (10 September), 24.

34 AIDS Project Los Angeles (10 September), 36.

35 Mauck, Division of Reproductive and Urologic Drug Products, FDA (9 September), 92–3.

36 Pearson, *National Women's Health Network* (9 September), 51, note 13, 52.

37 Yoder, American Leprosy Mission (4 September), 44, note 31, 43.

38 Mauck, Division of Reproductive and Urologic Drug Products, FDA (9 September), 92–3, note 35, 95.

39 Mauck, Division of Reproductive and Urologic Drug Products, FDA (9 September), 94.

40 Mauck, Division of Reproductive and Urologic Drug Products, FDA (9 September), 94.

41 Fishbein, University of Pennsylvania (10 September), 12, note 26, 10.

42 There was uncertainty regarding thalidomide's possible effects on sperm. The researchers decided that it was better to be cautious.

43 Fost, University of Wisconsin-Madison (9 September), 28.

44 Williams, Celgene Corporation (10 September), 30.

45 There is a large literature on precedents with similar outcomes. See, for example Adele Clarke, *Disciplining Reproduction: Modernity, American Life Sciences, and "the Problems of Sex"*, Berkeley, University of California Press, 1998; Sarah Franklin, *Embodied Progress: A Cultural Account of Assisted Conception*, London, New York: Routledge, 1997; Anne Donchin, "Feminist Critiques of New Fertility Technologies: Implications for Social Policy", *The Journal of Medicine and Philosophy*, Vol. 21(5), 1996, 475–98; Faye Ginsberg and Rayna Rapp (eds), *Conceiving the New World Order: The Global Stratification of Reproduction*, Berkeley: University of California Press, 1995.

46 Rapp, *Conceiving the New World Order*, p. 70.

47 Warren, Thalidomide Victim's Association of Canada (5 September), 54, note 15, 43.

48 J. Abraham and J. Sheppard, "International Comparative Analysis and Explanation in Medical Sociology: Demystifying the Halcion Anomaly", *Sociology*, 32, 1998, 141–62; US Congress, *Council on Competitiveness and FDA Plans to Alter the Drug Approval Process at the FDA* (Hearings before the Committee on Government Operations, Washington, DC, 1992); Andrulis, Andrulis Pharmaceuticals Corporation (10 September), 45.

49 S. Epstein, *Impure Science: AIDS, Activism, and the Politics of Knowledge*, Berkeley: University of California Press, 1996.

50 Abraham and Sheppard, "International Comparative Analysis", note 48.

51 S. Jasanoff, *The Fifth Branch: Science Advisors as Policymakers*, Cambridge, MA: Harvard University Press, 1990.

52 Warren, Thalidomide Victim's Association of Canada (9 September), 56.

53 Woodcock, Center for Drug Evaluation and Research, FDA (10 September), 86.

54 Bleakley Bleakley and P.C. McKeen (10 September), 57, note 19, 47.

55 R. D. Mann, *Adverse Drug Reactions: The Scale and Nature of the Problem and the Way Forward*, Camforth: Parthenon, 1987.

56 See, for example, J. Welsh, "Banned in US for Causing Birth Defects, Thalidomide Returns as an AIDS Drug", *The Wall Street Journal*, 2 June 1995.

57 Povar, George Washington University School of Medicine (10 September), 18, note 16.

58 Except for the drugs which are part of a system of mandatory restricted distribution.

59 Thomas, Celgene Corporation (5 September), 129.

60 For a similar case where such assumptions were unwarranted, see R. Rapp, "Refusing Prenatal Diagnosis: The Meanings of Bioscience in a Multicultural World", *Science, Technology, and Human Values*, 23, 1998, 45–71.

61 S. Timmermans and M. Berg, "Standardization in Action: Achieving Local Universality through Medical Protocols", *Social Studies of Science*, 27, 1996, 273–305.

62 Bleakley Bleakley and P.C. McKeen (10 September), 57, note 40, 50.

63 Woodcock, Center for Drug Evaluation and Research, FDA (10 September), 86, note 54, 86.

64 G. Bowker, "How to be Universal: Some Cybernetic Strategies, 1943–70", *Social Studies of Science*, 23, 1993, 107–27.

65 Vaughan, *The Challenger Launch Decision*, note 2.

Name index

Subject index